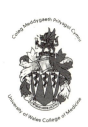

The Sir Herbert Duthie Library
University of Wales College of Medicine
Heath Park, Cardiff
Tel: (029) 2074 2875

This loan may be renewed

The Contextual Determinants of Malaria

Edited by
**Elizabeth A. Casman and
Hadi Dowlatabadi**

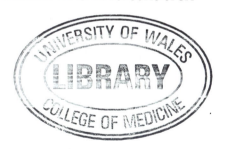

Resources for the Future
Washington, DC

Printed in the United States of America

An RFF Press book
Published by Resources for the Future
1616 P Street, NW, Washington, DC 20036–1400
www.rff.org

Library of Congress Cataloging-in-Publication Data
Casman, Elizabeth A.
    The contextual determinants of malaria / edited by Elizabeth A. Casman and Hadi Dowlatabadi.
        p.   cm.
    Includes bibliographical references and index.
    ISBN 1–891853–19–8 (lib. bdg. : alk. paper)
    1. Malaria—Environmental aspects. 2. Malaria—Social aspects. 3. Malaria—Economic aspects. I. Dowlatabadi, Hadi. II. Title.
RA644 .M2   C375   2002
616.9′362—dc21   2002017327

f e d c b a

This book was designed and typeset in ITC Stone Serif and Stone Sans by Betsy Kulamer. It was copyedited by Pamela Angulo. The cover was designed by Rosenbohm Graphic Design.

ISBN 1–891853–19–8 (cloth)

About
Resources for the Future
and RFF Press

Resources for the Future (RFF) improves environmental and natural resource policy-making worldwide through independent social science research of the highest caliber.

Founded in 1952, RFF pioneered the application of economics as a tool to develop more effective policy about the use and conservation of natural resources. Its scholars continue to employ social science methods to analyze critical issues concerning pollution control, energy policy, land and water use, hazardous waste, climate change, biodiversity, and the environmental challenges of developing countries.

RFF Press supports the mission of RFF by publishing book-length works that present a broad range of approaches to the study of natural resources and the environment. Its authors and editors include RFF staff, researchers from the larger academic and policy communities, and journalists. Audiences for RFF publications include all of the participants in the policymaking process—scholars, the media, advocacy groups, nongovernment organizations, professionals in business and government, and the general public.

Contents

Preface

Recent attempts to project the impacts of climate change on malaria often acknowledge the importance of social, economic, and other contextual variables but fail to explicitly incorporate them or consider how they may evolve along with demographic and environmental conditions. This problem is of critical interest to the climate policy community, which has been buffeted by claims and counter-claims concerning the impact of climate change on malaria.

While we hope that this book provides important advances to our understanding of the climate change–malaria linkage, we also intend it to address broader efforts to improve malaria control planning. There are many issues common to both assessing the impact of climate change on malaria prevalence and designing strategies for malaria control. In each line of investigation, it is important to consider why, as malaria has been eradicated in some parts of the world, the disease has persisted or reemerged in others. In each investigation, there is a need to identify the most successful interventions and to consider the factors that would allow the techniques to be transferred effectively from one setting to many others. And, in each domain, it is essential to consider the interaction of many dimensions of global change—and to consider the many stresses that will influence the course of malaria during the twenty-first century.

The origins of this book are in an international workshop that was held May 15–18, 2000, in Lausanne, Switzerland. The workshop was structured around developing a method for incorporating contextual factors into projections of the future incidence of malaria. Papers on the determinants of malaria prevalence around the world (including environmental, climatic, social, behavioral, demographic, land-use, economic, institutional, and technical factors) were presented and discussed, followed by papers on individual high-impact determinants and how they are expected to evolve over the next half-century, when the effects of climate change are expected to be more tangible. Workgroups were formed to synthesize this information into a conceptual framework that would assist those grappling with the problem of addressing the impact of climate change on the distribution of malaria. *The Contextual Determinants of Malaria* is the result of the refinement of the original papers in response to a two-year process of discussion and comment. Our objectives for the book are

- to provide a better understanding the role of global warming in malaria occurrence and to put climate effects in perspective with the other contextual variables, and
- to improve our understanding of the various factors controlling the incidence of malaria, their interactions and relative importance, and thereby to refocus attention on critical scientific and public health needs.

It is our hope that this book will be of value to those contemplating the effects of climate change on human health, to those devising malaria control programs and research initiatives, and to those trying to understand the global resurgence of malaria that has occurred in recent decades.

Acknowledgements

The Workshop on the Contextual Determinants of Malaria was made possible by the generous support of the ExxonMobil Foundation. Additional support was provided by the National Science Foundation (USA), the Electric Power Research Institute, the National Oceanographic and Atmospheric Administration (USA), and the American Petroleum Institute. The conference was organized by the editors, who are members of the Center for the Integrated Study of the Human Dimensions of Global Change at Carnegie Mellon University.

We wish to thank the World Health Organization, Geneva Office, for logistical and intellectual support. Also, we wish to express our gratitude to Baruch Fischhoff, Lester Lave, and M. Granger Morgan of Carnegie Mellon University for their valued assistance in conducting the workshop and to Ms Terri Jones, of the same institution, for secretarial assistance.

The papers and discussions from the workshop form the basis for this book, but the book, having been reviewed, edited, updated, and supplemented, is now much more than a proceedings. For their attention to detail and careful scrutiny we gratefully acknowledge the staff and associates at RFF Press, including Don Reisman, Sandra Hackman, Rebecca Henderson, and Gina Armento.

We are profoundly indebted to the distinguished group of public health professionals and academics who participated in the workshop. Their generous intellectual involvement accounts for the strengths of this volume. We would especially like to acknowledge the thoughtful contributions of two workshop participants whose names do not appear in the list of authors, Menno J. Bouma of the London School of Hygiene and Tropical Medicine and Steven W. Lindsay of the University of Durham, United Kingdom.

ELIZABETH A. CASMAN, *Carnegie Mellon University*
HADI DOWLATABADI, *University of British Columbia*

Contributors

Andrew Y. Au is affiliated with Raytheon Information Technology and Scientific Services and the National Aeronautics and Space Administration's Goddard Space Flight Center Geodesy Branch in Greenbelt, Maryland.

Reid E. Basher is director of applications at the New York–based International Research Institute for Climate Prediction, where he leads the development of integrative approaches to the use of climate information and seasonal predictions in key sectors such as agriculture, water, and health, especially in vulnerable developing countries. He has had senior roles in the activities of the Intergovernmental Panel on Climate Change (IPCC) and World Meteorological Organization and has published on climate variability and climate applications.

Andrei E. Beljaev is associate professor at the Chair of Tropical and Parasitic Diseases, Russian Academy of Postgraduate Medical Training, Moscow, Russia. His research has focused on the epidemiology and laboratory diagnosis of parasitic diseases, especially malaria. He has worked with the World Health Organization (WHO) on malaria in India, Southeast Asia, Africa, and the Middle East. His works recently appeared in WHO publications and among the teaching aids of the Russian Academy of Postgraduate Medical Training.

Martin Birley is co-director of IMPACT, the International Health Impact Assessment Consortium at the University of Liverpool. He is a senior lecturer in the Liverpool School of Tropical Medicine and manager of a WHO Collaborating Centre. His main interest is prospective health impact assessment of policies, programs, plans, and projects in developed and developing economies.

Robert Bos is executive secretary of the joint WHO/Food and Agriculture Organization/ United Nations Environment Programme Panel of Experts on Environmental Management for Vector Control and a scientist in the water, sanitation, and health unit at the headquarters of WHO in Geneva, Switzerland. His work focuses on health impact assessment of water resources development projects, environmental management for disease vector control, and the links between biodiversity and human health.

David J. Bradley, professor of tropical hygiene in the Department of Infectious and Tropical Diseases at the London School of Hygiene and Tropical Medicine, is a physician, epidemiologist, and zoologist. He serves as co-director of the U.K. Malaria Reference Laboratory and as head of a U.K. Department for International Development research group on applied aspects of tropical diseases, especially malaria.

Mark A. Cane is the G. Unger Vetlesen Professor of Earth and Climate Sciences at the Lamont–Doherty Earth Observatory of Columbia University. His current research centers on variations in the paleoclimate record, especially abrupt changes, and on the impact of climate variability on human activities, such as agriculture and health. With S.E. Zebiak, he built the first dynamical prediction model of El Niño, which was used to publicly forecast the 1986 El Niño event. Cane is the author of nearly 200 publications.

Elizabeth A. Casman is a member of the research faculty of the Department of Engineering and Public Policy at Carnegie Mellon University. Her research interests include the effects of global change on infectious disease incidence and risk modeling of infectious disease transmission.

Jonathan St. H. Cox is a research fellow in the U.K. Department for International Development–sponsored Malaria Programme at the London School of Hygiene and Tropical Medicine. In recent years, his research has examined linkages between the environment and malaria, especially in Africa. His current research is focused on the application of geographical information systems and remote sensing for malaria surveillance and epidemic early warning.

Robert S. Desowitz is professor emeritus of tropical medicine and medical microbiology at the University of Hawaii and adjunct professor of epidemiology at the School of Public Health, University of North Carolina. His major research has been on the epidemiology and immunology of malaria, particularly as related to pregnancy. He is a writer of popular books on infectious disease, including *Who Gave Pinta to the Santa Maria?* His book, *Kala-azar: Chroniques Indiennes d'une Epidemie,* was awarded the Prix Prescrire as the best French medical book for 2000–2001.

Hadi Dowlatabadi holds a Canada Research Chair in Applied Mathematics at the University of British Columbia and is a university fellow at Resources for the Future. Formerly, he was director of the Center for the Integrated Study of the Human Dimensions of Global Change at Carnegie Mellon University, where he and his colleagues developed integrated assessments of climate change and its impacts.

Baruch Fischhoff is university professor in the Department of Engineering and Public Policy and the Department of Social and Decision Sciences at Carnegie Mellon University, where he is also director of the Center for Integrated Study of Human Dimensions of Global Change. His research focuses on basic processes of judgement and decision-making relevant to managing environmental, health, and safety risks.

Ilya R. Fischhoff is a graduate student in the Department of Ecology and Evolutionary Biology, Princeton University, where he focuses on conservation biology. He has done research on public response to biotechnology, the precautionary principle, and animal behavior.

Dana A. Focks, recently with the Center for Medical, Agricultural, and Veterinary Entomology of the Animal Research Service, U.S. Department of Agriculture, is known for his numerical simulation models of dengue hemorrhagic fever transmission and mosquito density. He currently serves as a consultant to WHO and various U.S. government agencies on vector-borne diseases.

Duane J. Gubler is the director of the Division of Vector-Borne Infectious Diseases at the National Center for Infectious Diseases of the Centers for Disease Control and Prevention. He has spent 35 years working on the ecology, prevention, and control of vector-borne diseases and has coordinated major emergency epidemic responses, including the recent West Nile virus epidemic in the United States and the Indian plague epidemic in 1994. The author of 195 publications, he recently edited a book about dengue/dengue hemorrhagic fever.

Renato d'A. Gusmão is program coordinator for Communicable Diseases' Control of the Pan American Health Organization, which is a regional bureau of WHO. For the past 12 years, he has advised American countries regarding malaria control. Combining biomedical, environmental, and behavioral approaches, his work focuses on initiatives to promote better health conditions in Central and South America and the Caribbean.

Chev Kidson is a professor in tropical medicine at Mahidol University, Bangkok, and a professor at the Chinese Academy of Preventive Medicine, Beijing. He is also director of Science and Technology for Equitable Economic Development. His current research focuses on economic development policy and infectious disease surveillance strategy. Previously, he served as director of the Queensland Institute of Medical Research, Australia.

Anatole Kondrachine recently retired as chief of Malaria Control at WHO in Geneva. He has co-authored many manuals and textbooks on malaria prevention and control in the former Soviet Republics. His most recent book is *Malariology*.

R. Sari Kovats is a research fellow in the Department of Epidemiology and Population Health in the London School of Hygiene and Tropical Medicine. She was a lead author for the health chapter in the IPCC Third Assessment Report and has co-authored several reports on the health impacts of climate change and climate variability (particularly El Niño) for WHO and the United Nations Environment Programme.

Lester B. Lave is university professor and Higgins Professor of Economics at Carnegie Mellon University, with appointments in the Business School, Engineering School, and the Public Policy School. His research has focused on health, safety, and environmental issues, including the effect of air pollution on health, estimating the benefits and costs of automobile safety standards, risk analysis of carcinogenic chemicals, testing the carcinogenicity of chemicals, valuing natural resources, and global climate change.

Socrates Litsios retired from WHO in 1997 after 30 years of service. His career positions included chief of operational research in the Division of Research and Communications Science, chief of primary health care in the Division of Strengthening of Health Services, and senior scientist with the Control of Tropical Diseases Programme. His book publications are *The Tomorrow of Malaria* and *Plague Legends: From the Miasmas of Hippocrates to the Microbes of Pasteur*.

Janice Longstreth, a board-certified toxicologist, is president of the Institute for Global Risk Research, which she founded in 1998 and which is dedicated to the development of novel methods for risk assessment, risk management, and risk communication. She is a member of the Environmental Effects Panel of the United Nations Environment Programme and she was a lead author of the chapter on the human health effects of additional ultraviolet radiation for the 1991 and 1994 IPCC Assessments.

Wolfgang Lutz is leader of the Population Project at the International Institute for Applied Systems Analysis (IIASA), Austria; principal investigator of the Asian MetaCentre for Population and Sustainable Development Analysis, Singapore; coordinator of the Global Science Panel on Population and Environment; and secretary general of the International Union for the Scientific Study of Population. His main interests are population forecasting, family demography and population–environment interactions.

Pim Martens is a senior researcher at the International Centre for Integrative Studies, Maastricht University, the Netherlands, where he directs the Global Assessment Centre. His research focuses on globalization, environmental change, and human health. He was lead author of several IPCC assessment reports, as well as publications of WHO and the United Nations Environment Programme. He is editor-in-chief the international journal, *Global Change and Human Health*.

Penny Masuoka is an assistant professor at the Uniformed Services University and also is affiliated with the National Aeronautics and Space Administration's Goddard Space Flight Center in Greenbelt, Maryland.

Anthony J. (Tony) McMichael is director of the National Centre for Epidemiology and Population Health at the Australian National University in Canberra. His recent research focused on the health impacts of environmental changes, particularly climate change, and developing modeling approaches to estimate future impacts. He has chaired the health impact assessment team for IPCC since 1993 and advises organizations such as WHO and the World Bank on environmental health matters.

M. Granger Morgan is professor and head of the Department of Engineering and Public Policy at Carnegie Mellon University, where he also holds academic appointments in the Department of Electrical and Computer Engineering and in the H. John Heinz III School of Public Policy and Management. His research addresses a wide range of problems in technology and public policy, including risk assessment management and communication and the characterization and treatment of uncertainty.

Jean Mouchet was formerly chairman of the Microbiology, Parasitology, and Medical Entomology Division of the Institut de Recherches pour le Développement (IRD). Now retired, he serves as consultant for IRD and the French Ministry of Foreign Affairs. He is a member of the WHO Expert Panel on Malaria and he was WHO consultant in Asia and Africa on more than thirty missions. He has authored more than 350 scientific papers on vector-borne diseases and two books on malaria.

Paul Reiter is chief of the Entomology Section of the Centers for Disease Control and Prevention (CDC) laboratories in San Juan, Puerto Rico. Currently, he is directing a one-year CDC-funded research project on the biology and control of vectors of West Nile virus at the Harvard School of Public Health. He serves on the WHO Panel of Experts on Vector Biology and Control and has been a lead author for the U.S. Government Climate Change Research Program.

Donald R. Roberts is director of the Center for Applications of Remote Sensing and GIS in Public Health and professor of tropical public health at the Uniformed Services University of the Health Sciences in Bethesda, Maryland. He is also an adjunct professor in the emerging infectious diseases program. His research emphasizes malaria ecology and ecological issues of malaria control. He was the U.S. spokesperson for an international coalition that argued successfully for preserving options of developing countries to use DDT for malaria control.

Guido Sabatinelli is regional advisor for Roll Back Malaria in the WHO Office for the Eastern Mediterranean Region. Previously, he served as regional advisor for Roll Back Malaria in the WHO Regional Office for the European Region, where he established a malaria control program to address the resurgence of malaria in Turkey, the Caucasus, and the Central Asian countries of former Soviet Union. For 15 years, he worked on malaria epidemiology and control in Africa, and he has published more than 120 papers on malaria in international journals.

Allan Schapira is regional adviser on malaria at the WHO Regional Office for the Western Pacific. Previously, he has worked in Africa, at WHO headquarters, and in Vietnam, Cambodia, and Laos. His research has dealt mainly with management of malarial disease and drug resistance.

Michael E. Schlesinger is professor of atmospheric sciences, University of Illinois at Urbana–Champaign, where he directs the Climate Research Group. His research has focused on estimating the temperature sensitivity of the earth's climate system; determining the causes of temperature changes observed during the past 150 years; performing integrative assessments of climate change; and modeling the coupled climate-chemistry system.

Vinod Prakash Sharma, currently with the WHO South-East Asia Regional Office, New Delhi, previously served as director of India's Malaria Research Centre and as additional director general of the Indian Council of Medical Research. He has served in many organizations, including as president of the National Academy of Sciences, India (1999–2000); received many awards and honors, including the title of Padma Shree (given by the President of India for lifetime achievement) and the Darling Foundation Prize (given by WHO, Geneva); and authored many books, including *Indian Anophelines*.

Kenneth M. Strzepek is professor of civil and environmental engineering at the University of Colorado at Boulder and fellow of the International Water Management Institute. His recent research focuses on the economic impacts of climatic change on water, environmental, and agricultural systems. Recently, he served as the senior technical advisor for climate change impacts on water resources for the U.S. Country Studies Program. His book publications include *As Climate Changes: International Impacts and Implications*.

Tang Lin-hua is professor and director of the Institute of Parasitic Diseases of the Chinese Academy of Preventive Medicine, which is the WHO Collaborating Center for Malaria, Schistosomiasis, and Filariasis. His research focuses on the epidemiology of malaria and malaria control in the People's Republic of China.

Mark L. Wilson is associate professor of epidemiology (School of Public Health) and associate chair of ecology and evolutionary biology (College of Literature Science and the Arts) at the University of Michigan. His research addresses the environmental determinants of zoonotic and arthropod-borne diseases, the evolution of vector-host-parasite systems, and the analysis of transmission dynamics. He has served on many government advisory groups and is the author of more than 100 research articles, book chapters, and reports.

The Contextual Determinants of Malaria

Introduction

Elizabeth A. Casman and Hadi Dowlatabadi

One of our manuscript reviewers suggested we consider renaming this book *The Contextual Influences of Malaria*, because "Determinants" was too "deterministic." Yet, determinants are precisely what we are after. Various features of malaria epidemiology have long been given mathematical expression, and recent climate change impact studies have used such formulas as surrogates for future malaria risk. If we are to take such studies seriously, we must be convinced that their equations include the true controlling determinants.

To be able to predict future malaria risk, an understanding of the history of malaria and of its current contextual determinants is essential. Moreover, consideration of how the current determinants of malaria will evolve in the future, accompanied by a frank analysis of the uncertainty surrounding such predictions, is also necessary. We hope that the chapters in this volume will inform future malaria risk assessments by identifying the important contextual determinants and by making explicit the strengths, weaknesses, and conditionalities of the predictive relationships used in such assessments, especially those concerning the health impacts of global climate change.

Organization of the Volume

Because a desire to understand the effects and relative importance of future climate change on malaria largely motivated the development of the workshop, the book begins with a set of reports on the results of current malaria and climate change models and the role of the Intergovernmental Panel on Climate Change (IPCC; an investigative committee convened under the auspices of the World Meteorological Organization and the U.N. Environment Programme) in coming to grips with this issue (Part 1).

The discussions in Part 1 set the stage for the regional assessments presented in Part 2, which describe the factors that have controlled the retreat and spread of malaria in different parts of the world. Part 3 focuses on selected high-impact determinants and how we currently predict them to change over the next 50 years. Originally, we had thought that we would be able to distill a set of criteria from these reports that could be used together with the MIASMA malaria distribution model to better predict the risk of the spread of malaria in the twenty-first century. By the end of the workshop, however, it had become clear that an entirely new framing would be necessary; it is the focus of Part 4.

Overview of the Chapters

Part 1: Malaria and Climate Change

The well-established relationships between temperature and malaria parasite and vector maturation rates form the basis of the MIASMA malaria distribution model, which has played a central role in IPCC reports (Chapter 1 by McMichael and Kovats). The results and enhancements of the most recent version of this model are presented by the model's creator, Pim Martens, in Chapter 2. In Chapter 3, Casman elaborates on the concept of malaria risk and distinguishes it from transmission potential, reiterating the importance of contextual determinants in malaria risk calculations.

Part 2: Regional Assessments

The great malaria eradication campaigns of the mid-twentieth century form the backdrop for most of the current regional malaria situations. During those campaigns, malaria was eliminated from North America, Europe, the USSR, Australia, and most of India and China; it also was greatly reduced in Asia and Latin America. The eradication campaigns were massive, complex, and expensive—and, in countries that did not possess or create the public health infrastructure to continue these programs, ultimately doomed to failure. That said, most of the regions currently experience less malaria than they did before the eradication campaign. And because of the earlier eradication campaigns (which had reduced malaria to a focal disease in many places), today's malaria situation is often a story of radiation from isolated foci rather than widespread endemicity.

Central and South America fit this pattern. Like most other regions, this region experienced a period of fairly successful but incomplete suppression of malaria in the mid-twentieth century as a direct result of the global malaria eradication campaign. The termination of this effort was followed by a return of the disease to many of the places from which it had been eliminated. Roberts, the primary author of the regional assessment for the Americas presented in Chapter 4, maintains that the single most important contextual determinant of malaria in most parts of this region is the number of houses sprayed with DDT. He observes that the lowest malaria burden the Americas ever experienced was maintained during a period of warming temperatures, prolonged and unprecedented human population growth, poverty, urbanization, jungle colonization, population movement, social unrest, and government instability, all considered to be major determinants of malaria. Furthermore, he notes that, now that DDT house spraying has been greatly curtailed, the number of malaria cases is rapidly increasing in many parts of this region. He argues that DDT is still needed for malaria control in many areas, a view that is subsequently disputed by Gusmão in Chapter 5. (This debate is reminiscent of the ongoing schism between public health and medical approaches to malaria control under the constraint of funding inadequate to pursue both, the history of which is powerfully related in Chapter 17).

In Chapter 6, Sabatinelli describes the complex effects of political and economic decisions on the epidemiology of malaria in Europe, the Caucasus, and Central Asia. As mentioned before, the eradication campaigns of the mid-twentieth century eliminated malaria from Europe and from almost all the countries of the Soviet Union; however, malaria remained active in residual foci in the Asian part of Turkey and in Azerbaijan. By the end of the 1980s, malaria was nearly a forgotten disease in this region; however, since 1993, malaria has dramatically reemerged. Sabatinelli relates the disheartening story of how the fall of the Soviet Union contributed to the resurgence of malaria in the newly independent states, through a disintegration of infrastructures and the various ripple effects of economic disruption. He also discusses how large-scale agriculture and hydroelectric power development projects in Turkey led to malaria epidemics that spread throughout that country. Finally, the growing number and various types of imported malaria cases in western Europe are quantified.

Southeast Asia also has experienced the pattern of massive malaria control efforts, relaxation, and severe resurgence of malaria radiating from groups of people who did not benefit from the initial malaria control programs, cycling into new (more expensive, less effective) control efforts. Access to medical services is uneven in this region, and the ready availability of antimalaria drugs without proper quality control or patient supervision is blamed, in part, for the emergence of multiple-drug-resistant malaria strains in this region. In Indochina, malaria is kept in circulation among forest-dwelling ethnic minorities but is most lethal for the nonimmune temporary forest visitors: miners, loggers, farmers, and military personnel. In Chapter 7, Schapira explains how poverty and population pressure motivate nonimmune people to venture into the malarious forests and presents the various programs used to mitigate the risks.

The malaria situation in South Asia is also rooted in the worldwide eradication efforts. Malaria was nearly eradicated from India in the early 1960s, but now India is endemic for malaria except in some coastal and mountainous areas. Before the eradication era, an estimated 75 million cases and a million deaths were reported each year. After eradication programs (1946–1964), only about 100,000 cases a year were reported. The expensive, though successful, programs were deemphasized, resulting in the reemergence of malaria, which peaked at 6.5 million cases in 1976. A malaria control program begun in 1977 reduced cases to about 2 million by 1985, at which level it has stabilized. The malaria situation in this region is notable in the variety of "human-made" malarias present. In Chapter 8, Sharma describes the unintended effects of irrigation projects, industrial development, international borders, and the provision of intermittent piped drinking water to cities in enlarging vector habitat and amplifying malaria incidence. In addition to climate, factors such as widespread poverty, population growth, urbanization, population migration, drug resistance, pesticide shortages, and underfunded public health programs all contribute to the malaria problem in this region.

Although malaria has largely been suppressed in most of North Africa and the Middle East, warfare (and the attendant diversion of resources from public health) has created two large foci of malaria that are sources of malaria to their neighbors, enemies, and recipients of their refugees: Iraq and (from central Asia) Afghanistan. Smaller foci exist in Yemen and Syria, and the circulation of labor within the Middle East often brings cases of imported malaria. Beljaev reviews the malaria situation in this region and discusses hierarchies for the determinants of malaria in Chapter 9.

Unlike in the other regions, the malaria situation in Africa south of the Sahara has not improved relative to the pre-eradication days. Rather than the intense eradication programs instituted elsewhere, "pre-eradication studies" were undertaken in 1967–1969 to assess obstacles such as administrative, infrastructural, economic, and educational deficiencies that would have to be overcome to ensure the success of eradication, but full-scale eradication programs were never begun. In 1975, African malaria accounted

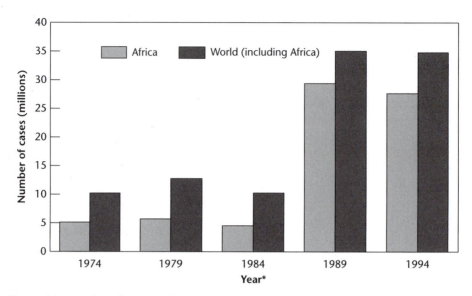

Figure I-1. Number of Reported Malaria Cases, WHO Africa Region, 1974–1994

Notes: See Chapter 10 of this book for a description of WHO Africa Region.

*Total for 1974 does not include China. 1994 data includes, for first time, both slide and clinically diagnosed cases. See original sources for further information about the collection and reporting of data; data collection methods shifted over time. Reported cases for 1974–1984 are from WHO data in Giles and Warrell 1993; 1989–1994 data are from WHO 1997.

for about one-half the world burden, but now approximately 90% of the world's 300–500 million cases occur in this region. It is not unrelated that less than 10% of antimalaria dollars are spent in Africa south of the Sahara. Figure I-1 contrasts *reported* cases of malaria in the region with the total world. Reported cases of malaria are an order of magnitude lower than estimated cases, with the greatest amount of underreporting considered to be in Africa.

In Chapter 10, Cox, Mouchet, and Bradley present a thoughtful discussion of what we do and don't know about the determinants of malaria in Africa and how this affects our predictive abilities. The key determinant of malaria transmission in Africa is the great efficiency of African vectors. This vector system is responsible for very high inoculation rates and is remarkably resilient in the face of a wide range of environmental conditions.

Stable malaria accounts for the bulk of malaria cases in Africa. With stable malaria, the consequences of environmental and social changes on transmission are damped by the immunity of the heavily infected population. Another category of malaria epidemiology—unstable, or epidemic malaria—occurs in Africa at the vectors' limits of altitude, latitude (surrogates for temperature), or rainfall. There, small changes in environmental or social variables may result in epidemics. Cox, Mouchet, and Bradley emphasize the importance of considering temperature and rainfall changes, background levels of immunity, population density, migration, contagious processes, land use, local entomology, the timing of the environmental change, and the availability of health-care and malaria-control measures when evaluating the effects of climate change in this region.

Part 3: A Changing Context

Part 3 is devoted to cross-cutting, high-impact global determinants and how we predict that they will change over the next 50 years. It strikes us as unbalanced to consider the impacts of climate change in isolation when other momentous global changes are predicted to simultaneously occur. The section begins with a report on the current state of the art in climate change prediction by Basher and Cane (Chapter 11), followed by chapters about the most important other global determinants of malaria and how they are expected to change in the near future.

The development of new, cheap, effective antimalaria treatments or vaccines could conceivably have a tremendous impact on the success of public health efforts and hence the distribution of malaria and the prospects for global eradication. In Chapter 12, Desowitz reviews the history of drug and vaccine development, its difficulties, and recent promising research directions. Vaccine research is currently very well funded, and several different vaccine strategies are being investigated. Desowitz warns, though, that it is prudent to assume that a cheap, effective vaccine will not be available in the next several decades. Therefore, the near-term strategy must rely on antimalaria drug developments, both drugs that can reverse drug resistance and new classes of drugs that attack unique *Plasmodium* organelles and metabolic pathways. Drug development is currently not as well funded as vaccine development, and as Desowitz points out, there are financial disincentives for pharmaceutical companies to engage in such research.

Urbanization is associated with increased malaria in some regions and decreased malaria in others, depending on how the cities and peri-urban slums affect vector habitat and on the ability of the health-care authorities to extend services to all inhabitants (see Chapters 7, 8, and 10). Thus, changing patterns of human density, especially urbanization, will change the malaria landscape in many places. Lutz provides an overview of current predictions of population growth, demographic changes, and urbanization in Chapter 13 and discusses the relationship between population growth, population growth policies, and climate change.

The predictor of success of past eradication programs and the best correlate to malaria's absence today is a country's ability to mount and sustain a sophisticated, thorough malaria-control effort that involves vector control, surveillance, and treatment. Such efforts are limited by the economic strength of the endemic and donor countries, among other variables. In Chapter 14, Lave and Dowlatabadi offer some thoughts on alternative economic futures for the world and how they might affect the future of malaria control.

Every one of the regional assessments identified population movement as a major determinant of malaria. In Chapter 15, Longstreth and Kondrachine discuss the relationship between malaria and population movements. Fischhoff presents a compilation of recent rate and trend data on major types of population movement (for example, internally displaced people, refugees, and vacation travelers) in Chapter 16.

Another major theme emerging from the regional assessments is the existence and sustainability of public health functions (public hygiene, disease prevention, epidemic detection and containment, and vector control) as distinct from medicine (which deals primarily with diagnosis and treatment). In Chapter 17, Litsios provides an insightful history of the evolution of public health infrastructures and malaria-control programs in the twentieth century, especially with respect to the activities and philosophies of the

World Health Organization and its predecessor, the World Health Assembly. Currently, malaria is receiving priority attention on many fronts; the World Health Organization's Roll Back Malaria initiative, which calls for a halving of the malaria burden by 2010, leads the way. Several multilateral and bilateral donor agencies and philanthropies have pledged of hundreds of millions of dollars for malaria suppression and research. Litsios fears that the mistakes (vertical, locally unsustainable, high-cost programs) of the past are about to be repeated with this infusion of resources and enthusiasm.

Part 4: Synthesis

Fischhoff and others begin Part 4 by attempting to organize the principles discussed throughout the book in a systematic integrated assessment framework (Chapter 18). The authors argue that even though doing so will add an even greater element of uncertainty to already uncertain projections, medical, economic, and sociopolitical change should be projected along with climate, demographics, and contagious processes in such assessments to ensure the inclusion of the dominant controlling variables that act on malaria distribution.

A workshop summary (Chapter 19) follows, in which the issue of the relationship between climate change and future malaria risk is revisited and the principal themes of the presentations are reviewed. One result of the presentations and discussions was the realization that malaria is influenced positively and negatively by numerous factors. Determinants are not identical in any two regions; however, in region after region, disease risks are associated with poverty, limited access to health services, population movement, under-resourced or negligent public health management by governments, marginalized populations serving as malaria reservoirs, and water management without adequate attention to health impacts.

As for the contribution of global warming to malaria risk, a less-than-unanimous consensus emerged during the drafting of the workshop summary (Chapter 19). The current determinants of malaria risk are expected to remain relevant into the next half-century, so a careful parsing of the risk attributable to these determinants should form the basis of future risk projections. Climate currently plays a central role in determining a region's underlying ecology and associated malaria potential, and climate variability influences the intensity of transmission. However, whether that potential is realized depends on an array of human actions. Analogously, the extent to which climate change will affect future malaria distribution can be evaluated only within the context of societal choices and actions.

References

Gilles, H.M., and D.A. Warrell (eds.). 1993. *Bruce-Chwatt's Essential Malariology,* 3rd edition. New York: Oxford University Press.

WHO (World Health Organization). 1997. World Malaria Situation in 1994. *Weekly Epidemiological Record* 72(36): 269–276.

PART 1

*Malaria and
Climate Change:
Issues and Analytic Tools*

Chapter 1

International Efforts To Understand the Link between Climate Change and Malaria

Anthony J. McMichael and R. Sari Kovats

In this chapter, we describe the Intergovernmental Panel on Climate Change (IPCC) and its process for evaluating the current science on the health impacts of climate change. IPCC is charged with carrying out systematic reviews and assessments of the relevant published scientific literature and with publishing formal reports of its assessments. Three reports have been published: in 1991, 1996, and 2001. Since the U.N. Framework Convention on Climate Change, forged at the 1992 U.N. Conference on Environment and Development in Rio de Janeiro, Brazil, IPCC has been the main source of scientific information and advice to governments within that convention.

Early IPCC assessments of changes in potential malaria transmission relied heavily on the results of the MIASMA model, which estimates how transmissibility would alter in response to changes in climate that affect the biology of mosquitoes and malaria parasites (Martens 1998). These assessments were influential in bringing the issue of the health implications of climate change into focus. This type of modeling, however, should be extended to take into account projections of social, economic, and demographic changes. For example, future assessments of health impacts could incorporate plausible scenarios of socioeconomic development (such as those as recently developed and proposed by IPCC) in a systematic effort to include these important contextual variables.

The IPCC Review Process

During the 1980s, several international conferences addressed the emerging prospect of global climate change occurring in response to the ongoing, accelerated buildup of anthropogenic greenhouse gases in the lower atmosphere (troposphere). Additional attention was focused on this issue by the newly forged international recognition of the hazards posed by human-induced stratospheric ozone depletion and by the emerging commitments to multilateral action to curb the release of ozone-destroying gases, especially chlorofluorocarbons. The Montreal Protocol was adopted in 1987 for the control of ozone-destroying substances.

The manifest complexity of the anticipated global climate change process and of the mechanisms by which it might affect various natural and societal systems suggested the need for an international, multidisciplinary scientific review and assessment. This

9

endeavor would be a source of continuing information for national governments and policymakers. IPCC was thus established in 1988 and exists under the aegis of the World Meteorological Organization (WMO) and the U.N. Environment Programme. Its secretariat is located within the WMO in Geneva, Switzerland.

Approximately 2,000 scientists contribute to the IPCC reports as lead authors in chapter teams; they work on a volunteer basis, and national governments pay their participation costs. These scientists are organized in three working groups. Working Group I addresses the science of the climate change process and the modeled predictions of future climate scenarios in response to various scenarios of future greenhouse gas emissions. Working Group II addresses the impacts of climate change and the prospects for adaptive reduction of those impacts. Working Group III addresses the social, economic, and policy dimensions of climate change impacts and their mitigation.

The chapter teams are assembled by the co-chairs of the IPCC Working Groups from nominations received from national governments. This process must weigh the need for topic and disciplinary expertise against the need for balanced international representation. Various contributing authors (identified primarily but not exclusively via the network of lead authors) also make specific expert contributions to the text drafts.

The IPCC review process is open, participatory, and accountable. The essential task is scientific review by consensus. The IPCC chapter teams do not carry out research in their own right. Their task is to review the published scientific literature, a process which takes approximately two years for each review cycle. The draft chapters are eventually sent to a wide range of scientists, who serve as external peer reviewers. The reviewers' comments are then systematically considered by the lead authors in the presence of the chapter's two review editors, who must confirm to the Working Group that the review comments have been responded to satisfactorily. The development of this broad-based, peer-reviewed, and increasingly transparent procedure of consensual scientific review provides a workable model of how to minimize the influence of vested interests in the assessment of such intrinsically complex, political, and commercially sensitive topics. The IPCC review process has thus effectively neutralized the partisan influence of "bought science," that is, the substantial conservative interests of the coal, oil-producing, petrochemical, and automotive industries. This neutralization is achieved not by exclusion but by dilution of the full spectrum of partisan views within a broad-based, open process.

In its recent work, IPCC has sought to standardize the work of the various chapter teams by specifying crosscutting issues or themes that should be addressed. Within Working Group II, for example, the Third Assessment Report pays systematic attention to the handling and communication of scientific uncertainty; to considerations of how anticipated impacts and their avoidance could affect sustainable development and international equity; to the implications for social decisionmaking (within a decision-analytic framework); and, where possible, to the estimation of the economic costs of impacts and adaptive strategies.

The IPCC Analysis of Health Impacts

The First Assessment Report had relatively little to say about the potential impact of climate change on human health. That topic evidently was a blind spot in the collective eye of climate change science in the late 1980s. However, by the early 1990s, recognition of the potential importance of this topic was growing. Consequently, both the Second and Third Assessment Reports have contained stand-alone chapters on human health impacts.

The published scientific literature on the health impacts of climate change was relatively modest throughout the 1990s. Indeed, over previous decades, epidemiologists had carried out relatively few conventional studies of how natural variations in climatic conditions affected human health. Because the weather is always with us and is not substantively modifiable by human intervention, it drew little interest from public health scientists. However, the dual stimuli of the prospect of global climate change and of the rapidly accruing new knowledge about the quasiperiodic cycles of the El Niño system and other regional climatic oscillations (see Chapter 11) drew attention to the importance of studying climate variation, climate change, and human health.

The recognized range of likely health impacts of climate change is considerable and diverse. It includes the direct impacts of thermal stress (heat waves and cold spells), meteorologically modulated air pollution, and weather disasters (tropical cyclones, storms, floods, and droughts). It also includes a wider range of less direct, often ecologically mediated impacts such as geographic and temporal changes in the transmission patterns of vector-borne and other infectious diseases; changes in regional yields of agriculture and, perhaps, ocean fisheries (and hence in the nutrition and health of local dependent populations); and the diverse health consequences of population displacement (for example, due to a rise in sea level or to declining agroecosystems) and economic dislocation.

For only several of these health outcomes had the likely impacts of climate change been systematically and quantitatively assessed. By the mid-1990s, early attempts at modeling health impacts had been published for heat wave–associated mortality, malaria, and dengue fever (Martens et al. 1995; Martens, Jetten, and Focks 1997). Perhaps not surprisingly, in the health impact chapters of the IPCC reports, considerable emphasis has been placed on the issue of how climate change is likely to affect potential patterns of malaria transmission. It is, after all, one of the world's great (and currently increasing) public health problems, affecting several hundred million people every year and causing approximately 1 million deaths, mostly in children. Furthermore, the basic relationship of malaria transmission to temperature and humidity was worked out in the 1950s (Macdonald 1957), and it has long been understood that climatic conditions set the ultimate boundaries for malaria transmission and that shorter-term climate variations affect the local patterns and cycles of transmission.

The IPCC Analysis of Malaria Transmissibility

Each IPCC health impact team reviews three categories of scientific evidence for each health outcome:

1. the accrued empirical evidence that describes the climate-disease relationship and any associated theory that has evolved around that knowledge;
2. any evidence that recent climatic trends (regardless of whether they are human-induced) have been associated with changes in health outcome patterns; and
3. the results of formal scenario-based modeling of potential future changes in the geography, seasonality, or rates of occurrence of the health outcome.

Because of space constraints within each IPCC chapter, a detailed review of the evidence is not possible. Typically, the first category above has been dealt with summarily in the chapter text, even though the lead authors for each particular health outcome category are usually knowledgeable about that dimension of evidence.

Historically, for malaria, a great deal of evidence has been published about its relationship to climatic and environmental conditions. However, much of this reporting has been local and episodic. Few systematic analyses exist of historical patterns and trends in malaria transmission in relation to climatic variation or climate change.

In the Second Assessment Report, considerable emphasis was paid to several early mathematical modeling studies of the impact of climate change on future potential malaria transmission (IPCC 1996). These comprised both statistical and process (or biological) models that produced estimates of how the geographic boundaries of potential malaria transmission would change under specified climate change scenarios. From this basis, it was possible to discuss the approximate shift in the proportion of the world population living in geographic zones of potential transmission.

Since the mid-1990s, attempts to improve and extend the modeling of climate change impacts on malaria transmission using the MIASMA model (see Chapter 2) have been intensive. The IPCC process has generated positive feedback and has stimulated the following developments in modeling climatic impacts on malaria transmission:

- replacement of a global "world standard mosquito" with 19 regionally dominant anopheline species and their associated temperature-sensitive parameter values,
- the modeling of regional changes in seasonal transmission patterns,
- the estimation of additional numbers of people at risk under alternative emissions scenarios (unconstrained and constrained), and
- the modeling of how alternative socioeconomic development scenarios would modulate the impact of climate change on potential malaria transmission.

The last development listed above highlights the tension between seeking clarity of scenario-based modeling, with minimum specified change in the future, and seeking to incorporate as many of the important, plausible, modulating influences as technically possible. The minimalist approach, in the tradition of classical experimental science, says, "If we hold constant everything else, how would a change in world climate affect malaria transmission?" The expansionist approach says, "Yes, but that is unrealistic. We live in a changing world—and, furthermore, we have the capacity to enact various purposeful changes that might reduce the incidence of malaria. So, the more interesting question is, 'What residual impacts would climate change have on malaria transmission patterns, once we have allowed for those additional social, economic, technological, and political changes?'"

IPCC recently produced a set of emission scenarios; each scenario is a different configuration of parameter values on key economic, social, and political axes (IPCC 2000). For example, a two-by-two matrix based on two axes—local versus global, and market-driven consumerism versus community-based conservationism—yields four possible future worlds (Figure 1-1). These four worlds (and one typical model-based estimate of their associated emission-dependent temperature increases by 2050) are referred to as:

A1: World markets (+1.6 °C),
A2: Provincial enterprise (+2.2 °C),
B1: Global sustainability (+0.8 °C), and
B2: Local stewardship (+1.6 °C).

Conclusion

The plan is that, in future IPCC modeling of global climate change, researchers will use some or all of this family of socioeconomic scenarios and their estimates of greenhouse gas emissions. Furthermore, these scenarios also can be used to estimate the modulating

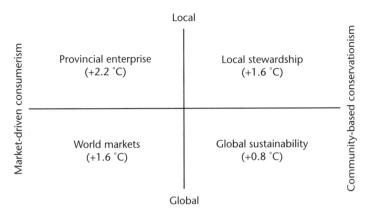

Figure 1-1. Future Worlds Using the IPCC Emissions Scenario

effects of social, economic, and political changes on population vulnerability to health impacts.

Tackling those issues is a primary focus of the chapters that follow.

References

IPCC (Intergovernmental Panel on Climate Change). 1996. *Climate Change 1995: Impacts, Adaptations and Mitigation of Climate Change: Scientific-Technical Analysis,* edited by R.T. Watson, M.C. Zinyowera, and R.H. Moss. Contribution of Working Group II to the Second Assessment Report of the Intergovernmental Panel on Climate Change. New York: Cambridge University Press.

———. 2000. *Special Report on Emission Scenarios,* edited by N. Nakićenović and R. Swart. New York: Cambridge University Press.

Macdonald, G. 1957. *The Epidemiology and Control of Malaria.* London, U.K.: Oxford University Press.

Martens, P. 1998. *Health & Climate Change: Modelling the Impacts of Global Warming and Ozone Depletion.* London, U.K.: Earthscan.

Martens, P., T.H. Jetten, and D.A. Focks. 1997. Sensitivity of Malaria, Schistosomiasis and Dengue to Global Warming. *Climatic Change* 35: 145–56.

Martens, P., T.H. Jetten, J. Rotmans, and L.W. Niessen. 1995. Climate Change and Vector-Borne Diseases: A Global Modelling Perspective. *Global Environmental Change* 5(3): 195–209.

Chapter 2

Of Malaria and Models

Challenges in Modeling Global Climate Change and Malaria Risk

Pim Martens

Malaria is a major cause of illness and death worldwide. About 2.4 billion people are at risk of contracting the disease; malaria is currently endemic in 92 countries, and pockets of malaria transmission exist in 8 additional countries (WHO 1997). There are 300–500 million clinical cases of malaria, more than 90% of which occur in sub-Saharan Africa. Worldwide, malaria accounts for about 2 million deaths per year, and the majority of these deaths are of children under five years of age. Of all infectious diseases, malaria continues to be one of the biggest contributors to the global disease burden in terms of death and suffering.

Malaria risk is determined by many factors, especially the abundance of anopheline mosquito species, human behavior, and the presence of malaria parasites. A change in any of these factors, therefore, will affect the risk of attracting the disease. Only recently has attention been paid to the potential impact of global changes on malaria risk. The geographic range of malaria may change in response to changes in climate, land-use patterns, biodiversity, and sociodemographic structures (including urbanization). Large-scale migration of populations from areas in which malaria is endemic into receptive areas—or vice versa—also may become important (Martens and Hall 2000). In addition, certain human activities can help to prevent the spread of pathogens and reduce mosquito populations; these activities restrict the distribution of malaria in countries that can afford them.

The assessment of the future impact of global changes on malaria is a complex task, because many relationships between changes in global natural and socioeconomic systems and malaria risk are not known, or are insufficiently known. Global changes would not affect malaria in isolation but simultaneously and in conjunction with other ecological and socioeconomic changes occurring on smaller scales. Furthermore, the net impact of global changes would depend on various interactive phenomena: multiplicative exposure effects, feedback pathways, and differences in the vulnerability of local populations. Therefore, a health risk assessment must accommodate the multiple uncertainties across these ecological, economic, and social changes on different spatial and temporal scales (McMichael and Martens 1995).

Of the various global change processes that would affect malaria, most scientific attention to date has focused on climate change and its consequences. In this chapter, I discuss the main models that have been developed to explore this risk (see also McMichael et al. 2000) and the remaining challenges to improving our insight into how global climate change will affect malaria.

Modeling

Kinds of Models

Epidemiologists often use modeling to gain insight into the dynamics of infectious disease epidemics. In estimating the future impacts of climate change on health, several modeling approaches are used. Among the most important ones are empirical–statistical models, process-based models, and integrated models (Parry and Carter 1998).

Empirical–statistical models are based on the statistical relationships observed between climate and health (or health-related) outcomes. They may range from applying simple indices of risk (e.g., identifying the minimum temperature threshold for malaria transmission) to using complex, multivariate models that combine various important environmental factors that affect risk. When these models are founded on good knowledge and when there are good grounds for extrapolation, they can be useful tools for assessing the impact of climate change on health. Empirical–statistical models often are easier to use and less data-demanding than process-based models.

Process-based models draw entirely or substantially on accepted theory (the product of previously accumulated, coherent research findings). They incorporate mathematical equations that represent processes that can be applied universally to similar systems in different environments. For example, an index that encapsulates many of the important processes in malaria transmission is the basic reproduction rate (see next section) or the related vectorial capacity, which may apply to a range of vector-borne diseases and circumstances. Although process-based models provide more insight into the underlying processes than do empirical–statistical models, they are also more data-demanding.

An *integrated modeling approach* is the most comprehensive treatment of the interactions between atmospheric changes and society (Carter et al. 1994). In general, integrated assessment (IA) models try to describe as quantitatively as possible the cause-and-effect relationship of a phenomenon (vertical integration) as well as the cross-linkages and interactions between different contextual circumstances and processes (horizontal integration), including feedback and adaptation. Feedback processes can amplify or dampen important aspects of the system. For example, one important determinant of the number of people infected by malaria is the level of temporary immunity within the target population. Hence, in highly endemic regions where immunity prevalence is high, the impact of a climate-related increase in the malaria transmission potential of the mosquito population will be low (and will soon be counteracted by the additional boost in immunity). Although the modeling approaches are discussed separately, process-based models often draw on relationships derived from empirical–statistical models, and integrated models use all of these methods.

The Impact of Climate Change on Malaria

Models that incorporate a range of meteorological variables have been developed to describe a specific bioclimate "envelope" for malaria. Empirical–statistical models may use multivariate statistical techniques to select predictive variables (whether meteorological or environmental, ground-based or remotely sensed).

Some mosquito species have been successfully mapped in Africa using meteorological data (Lindsay, Parson, and Thomas 1998). Satellite data are often used as a substitute for instrumental meteorological data; weather variables are usually measured at ground level, but coverage can be relatively sparse or inappropriate, especially in developing countries (Hay et al. 1996). In addition, more complex indices may be useful: the normalized difference vegetation index correlates with the photosynthetic activity of plants, rainfall, and saturation deficit. The changes of three important disease vectors (ticks, tsetse flies, and mosquitoes) have been mapped in southern Africa under three climate change scenarios (Hulme 1996). Results indicate that changes in areas suitable for each vector species would be significant, with a net increase for malaria mosquitoes (*Anopheles gambiae*). The final objective of such work is to map human disease risk, but the relationship between vector-borne disease incidence and climate variables is complicated by many socioeconomic and environmental factors.

Another example of an empirical–statistical model is CLIMEX, developed by Sutherst, Maywald, and Skarratt (1995). This model maps the translocation of species between different areas as they respond to climate change. The assessment is based on an ecoclimatic index governed largely by the temperature and moisture requirements of the malaria mosquito. CLIMEX analyses conducted in Australia indicate that the indigenous vector of malaria would be able expand its range 330 kilometers south under one typical scenario of climate change. However, these studies clearly cannot include all factors that affect species distributions. For example, local geographic barriers as well as interaction or competition between species are important factors that determine whether species colonize the full extent of suitable habitat (Davis et al. 1998). Assessments also can include additional dynamic population (process-based) models (e.g., DYMEX, discussed in Sutherst 1998).

In a similar approach, Martin and Lefebvre (1995) developed a malaria potential-occurrence zone model. This model was combined with five general circulation models (GCMs) to estimate the changes in malaria risk based on moisture as well as minimum and maximum temperatures required for parasite development. It corresponded fairly well with the distribution of malaria in the nineteenth century and in the 1990s (the time periods used in the model), after allowing for areas where malaria had been eradicated. An important finding of this modeling exercise was that all simulation runs indicated an increase in seasonal (unstable) malaria transmission at the expense of perennial (stable) transmission.

To assess the health impacts related to climatic changes, the eco-epidemiological modeling framework MIASMA (Modeling Framework for the Health Impact Assessment of Man-Induced Atmospheric Changes) was developed at Maastricht University. MIASMA consists of five models: the thermal stress model, the skin cancer model, the malaria model, the dengue model, and the schistosomiasis model. The models are driven by scenarios of population figures and atmospheric changes, superimposed on baseline data regarding disease incidence, climatic conditions, and ozone-layer thickness.

Martens and colleagues developed an integrated mathematical model for estimating the climate change impacts on malaria that is part of the MIASMA modeling framework (Martens, Jetten, et al. 1995; Martens, Niessen, et al. 1995; Martens, Jetten, and Focks 1997; Martens et al. 1999). MIASMA differs from the other models in that it takes a broad approach in linking GCM-based climate change scenarios with a module that uses the formula for the basic reproduction rate (R_0) to calculate the transmission or epidemic potential of a malaria mosquito population. The use of R_0 is defined as the number of new cases of a disease that will arise from one current case when introduced into

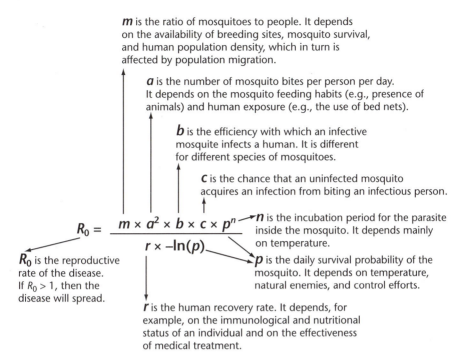

Figure 2-1. Basic Reproduction Rate (R_0) of Malaria

Source: Levins et al. 1993.

a nonimmune host population during a single transmission cycle (Anderson and May 1991). It goes back to classical epidemiological models of infectious disease (Figure 2-1). Model variables within R_0 that are sensitive to temperature include mosquito density, feeding frequency, survival, and extrinsic incubation period. The extrinsic incubation period (i.e., parasite development in the mosquito) is particularly important. The minimum temperature for parasite development is the limiting factor for malaria transmission in many areas.

Tol and Dowlatabadi (1999) integrated the results of MIASMA within FUND (the Climate Framework for Uncertainty Negotiation and Distribution) to estimate the trade-off between climate change and economic growth for malaria risk. The first results of this exercise show the importance of economic variables in estimating changes in future malaria risk.

Challenges

All of the models discussed above have specific advantages and disadvantages (see also Lindsay and Birley 1996), and any attempt to fully represent the complexity of malaria epidemiology and its numerous linkages with other factors in a quantitative model is doomed to failure. However, when dealing with complex, long-term issues surrounded with uncertainties, IA models seem to be appropriate tools. There are multiple approaches to IA (e.g., see Rotmans and Dowlatabadi 1998). The simultaneous use of various methods may improve the quality of an assessment considerably. Even a simplified but integrated model can provide a useful guide to complex issues and complement highly detailed models that cover only some parts of the complexity of malaria epidemiology.

However, to improve health risk assessment by means of integrated modeling, several challenges require our attention. First, highly aggregated assessment models, such as the MIASMA model, clearly need to be validated on a local or regional scale. The equations within a global model may well be inappropriate for particular local conditions. Second, the unavoidable uncertainties introduced within these models must be treated adequately. Finally, model projections must move from looking at climate as the only factor to introducing additional components that influence malaria risk. The challenge lies in the consideration of an evolving context of exposure (McMichael 1996; Dowlatabadi 1997). All of these challenges are intertwined with the level of scale of analysis.

Validation in the Absence of Good Data

For the purposes of this discussion, *validation* is defined as the procedure for testing the adequacy of a given mathematical model (Rotmans et al. 1994). However, two major problems plague the validation of integrated models. First, complete validation of simulation models is impossible because the underlying systems are never closed; that is, they lack essential components (Oreskes, Shrader-Frechette, and Belitz 1994). Second, validation often is not possible because the requisite data and scientific knowledge are not available. One problem often encountered in applying process-based models is that the models—often adequately validated in the data-rich developed world—are found to be ill-suited to, or poorly calibrated for, use in less-developed countries. A paucity of data for validation generally means that data-demanding models often cannot be used under such circumstances (Carter et al. 1994). Unavailability of data will necessitate a reliance on simplified assumptions to generate an initial framework for analysis; this framework can be used to focus interdisciplinary communication on assessing health risks and identifying priorities for future research. Although the use of such assumptions and simplifications will potentially decrease the quantitative accuracy of the assessment, it should still allow for adequate prioritization and estimation of relative risk (Patz and Balbus 1996).

Validation can be divided into different types (Rodin 1990; Rykiel 1996). *Data or pragmatic validation* requires concordance of the model's projections with observational data sets; this concordance often can be assessed by testing the model on historical data sets. However, as mentioned above, the relative inaccuracy and imprecision of ecological and epidemiological data places limits on the model's testability in this way. *Conceptual validation* requires that the hypotheses and the theoretical structures of the model reasonably describe the perceived real world. By implication, the model structure, relations, parameters, and dynamic behavior reflect the prevailing theoretical insights and the key facts relating to the part of reality that the model is supposed to represent.

Although the underlying model relationships may well reflect the prevailing theoretical insights (e.g., the use of the R_0 or its derivatives to estimate malaria transmission dynamics), a conceptually valid model will not necessarily make accurate projections. The highly aggregated outcomes of the global models presented earlier remain difficult to validate, because great uncertainty surrounds the natural limits of malaria distribution (Molineaux 1988). This uncertainty is partly due to the lack of historical records describing the presence of malaria and partly due to the high instability of malaria transmission at the fringes; only infrequent transmission occurs.

However, more confidence in global model outcomes can be obtained by validating the models on a local or regional scale, where data are available. For example, the malaria model developed by Martens and colleagues has been partially validated at the national and regional levels (Martens, Jetten, et al. 1995; Martens, Niessen, et al. 1995; Martens, Jetten, and Focks 1997; Martens et al. 1999). For Africa, and more specifically for Zimbabwe, the model simulated both a seasonal pattern of transmission and the distribution of transmission intensity by altitude within the country (Lindsay and Martens 1998). The model also was validated by using a time series of malaria cases in Colombia. The model output reproduced the interannual variation in malaria cases and the historical peaks (Poveda et al. 1999).

Both exercises showed a qualitative agreement of the model and the observed risk of malaria, illustrating the role of temperature variability in modulating malaria transmission in these regions. Nevertheless, the results must be interpreted with caution; in other regions, climate may not be as dominant in determining the seasonality of malaria transmission.

In this context, Root and Schneider (1995) propose an interesting approach: the so-called strategic cyclical scaling (SCS) method, which involves continuous cycling between large- and small-scale assessments. Such an iterative scaling procedure implies that a specific global model is disaggregated and adjusted for a specific region or country. The new insights are then used to improve the global version, and implementation for another region or country follows. In malaria modeling, some progress has been made (Lindsay and Martens 1998). The SCS method also can be used for the conceptual validation of models.

Cumulative Uncertainties

Any exploration of future developments inevitably involves a considerable degree of uncertainty. The cross-disciplinary character of IA modeling necessarily includes many kinds and sources of uncertainty. Because IA models are end-to-end approaches, they also contain an accumulation of uncertainties (Figure 2-2). Uncertainties may arise from incomplete knowledge of key physiological, chemical, and biological processes. Many uncertainties are of a socioeconomic nature and reflect inadequate knowledge with respect to the driving forces of human behavior.

Various attempts have been made to classify the different types and sources of uncertainty. Morgan and Henrion (1990) distinguish uncertainty about empirical quantities and uncertainty about the functional form of models, which may have arisen from subjective judgement, disagreement among experts, systematic errors, approximation, and inherent randomness. Funtowicz and Ravetz (1990) classify uncertainties in three categories: technical uncertainties concerning observations versus measurements, methodological uncertainties concerning the right choice of analytical tools, and epistemological uncertainties concerning the conception of a phenomenon.

The various types and sources of uncertainty are aggregated into two categories (Rotmans et al. 1994) (Figure 2-3). *Scientific uncertainties* arise from the degree of unpredictability of global climate change processes and their impact on human health, and they may be narrowed as a result of further scientific research or more detailed or appropriate modeling. These uncertainties include, for example, incomplete knowledge about the relationship between precipitation patterns and mosquito abundance. *Social and economic uncertainties* arise from the inherent unpredictability of future geopolitical, socioeconomic, demographic, and technological evolution. Examples of these future eventualities are vaccine development, trends in urbanization, and levels of poverty, all of which affect the vulnerability and response of human populations to global changes.

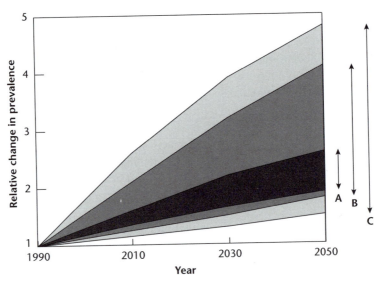

Figure 2-2. Cumulation of Uncertainties Associated with Climate Change Projections, the Dynamics of Malaria Transmission by Vector Mosquitoes, and Malaria Prevalence

Notes: Variations of only some crucial parameters are shown. This example, for *Plasmodium falciparum* in regions of low endemicity, shows how the uncertainty range widens as one moves toward more remote parts of the cause-and-effect chain. Uncertainties in the estimates of changes in malaria prevalence are influenced by uncertainties in the outcomes of climate change models (A), cumulated with uncertainties in the climate-related change of the transmission potential of a vector population (B), and cumulated with uncertainties in the spread of the disease in the human population (C).

The various types and sources of uncertainties in IA models need to be adequately addressed. One simple way of presenting uncertainties is by specifying a set of future scenarios, where the scenarios selected are expected to span a range of plausible, representative futures. The Intergovernmental Panel on Climate Change, for example, adopted this approach for its greenhouse gas emissions scenarios. The difficulty with this approach is that it does not indicate the cumulative uncertainty as well as the origin and meaning of the uncertainty range.

Another approach is the probabilistic method, using a subjective probability distribution for empirical quantities. In this method, a large number of inputs are specified as probability distribution functions, and many model runs are done to determine the uncertainties surrounding the output(s), as shown in Figure 2-2. The major difficulty with this method is that it requires specific knowledge about the nature of the distribution functions and the number of runs required. Furthermore, probability density functions are used merely to address technical uncertainties. These techniques are not suitable for analyzing methodological and epistemological uncertainties, which arise primarily from subjective judgements and fundamental disagreement among experts. Another problem is that classical uncertainty analysis methods address only uncertainties in model inputs and neglect the interactions among multiple, simultaneous uncertainties that are crucial in IA modeling. Therefore, new methods are needed, for example, methods in which not only parameters but also relationships within the model are varied according to the bias and preference of a particular perspective (van Asselt and Rotmans 1996; Janssen 1998).

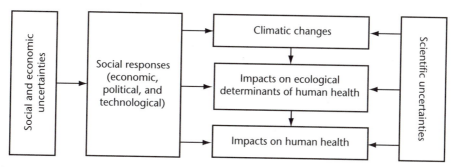

Figure 2-3. Layers of Uncertainty Underlying the Health Impact Assessment of Global Climate Change

Compounding Factors: From Sensitivity to Vulnerability

Early estimates of the impacts of climate change on health focused on climate-determined ranges of disease vectors. These models recognized the importance of temperature in regulating the pace of development for both the malaria parasite and its vector. Put simply, if temperature is too low, the parasite does not complete its development stages in the mosquito. If temperature is too high, the parasite develops, but the mosquito suffers higher mortality and does not live to bite another host. This *climate optimum* is the underpinning of early assessments linking climate change to the spread of malaria.

Recently, there have been significant refinements to the simple model above. The new models reflect species-specific ecological optima in place of a global climate optimum. The new models also acknowledge the ability of mosquitoes to seek microclimates to their liking. These refinements deemphasize the previously assumed linear relationship between temperature and the natural risk of malaria.

There is now also an appreciation of how socioeconomic factors drive a wedge between the natural risk of malaria and its actual manifestation. Thus, while malaria occurred naturally in most temperate regions of the world (e.g., throughout North America and Europe), land use change, industrialization, and isolation of infected individuals led to its eradication (Hamoudi and Sachs 1999). Tol and Dowlatabadi (2001) suggested a simple approach to incorporating the importance of economic development in malaria assessment models. According to this simple paradigm, even where a climate optimum exists, if income per capita is over some $3,000 (in 1999 dollars), malaria has been wiped out. This is a gross oversimplification, but it is another step toward developing more realistic estimates of the global risk of malaria in the next century.

Figure 2-4 displays the results from the latest model by Martens and colleagues (1999). The model projects the population that, in the absence of any interventions, is at risk of getting malaria. This population more than doubles from about 4 billion in 2000 to over 9 billion in 2080. This doubling stems from population growth where malaria risk is present, as well as climate change expanding the range of malaria risk. Concurrent with these changes, the model assumes that socioeconomic development occurs throughout the world, and that more people reach the threshold of annual incomes above $3,000. The population that is at risk of malaria and has not reached the $3,000 income threshold rises initially but then falls as more and more people where malaria would naturally have found a foothold enjoy standards of living, managed environments, and lifestyles that suppress manifestation of this disease.

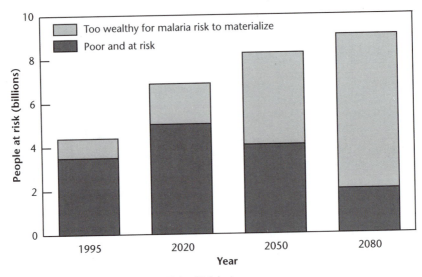

Figure 2-4. Projected Population at Risk of Malaria

Note: Each overall bar shows the projected population at risk of malaria assuming population growth and climate change, from Hadley Centre computer models (HadCM2). A rising proportion of the at-risk population would benefit from socioeconomic development, allowing them to overcome conditions suitable for transmitting malaria. People who remain poor would be more likely to actually contract the disease.

Of course, malaria is determined by a complex array of ecological, social, and economic factors that account for its tenacious hold in tropical regions. Therefore, malaria in tropical countries cannot be compared with the past malaria situation in temperate regions. Furthermore, development trajectories that already compromise overall sustainability (as is the case in most poor countries) will leave the burden of disease as a result of climate change either unmitigated or mitigated only at a high cost to the economy.

A Matter of Scale

In addressing the challenges of validation, uncertainty, and compounding factors, the critical issue is the level of aggregation. The problem of modeling the impact of global change processes on malaria risk is that modeling must cope with many processes that operate on different temporal and spatial levels and that differ in complexity. Looking at Figure 2-5, it is apparent that climate, human, and mosquito systems vary in their spatial and temporal scale—mosquito larvae develop at the level of puddles and at time scales varying from days to weeks, whereas climate change influences the global climate system in time frames from years to centuries or more and economic processes operate on short to medium time scales. Furthermore, short-term needs and interests of stakeholders have to be considered.

Although the assessment of malaria risk may be done on various geographic scales—varying from a village to a country, a region, or the entire world—so far, experience in experimenting with scale levels in modeling is sparse. Downscaling or upscaling the spatial level of a model has profound consequences related to the extent to which the processes considered are generic or distinctly spatially bound in character, that is, whether a relationship holds at larger- or smaller-scale levels. For instance, an early version of the malaria model developed by Martens, Jetten, and colleagues (1995) uses a composite measure of different *Anopheles* species. This globally aggregated model

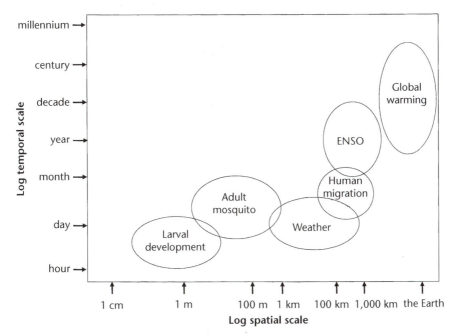

Figure 2-5. Effect on Malaria Epidemiology of Processes on Different Temporal and Spatial Scales

Note: ENSO = El Niño–Southern Oscillation (see Chapter 11).

assumed universal relationships that are sufficiently dominant to ensure a valid approximate overall forecast. Subsequent versions of the model (Martens et al. 1999) include species-specific relationships (as far as were available in literature) between climate and transmission dynamics. Even so, the equations within a global model may well be inappropriate for particular local conditions.

The trend in current IA modeling is to move toward greater regional disaggregation, assuming that it yields better models (Rotmans and van Asselt 1999). Past decades of model building have indicated that small, transparent models are often superior in that they provide similar results to large models yet are faster and easier to use. In this respect, it is useful to distinguish between complicated models and complex models. *Complicated models* include many processes, many of which may be linked. If incremental changes in these processes generally lead to incremental changes in model output, then the dynamics of the model are almost linear and not complex at all. The more complicated the model, the higher the possibility of errors and bugs. It requires thorough testing to eliminate most, if not all, errors and bugs; this activity is, unfortunately, severely underrated. *Complex models,* however, may contain relatively few processes, but incremental changes in these processes may result in considerable changes in the results of the overall model. This nonlinear behavior may be due to the inclusion of feedback, adaptation, self-learning, and chaotic behavior and is often unpredictable.

Practically speaking, the disaggregation of IA models has profound consequences for the dynamics of the model. Breaking down a global model into various regions implies that the regional dynamics should be dealt with in an adequate manner. Regional IA models use grid cells or classes for representing geographic differences and heterogeneities. However, they do not capture the regional dynamics with regard to population growth, economic development, resource use, and environmental degradation, let alone regional interactions through migration and trade.

Conclusion

With respect to the models described in this chapter, aggregating data about the natural world (including humans) necessarily involves simplification and averaging. An additional difficulty of implementing an integrated modeling approach is that vulnerability to global changes will vary greatly among different segments of the world's population. Poor populations, such as those in Bangladesh and sub-Saharan Africa, will be more vulnerable to climate change impacts than populations in rich nations. Globally aggregated models average across all populations, but specific projections often are required for more localized populations. Furthermore, the complexity of influences of various factors on malaria defies a ready quantitative analysis of net effects. For example, the distribution of malaria is strongly influenced by the use of pesticides, the availability of vaccination, and the emergence of drug resistance in the *Plasmodium* parasite that causes malaria.

Because the full complexity of the interaction between global developments and malaria epidemiology cannot satisfactorily be reduced to modeling, what is the role of such modeling? Despite the difficulties and limitations of the modeling process, the models discussed in this chapter draw attention to the potential health impact of these global changes. They also can indicate the relative importance of the factors that influence such outcomes to enhance public discussion, education, and policymaking. However, even more important is the role of integrated modeling in the systematic linkage of multiple cause-and-effect relationships based on available knowledge and reasoned guesses. This should increase our understanding of the health impacts of global changes and identify key gaps in data and knowledge needed to improve the analysis of these effects.

Therefore, considerable scientific effort is now being applied to the development of integrated models and to imbuing top-down models with the capacity for downscaled application to regions and countries that takes into account local physical, ecological, and demographic data. Assessment of future health risk attributable to climate change ultimately will need to integrate the global climate change scenarios with local socioeconomic and environmental factors into an integrated modeling framework that is based on variables that represent climate, vectors, parasites, humans, and health impact (McMichael et al. 2000). Recently, the need for integrated mathematical models to take account of feedback processes within and between linked systems has been recognized; in other words, complex systems may often need to be modeled as complex adaptive systems, displaying spontaneous or socially based adaptive responses. The use of genetic algorithms (Janssen and Martens 1997) and artificial neural networks (Sethi and Jain 1991), which incorporate a capacity for adaptive change and learning processes, holds much promise for this purpose.

Acknowledgements

Many thanks to the participants of the Contextual Determinants of Malaria workshop (May 15–18, 2000, in Lausanne, Switzerland) for stimulating discussion. Also thanks to Sari Kovats and Piebe de Vries for comments on drafts of this chapter.

References

Anderson, R.M., and R.M. May. 1991. *Infectious Diseases of Humans: Dynamics and Control.* New York, NY: Oxford University Press.

Carter, T.R., M.L. Parry, H. Harawasa, and S. Nishioka. 1994. *IPCC Technical Guidelines for Assessing Climate Change Impacts and Adaptations.* London, U.K./Tsukuba, Japan: University College London/Centre for Global Environmental Change.

Davis, A.J., L.S. Jenkinson, J.H. Lawton, B. Shorrocks, and S. Wood. 1998. Making Mistakes When Predicting Shifts in Species Range in Response to Global Warming. *Nature* 391: 783–86.

Dowlatabadi, H. 1997. Assessing the Health Impacts of Climate Change: An Editorial Essay. *Climatic Change* 35: 137–44.

Funtowicz, S.O., and J.R. Ravetz. 1990. *Uncertainty and Quality in Science for Policy.* Dordrecht, the Netherlands: Kluwer Academic.

Hamoudi, A., and J.D. Sachs. 1999. The Changing Global Distribution of Malaria: A Review. CID Working Paper no. 2. Boston, MA: Harvard University.

Hay, S.I., C.J. Tucker, D.J. Rogers, and M.J. Packer. 1996. Remotely Sensed Surrogates of Meteorological Data for the Study of the Distribution and Abundance of Arthropod Vectors of Disease. *Annals of Tropical Medicine and Parasitology* 90: 1–19.

Hulme, M. (ed.). 1996. *Climate Change and Southern Africa: Exploration of Some Potential Impacts. Implications for the SADC Region.* Report commissioned by WWF International, Climatic Research Unit. Norwich, U.K.: University of East Anglia, 49–55.

Janssen, M.A. 1998. *Modelling Global Change: The Art of Integrated Assessment Modelling.* Cheltenham, U.K.: Edward Elgar.

Janssen, M.A., and P. Martens. 1997. Modelling Malaria as a Complex Adaptive System. *Artificial Life* 3: 213–36.

Levins, R., C. Albuquerque de Possas, T. Awerbuch, et al. 1993. Preparing for New Infectious Diseases. Working Paper no. 8, June. Boston, MA: Harvard School of Public Health, Department of Population and International Health.

Lindsay, S.W., and M.H. Birley. 1996. Climate Change and Malaria Transmission. *Annals of Tropical Medicine and Parasitology* 90(6): 573–88.

Lindsay, S.W., and P. Martens. 1998. Malaria in the African Highlands: Past, Present and Future. *Bulletin of the World Health Organization* 76(1): 33–45.

Lindsay, S.W., L. Parson, and C.J. Thomas. 1998. Mapping the Ranges and Relative Abundance of the Two Principal African Malaria Vectors, *Anopheles gambiae sensu stricto* and *An. arabiensis,* Using Climate Data. *Proceedings of the Royal Society of London* 265: 847–54.

Martens, P., and L. Hall, L. 2000. Malaria on the Move: Human Population Movement and Its Impact on Malaria Transmission. *Emerging Infectious Diseases* 6(2): 7–13.

Martens, P., T.H. Jetten, and D.A. Focks. 1997. Sensitivity of Malaria, Schistosomiasis and Dengue to Global Warming. *Climatic Change* 35: 145–56.

Martens, P., T.H. Jetten, J. Rotmans, and L.W. Niessen. 1995. Climate Change and Vector-Borne Diseases: A Global Modelling Perspective. *Global Environmental Change* 5(3): 195–209.

Martens, P., L.W. Niessen, J. Rotmans, T.H. Jetten, and A.J. McMichael. 1995. Potential Impact of Global Climate Change on Malaria Risk. *Environmental Health Perspectives* 103(5): 458–64.

Martens, P., R.S. Kovats, S. Nijhof, P. De Vries, M.T.J. Livermore, D.J. Bradley, J. Cox, and A.J. McMichael. 1999. Climate Change and Future Populations at Risk of Malaria. *Global Environmental Change* S9: 89–107.

Martin, P.H., and M.G. Lefebvre. 1995. Malaria and Climate: Sensitivity of Malaria Potential Transmission to Climate. *Ambio* 24(4): 200–7.

McMichael, A.J. (ed.). 1996. Human Population Health. In *Climate Change 1995: Impacts, Adaptations, and Mitigation of Climate Change: Scientific-Technical Analysis,* edited by R.T. Watson, M.C. Zinyowera, R.H. Moss, and D.J. Dokken. Contribution of Working Group II to the Second Assessment Report of the Intergovernmental Panel on Climate Change. New York, NY: Cambridge University Press, 563–84.

McMichael, A.J., and P. Martens. 1995. The Health Impacts of Global Climate Change: Grappling with Scenarios, Predictive Models and Multiple Uncertainties. *Ecosystem Health* 1: 23–33.

McMichael, A.J., P. Martens, R.S. Kovats, and S. Lele. 2000. Climate Change and Human Health: Mapping and Modelling the Potential Impacts. In *Spatial Epidemiology: Methods and Applications,* edited by P. Elliott, J.C. Wakefield, N.G. Best, and D.J. Briggs. Oxford, U.K.: Oxford University Press.

Molineaux, L. 1988. The Epidemiology of Human Malaria as an Explanation of Its Distribution, Including Some Implications for Its Control. In *Malaria: Principles and Practice of Malariology,* Volume 2, edited by W.H. Wernsdorfer and I. McGregor. New York, NY: Churchill Livingstone, 913–98.

Morgan, G.M., and M. Henrion. 1990. *Uncertainty: A Guide to Dealing with Uncertainty in Quantitative Risk and Policy Analysis.* New York, NY: Cambridge University Press.

Oreskes, N., K. Shrader-Frechette, and K. Belitz. 1994. Verification, Validation, and Confirmation of Numerical Models in the Earth Sciences. *Science* 263: 641–46.

Parry, M.L., and T.R. Carter. 1998. *Climate Impact and Adaptation Assessment.* London, U.K.: Earthscan.

Patz, J.A., and J.M. Balbus. 1996. Methods for Assessing Public Health Vulnerability to Global Climate Change. *Climate Research* 6: 113–25.

Poveda, G., N.E. Graham, P.R. Epstein, W. Rojas, I.D. Velez, M.L. Quiñones, and P. Martens. 1999. Climate and ENSO Variability Associated to Malaria and Dengue Fever in Colombia. Presented at the 10th Symposium on Global Change Studies, January 10–15, 1999, Dallas, TX.

Rodin, E.Y. (ed.). 1990. *Mathematical Modelling: A Tool for Problem Solving in Engineering, Physical, Biological and Social Sciences.* Oxford, U.K.: Pergamon Press.

Root, T.L., and S.H. Schneider. 1995. Ecology and Climate: Research Strategies and Implications. *Science* 269: 334–41.

Rotmans, J., and H. Dowlatabadi. 1998. Integrated Assessment Modelling. In *Human Choice and Climate Change. Volume 3: Tools for Policy Analysis,* edited by S. Rayner and E.L. Malone. Columbus, OH: Battelle, Chapter 5, 291–377.

Rotmans, J., and M.B.A. van Asselt. 1999. Integrated Assessment Modelling. In *Climate Change: An Integrated Perspective,* edited by P. Martens and J. Rotmans. Dordrecht, the Netherlands: Kluwer Academic, Chapter 7, 239–75.

Rotmans, J., M.B.A. van Asselt, A.J. de Bruin, M.G.J. den Elzen, J. de Greef, H. Hilderink, A.Y. Hoekstra, M.A. Janssen, H.W. Koster, P. Martens, L.W. Niessen, and H.J.M. de Vries. 1994. *Global Change and Sustainable Development: A Modelling Perspective for the Next Decade.* GLOBO Report Series no. 4. RIVM Report no. 461502004. Bilthoven, The Netherlands: RIVM.

Rykiel, E.J., Jr. 1996. Testing Ecological Models: The Meaning of Validation. *Ecological Modelling* 90: 224–9.

Sethi, I., and A.K. Jain (eds.). 1991. *Artificial Neural Networks and Pattern Recognition: Old and New Connection.* Amsterdam, the Netherlands: Elsevier.

Sutherst, R.W. 1998. Implications of Global Change and Climate Variability for Vector-Borne Diseases: Generic Approaches to Impact Assessments. *International Journal of Parasitology* 28: 935–45.

Sutherst, R.W., G.F. Maywald, and D.B. Skarratt. 1995. Predicting Insect Distributions in a Changed Climate. In *Insects in a Changing Environment,* 17th Symposium of the Royal Entomological Society of London, edited by R. Harrington and N.E. Stork. London: Royal Entomological Society, 60–91.

Tol, R.S.J., and H. Dowlatabadi. 2001. Vector-Borne Diseases, Economic Growth, and Climate Change. *Integrated Assessment* 2: 173–181.

van Asselt, M.B.A., and J. Rotmans. 1996. Uncertainty in Perspective. *Global Environmental Change* 6(2): 121–57.

WHO (World Health Organization). 1997. World Malaria Situation in 1994. *Weekly Epidemiological Record* 72: 269–76.

World Bank. 2000. *World Bank Atlas 2000,* 32nd edition. Washington, DC: World Bank.

Chapter 2 Discussion

The Proper Use of Malaria Models
Duane J. Gubler

Martens addresses the problems associated with modeling malaria and other vector-borne diseases. As he correctly points out, complex transmission cycles are climate sensitive and, therefore, are strongly influenced by temperature, precipitation patterns, and extreme weather events. However, many other demographic, social, technological, and biological factors have a profound influence on the transmission dynamics (or transmission potential) and thus the incidence of malaria and other similar diseases. The influence of these factors is not fully understood, but it involves complex ecological interactions among the host, the parasite, the mosquito vectors, and the environment at regional and local levels. Some of these factors include

- unprecedented population growth in tropical developing countries, which is a major driving force for the resurgence of vector-borne diseases such as malaria and dengue;
- population movement and migration;
- changing patterns of land use and deforestation;
- biological variation among geographic strains of vector, parasite, and host;
- climate change; and
- social, cultural, and economic issues or decisions that directly affect transmission.

The last factor includes policy decisions that shift priorities for limited resources, thereby changing the forms of programs that have influenced the emergence of drug resistance among malaria parasites and insecticide resistance among mosquito vectors. These decisions, subsequent to successful malaria, dengue, and yellow fever control programs in the 1950s and 1960s, resulted in general complacency and apathy as well as a decay in the public health infrastructure for vector-borne diseases in many countries of the world.

To date, little scientific evidence has indicated that global warming or climate change has played a significant role in the recent resurgence of malaria. This does not mean that climate change is not or will not be important. It is, but the numerous biological, demographic, social, economic, and public health factors listed above are more important. An understanding of how these complex interactions influence transmission dynamics will directly influence our ability to control malaria. The most cost-effective way to mitigate the future effects of projected climate change is to develop and implement effective regional and local prevention and control programs in endemic countries around the world. Thus, global climate change should not adversely impact malaria transmission if the appropriate public health infrastructure and programs are developed. To ignore this adaptation option and focus on climate change alone is negligent on the part of public health officials.

How does this affect malaria modeling? Modeling is an important approach to a better understanding of the transmission dynamics of malaria. Models should be used to identify and answer specific questions about malaria biology. However, they should not be used to predict future disease scenarios, because the input data are not validated and inaccurate input data will lead to erroneous conclusions. Policymakers and government officials must be educated about the complexities of this disease. It is especially important that policymakers not be allowed to use modeling results out of context and thus draw conclusions that are not valid.

Chapter 3

Malaria Potential and Malaria Risk

Elizabeth A. Casman

The purpose of this chapter is to highlight the differences between malaria risk and what is calculated by MIASMA, the climate change–health impact model cited extensively in assessments by the Intergovernmental Panel on Climate Change (IPCC; see Chapter 1). The MIASMA model does not actually calculate malaria risk but transmission potential (TP). In this chapter, I examine TP—its meaning, assumptions, and limitations—and argue that TP calculations capture only aspect of malaria risk.

The MIASMA model has contributed immensely to the discussion of how climate change may affect the spread of malaria in the next century (Martens 1998; Chapter 2). Results of the model, however, may overstate the magnitude of increased risk of malaria under global warming conditions for several reasons.

- MIASMA is "hard-wired" to show increased malaria risk with global warming. Because the only external driver of the model is temperature, the model can predict only that future warming will affect TP (see Reiter 1998).
- Malaria "risk" due to population growth has been attributed to climate. A fraction of predicted future malaria cases (modeled or actual) will be due to simple population growth. Attributing these cases to global warming is misleading. Tol and Dowlatabadi (2001), using MIASMA predictions and assumptions within a broader modeling framework, have differentiated increased malaria incidence due to population growth from that due to climate change. They show that 50% of the predicted increases in cases in 2050 and 75% of the increase in cases in 2100 are due to population growth in vulnerable regions.
- The measure of risk calculated by the TP model does not really estimate risk in the traditional understanding of the term.

This chapter is devoted to a closer examination of the third issue—that malaria TP is not the same as malaria risk.

What Is Risk?

The terms *malaria risk* and *malaria potential* have been used interchangeably in both popular and scientific writings, even though they are not equivalent. The distinction is clear to modelers who calculate such things, but has been blurred in the minds of the lay audience.

Malaria risk is the probability of contracting malaria. It typically is calculated either over a short period of time or over a lifetime. Generically, an individual's risk of infection is some function of a dose–response relationship evaluated at a delivered dosage multiplied by the probability of exposure. These concepts, in turn, rely on entities such as the size of the vector population, the probability of a vector being infectious, the existence and prevalence of a vector-compatible parasite reservoir within the human population, the probability of receiving infective bites, and the effectiveness of antimalaria strategies used locally. Malaria risk deals with the probability of infection; this is quite different from TP, which focuses on the speed of mosquito and parasite maturation.

There is concern that in the future, as a result of global warming, malaria will become endemic in currently nonmalarious regions. This kind of geographic risk of introduction is distinct from an individual's risk of contracting malaria. It describes the crossing of a threshold and the establishment of sustained autochthonous transmission (without reference to intensity). Because of the complexity, contingency, and multiplicity of events and conditions that can influence this risk, it is impossible to credibly model it based on mosquito and parasite maturation dynamics alone. One purpose of this book is to identify the major climatic and nonclimatic forces that contribute to this kind of risk and attempt to systematize them in a modeling framework.

What Isn't Risk?

MIASMA results have been reported as the increase in numbers of people living in areas that are climatically permissive of malaria transmission. The number of people living in areas where malaria is climatically permitted is not an estimate of risk. This assertion is empirically supported by the current absence of malaria in regions with permissive climates (Dowlatabadi 1997; Reiter 2001).

In the current version of MIASMA, malaria risk in areas with a current income of more than US$3,030 per capita is considered to be negligible. This improves the agreement of the model output with the current malaria distribution pattern. Although per capita income cannot capture all the socioeconomic and political variables that affect malaria status, it does correlate well with nutritional status; personal health care; living conditions; and, to a lesser degree, the quality of public health services. This means test does not change the basic distinction between MIASMA model output and risk, although its beneficial effect on MIASMA's baseline calibration does suggest that socioeconomic determinants dominate TP in determining malaria distribution in many parts of the globe.

What Is Transmission Potential?

Malaria *transmission potential* is an index of the maximum transmission intensity permitted by local temperature conditions. This index (coupled with annual precipitation and gross national product [GNP] per capita tests) is used in the MIASMA model to demarcate areas conducive to malaria spread in the twenty-first century. This area is larger than the area where people will be at risk of malaria, because an area can be at once climatically conducive to malaria and at low risk of becoming endemic.

TP is derived from the basic reproduction rate (R_0), the expected number of secondary infections arising when a single infectious individual enters a completely susceptible population (Macdonald 1957):

$$R_0 = \frac{ma^2bcp^n}{-\ln(p)r} \tag{3-1}$$

where

$m =$ the number of biting mosquitoes per person
$a =$ the number of bites per mosquito per day
$b =$ the efficiency of infection, mosquito to human
$c =$ the efficiency of infection, human to mosquito
$p =$ the daily probability of mosquito survival
$n =$ the maturation time for the parasite in the mosquito
$r =$ the rate of human recovery

A simplified version of this relationship, setting b, c, and r equal to 1, is the vectorial capacity (VC), the expected maximum number of people bitten (not infected) by competent vectors feeding on a single infectious human per day:

$$VC = \frac{ma^2p^n}{-\ln(p)} \tag{3-2}$$

Equations 3-1 and 3-2 are not used in MIASMA because estimating m requires detailed local knowledge of the density of the human and mosquito populations. Instead, TP is used to circumvent this necessity. TP is derived by first calculating the critical mosquito density (m_c) when $R_0 = 1$:

$$m_c = \frac{-\ln(p)r}{bca^2p^n} \tag{3-3}$$

Its inverse, the number of people per mosquito when $R_0 = 1$, is TP:

$$TP = \frac{1}{m_c} = \frac{bca^2p^n}{-\ln(p)r} \tag{3-4}$$

Setting b, c, and r to 1 gives the simplified equation used in MIASMA, the number of people per mosquito when VC = 1:

$$TP \approx \frac{a^2p^n}{-\ln(p)} \tag{3-5}$$

Malaria should spread more easily in places with higher values for TP because it takes fewer mosquitoes per person to have the same hypothetical effect (of VC = 1). Thus, TP provides a way to compare epidemic-prone areas.

When Does TP Correlate with Risk?

Where vector control and disease surveillance and treatment capabilities are insignificant, where the mixing of infected and susceptible humans with competent infectious *Anopheles* mosquitoes is unimpeded, and where most people are nonimmune, TP may correlate with malaria transmission intensity in endemic situations. Where other conditions prevail, TP does not track malaria transmission intensity. Therefore, TP is not a suitable surrogate for malaria risk in all parts of the globe.

In holoendemic situations (nonepidemic, stable malaria), TP does not correlate with individual risk because the nonimmune population is small (violating one assumption of the derivation of TP). Nor does TP correlate with risk in regions where malaria eradication programs have succeeded and are maintained or where control programs have made significant progress.

Though it may be correlated with risk in some situations, TP is not equivalent to either kind of malaria risk commonly discussed—that is, the probability of an individual's contracting malaria or the probability of a region's becoming endemic, both of which rely on quantitative estimates of factors such as the size of the vector population, the probability of a vector being infectious, the existence of a compatible parasite reservoir within the human population, the probability of receiving infective bites, the level of immunity in the population, and the effectiveness of antimalaria strategies used locally.

Toward an Alternative to TP for Risk Assessment

Theoretically, R_0 calculations (but not TP) could incorporate various contextual determinants of malaria, such as the degree and type of mosquito control operation and standard-of-living qualities that reduce human–mosquito contact (Figure 3-1). Embedded in some broader assessment framework, this calculation may be able to capture more of the elements of malaria risk (see Chapter 18).

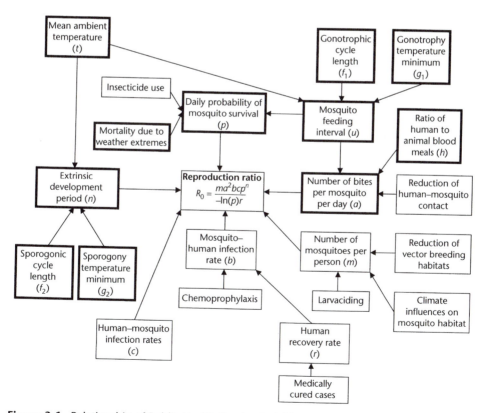

Figure 3-1. Relationship of Public Health Service Activities to the Variables of R_0

Note: Variables that are included in MIASMA Transmission Potential calculations appear in nodes with thicker borders.

Certain antimalaria activities have clear relationships to the parameters in the R_0 equation. Imagociding (adulticiding) affects p (daily mosquito survival probability). Bed nets, screens, and repellents reduce a (the number of bites per mosquito per day). Larvaciding and engineering modifications of the landscape reduce m (the number of mosquitoes per person). Medical treatment affects r (the human recovery rate). Chemoprophylaxis (preventive drug therapy) affects b (the mosquito-to-human infection rate).

Conclusion

The venerable epidemiological indices of vectorial capacity and related derivatives are not suitable for estimating future malaria risk. Furthermore, the past neglect of contextual variables other than climate change has resulted in an overstatement of the effects of temperature on future malaria distribution.

References

Dowlatabadi, H. 1997. Assessing the Health Impacts of Climate Change: An Editorial Essay. *Climatic Change* 35(2): 137–44.

Macdonald, G. 1957. *The Epidemiology and Control of Malaria*. London, U.K.: Oxford University Press.

Martens, P. 1998. *Health & Climate Change: Modelling the Impacts of Global Warming and Ozone Depletion*. London, U.K.: Earthscan.

Reiter, P. 1998. Correspondence Concerning Global Warming and Vector-Borne Disease. *The Lancet* 351(9117): 1737.

———. 2001. Climate Change and Mosquito-Borne Disease. *Environmental Health Perspectives* 109(Suppl. 1): 141–61.

Tol, R.S.J., and H. Dowlatabadi. 2001. Vector-Borne Diseases, Development, and Climate Change. *Integrated Assessment* 2: 173–181.

PART 2

Regional Assessments

Chapter 4

Determinants of Malaria in the Americas

Donald R. Roberts, Penny Masuoka, and Andrew Y. Au

Developing countries of the Americas are experiencing a long-term increase in the number and geographical distribution of cases of malaria and other arthropod-borne diseases (Roberts et al. 1997; Guarda, Asayag, and Witzig 1999). To varying degrees, human experiences with these diseases share a common history. Before the advent of the pesticide DDT, no broadly applicable, affordable, long-acting, and effective methods of arthropod-borne disease control were available. Then, beginning around 1945, specific applications of DDT resulted in 20–40 years of spectacular and sustained disease control (Brown, Haworth, and Zahar 1976). The era of vector control through persistent pesticides has now passed; in developing countries, the use of insecticides by public health authorities is declining, and diseases are reemerging.

Modern ecology-based explanations for increasing disease are anchored in popular belief that increased disease in human populations is linked to increased pollution, environmental degradation, and global warming. These anthropogenic effects, in turn, are held responsible for the increased burden of arthropod-borne diseases (Pimentel et al. 1998). Warmer temperatures certainly could increase the potential environmental capacity for malaria transmission (Martin and Lefebvre 1995). Yet the ecological explanations fail to consider that, during the 1950s and 1960s, the malaria burden was reduced in the Americas—even eliminated in some areas—and maintained under variable levels of control during conditions of warming temperatures and prolonged periods of unprecedented growth in human populations. Indeed, the rate of population growth actually reached its zenith during the years of maximum reduction in disease burden (U.S. Bureau of the Census 1996). The decades of reduced malaria also were characterized by poverty, increased urbanization, movements of migrant laborers, colonization of frontier areas, social unrest, unstable governments, extensive deforestation, and gold mining. Inexplicably, many people attribute the modern growth in disease burden to these conditions even though the same factors were abundantly present during the decades when malaria was controlled (see "Influence of Anthropogenic Environmental Changes" later in this chapter).

Malaria rates can decrease as well as increase in response to environmental or sociological upheavals. Malaria is essentially a rural disease, and during periods of control, the disease was pushed back to mostly rural settings in the Americas (see "Environmental Capacity for Malaria in the Americas" later in this chapter). If control measures are held constant, then increased poverty, temporary housing, mobile labor or refugee populations, and movements of rural populations to urban areas exacerbate malaria problems. Improved standards of living and house construction that accompany economic improvement reduce malaria rates. There have been economic improvements: the real gross domestic product in South America increased from 4% of the world total in 1970 to 5% in 1998 (U.S. DOE 2000). On a hemispherical basis, there is no reason to believe that social conditions have uniformly deteriorated over time in such a way as to continually produce more malaria. In fact, increases in malaria transcend, in both space and time, such factors as government-sponsored colonization, phases of population migration, and episodic wars and guerrilla actions. Ecological causes offer only a partial explanation for increased malaria. The primary correlate (negative in sign) with population-based malaria rates across malaria-endemic regions of South America is the number of houses sprayed with DDT (Roberts et al. 1997).

As stated above, there are some commonalties in the reemergence of certain major disease threats. As with malaria, the reemergence of uta (a form of New World leishmaniasis) in the Andes, the reinvasion of dengue fever (accompanied by dengue hemorrhagic fever), and the increasing threat of urban yellow fever in the Americas are attributable to reduced emphasis on vector control. Uta was reduced in villages of the Andes by malaria control. Risks of dengue fever and urban yellow fever were controlled or eliminated through the *Aedes aegypti* eradication program. *Ae. aegypti* was rapidly eliminated from most countries with the startup of the Pan American Health Organization's eradication program in 1947. (For details on control programs, see Gubler 1998, Severo 1955, and Davies et al. 1994.)

Major achievements in disease control were maintained until the 1970s, when growing environmental concerns in developed countries increasingly led to international pressure to stop the public health use of insecticides (Roberts et al. 1997; Tren 2000). The *Ae. aegypti* eradication program was stopped (Gubler 1998). Achievements in malaria control were generally sustained until the late 1970s, when the World Health Organization formally deemphasized the vector control approach to malaria control. Both malaria control and *Ae. aegypti* eradication were based on public health use of DDT.

In the 1940s, dengue and urban yellow fever were present in the Americas; but the life-threatening form of dengue (dengue hemorrhagic fever) was not. The *Ae. aegypti* eradication effort was initiated because yellow fever immunizations did not stop deadly outbreaks of urban yellow fever. The eradication program entailed spraying DDT on and around larval habitats (referred to as peri-focal spraying) specifically for eliminating vectors. A single spraying cycle with DDT in a village of 5,000 was sufficient to eradicate *Ae. aegypti* (Severo 1955).

Spraying houses with DDT controlled malaria transmission over large geographical regions, but often the environmental capacity for malaria was unchanged. In other words, the regions were still receptive to malaria because the vectors were still present (but less common), and only the presence of DDT-sprayed walls and the concomitant low number of gametocyte donors (i.e., malaria-positive individuals) afforded protection from malaria. The situation was different for dengue and urban yellow fever. Environmental capacities for these viral diseases were eliminated when *Ae. aegypti* was eradicated. Most countries of the Americas did not become receptive to disease transmission again (generally true for urban yellow fever, but not for jungle yellow fever) until peri-focal spraying was stopped and countries became reinfested with *Ae. aegypti* populations.

The type, seasonality, and amount of malaria vary from one geographical area to another. This diversity in disease distribution reinforces the idea that a complex set of conditions determines where and when malaria and malaria vectors might occur. Important variables include climate, physical geography, ecology and behavior of native vector species, biology of malaria parasites and their drug susceptibilities, and time–space distributions of human populations and their sociocultural characteristics. We can unite these variables into a single concept of a *regional environmental capacity* for malaria and malaria transmission. Regional environmental capacity can be subdivided into capacity of the natural environment versus an altered capacity due to human-made environmental changes. The term *altered capacity* is used because anthropogenic environmental changes can increase, decrease, or simultaneously increase and decrease malaria transmission.

The preceding comments provide perspective for discussing the contextual determinants for malaria in the Americas. Human malaria is a highly preventable disease. As such, applications of preventive measures govern the amount of malaria within any environment. However, vector efficiency, behavior, and ecology influence the impact of preventive measures. Without doubt, these factors strongly influence the effectiveness of residual spraying.

In this chapter, we first describe the characteristics that are determinants of malaria (demography, physical geography, and climate) and the malaria vectors, ecoregions, and climatic zones of the Americas—focusing on South America. Next, we examine more closely the presence of malaria in the Americas, including disease distribution, the area's environmental capacity, and the influences of human-made environmental changes. Then, we consider issues of malaria control, including the use of DDT, the connection between malaria control and epidemiology, insecticide resistance, and options. Finally, we summarize the present status of malaria in the Americas, discussing current research findings and several policy recommendations.

Geographical Analysis of Determinants of Malaria

This section is an overview of conditions in the Americas, especially South America. Although we used a 10-year average for weather data and a 1992–1993 derived land cover map, all parameters (land cover, population, temperature, and precipitation) except elevation can change on a short time scale.

Demography

Distributions of human populations in South America are illustrated in Plate 4-1.* In general, humans are largely concentrated in the coastal regions. Because of this clustering around South American coastal centers, the continent has been described as "hollow" (ASI Global 1997). This demographic pattern is expected to continue as interior populations level off and, in some areas, decline. Before European settlers arrived, most indigenous people lived in the Andes, especially in Incan cities. Later, the slave trade was centered in northeast Brazil, and settlers amassed around sources of labor near the

*Color plates for this chapter appear following page 46.

Atlantic Ocean. Meanwhile, inland indigenous populations declined under the pressure of diseases and lack of economic opportunities. This pattern persisted until the mid-twentieth century.

Death rates in the Americas began a steep decline in the 1940s that continued through the 1970s (U.S. Bureau of the Census 1996; U.S. DOE 2000). This decline in death rates corresponds with success in controlling infectious diseases, including malaria and other arthropod-borne diseases. Average population growth rates reached their zenith in the 1960s. Since then, the growth rate has been declining. For example, the population of Brazil almost doubled between 1950 and 1970, from 53.4 million to 95.7 million. Today, Brazil's population is 155.9 million, representing progressively slower growth over the past 30 years (U.S. Bureau of the Census 1996).

Physical Geography

Plate 4-2 is an image of a digital elevation model of South America. Three general topographic regions are visible:

- the high elevations of the Andes Mountains along the Pacific coast;
- the lower-elevation areas of the Guiana shield in the north central region of the map, the central eastern region below the Amazon River, and the southern extensions of the Andes Mountains in Chile and Argentina; and
- the lowest areas, along the northern stretches of the Pacific coast (south to northern Peru), encircling the northern sector of the Guiana shield, the central area of the Amazon Basin, along the Amazon River as it travels to the Atlantic Ocean, and in Paraguay, Uruguay, southern Brazil, and northern Argentina.

Climate

Plate 4-3 illustrates rainfall, temperature, and relative humidity for South America; specific data are presented later, in the descriptions of ecological zones. The area of high precipitation on the Pacific coast of Colombia (near the isthmus of Panama) is for January–March and July–September. The area of high precipitation for January–March on the Atlantic coast of Brazil, however, is much drier than for July–September. This zone of high precipitation also extends inland and far south into Brazil. Otherwise, the pattern of high to moderate rainfall that is characteristic of the Amazon Basin during January–March generally corresponds to low elevations; the same low-lying areas are less wet during July–September (winter in the southern latitudes). The Guiana shield countries, as well as northern Colombia and Venezuela (i.e., areas north of the equator), are generally dry from January to March and wet from July to September. In contrast, areas south of the Amazon Basin are wet from January to March and exceedingly dry (characterized by variable but low relative humidity and rainfall) from July to September. Similarly, the isolated belt of high rainfall along the eastern side of the Andes in Bolivia and Peru is exceptionally wet from January to March and much drier from July to September.

Based on estimates of average temperatures, most regions of South America are hotter during January–March than during July–September. The 6:00 a.m. temperatures (approximately the minimum ambient temperatures) are low at higher elevations of the Andes during both three-month intervals. Additionally, low elevation and low minimum temperatures from July to September extend northward into southern Brazil.

Malaria Vectors

Several important vectors of malaria can be identified in North, Central, and South America. For any given locality, one or more of these species could be involved in disease outbreaks. We discuss only four of several vector species because of their overall importance and because each represents interesting facets of geographical distribution, ecology, and vector behavior.

Anopheles darlingi is by far the most important vector in inland areas of South America and is also important in areas of Central America. It is the primary vector throughout the Amazon Basin (Forattini 1962; Gabaldon 1949b; Rubio-Palis and Zimmerman 1997). The ecology of larval habitats has been reviewed previously (Rozendaal 1992; Manguin et al. 1996). In general, the larvae are found in the flowing water of rivers and streams and in pools and lagoons along major waterways. Human settlements along major waterways bring humans into close contact with this dangerous species. The distribution of this species is discontinuous. It is found from Venezuela to northern Argentina and also is present in Belize, Guatemala, Honduras, and southern Mexico. *An. darlingi* does not seem to be a species complex (Manguin et al. 1999). It is characteristically endophagic; that is, it aggressively enters houses to bite humans indoors. *An. darlingi* seems capable of traveling considerable distances (for example, up to seven kilometers) to arrive at a house (Charlwood and Alecrim 1989). The construction of ponds for fish production is a human-made environmental change that seems to favor the production of *An. darlingi* mosquitoes (Guarda, Asayag, and Witzig 1999).

Anopheles pseudopunctipennis is an important vector in many areas of Central and South America, from Mexico to Argentina. Larvae of *An. pseudopunctipennis* occur in patches of filamentous algae in sun-exposed pools of water in drying rivers and streams. Populations are most common in foothill areas and have been found as high as 3,200 meters above sea level. The distribution of Andean malaria is practically defined by the distribution of this vector. Transmission of malaria by *An. pseudopunctipennis* is more influenced by ambient temperatures than most other species because of the mosquito's presence at high altitudes and because of its distribution in colder southern latitudes. This species is recognized as anthropophilic (prefers to bite humans) and endophagic. Manguin and colleagues (1995) used isozyme techniques to define three geographic populations of *An. pseudopunctipennis* from the West Indies, Central America, and South America. More recently, Coetzee et al. (1999) reported cytogenetic evidence that at least two of the populations (Grenada versus Central America) represent different species.

Anopheles aquasalis is an important coastal species that seldom penetrates beyond 10 kilometers from the seashore. It is found from the state of São Paulo in Brazil north along the coast to the Gulf of Guayaquil in Ecuador. It is zoophilic (prefers to bite animals) and seldom becomes important as a malaria vector for humans in the presence of domestic animals. Compared to *An. darlingi*, *An. aquasalis* is not strongly endophagic.

Anopheles albimanus is widely distributed and an important malaria vector in the coastal areas of Central and South America. In Central America, it is found on both the Pacific and Atlantic coasts. In South America, it is found in the Pacific coastal zone. It is also important along the Caribbean coasts of northern Colombia and Venezuela. Normally not found at altitudes above 500 meters, *An. albimanus* prefers temperatures above 25 °C. Its larvae are commonly found in sunlit grassy pools. This mosquito exhibits considerable variability in host-seeking behavior but is generally considered to be weakly endophagic, strongly zoophagic, and capable of producing many cases of malaria only when it is highly abundant. *An. albimanus* will proliferate in irrigated areas, thus irrigation agriculture is one way that geographical and seasonal distribution of this important vector can be altered by anthropogenic environmental changes.

Ecoregions

Many attempts have been made to develop useful ecological zones that express variable potentials for malaria transmission. The five ecoregions for Central and South America, as defined by Rubio-Palis and Zimmerman (1997), are described and referred to in this chapter. These ecoregions are coastal, savanna, piedmont, interior lowland forest, and high valley (Plate 4-4).

From a land cover map distributed by EROS Data Center, we developed a simplified land cover map of South America that provides additional information on the five ecoregions (Plate 4-5). Four broad categories of land cover are classified: forest, savanna, barren or sparsely vegetated, and cropland/vegetation mosaic. The fifth classification (blue) is a composite of all other types of ground cover. Malaria is less likely to occur in areas above 2,600 meters; however, humans in widely distributed high valley environments might still be host to *An. pseudopunctipennis* mosquitoes as well as *Plasmodium vivax* or *Plasmodium malariae* parasites (Hackett 1949; Gabaldon 1949b; Rubio-Palis and Zimmerman 1997).

Along the Pacific coast are two zones, represented as green in the north and orange in the south in Plate 4-5. The northern zone is variably characterized by forest and a mosaic of cropland and vegetation. The dominant vector in this zone is probably *An. albimanus,* and its presence is probably greatest in areas of irrigated agriculture. *An. pseudopunctipennis* is also an important vector in the foothill areas of this zone. The southern zone of barren or sparsely vegetated ecology is arid. Malaria occurs in this zone in isolated mountain valleys in association with *An. pseudopunctipennis* (Hackett 1949).

The large area of forest in the Amazon Basin defines an extensive region where *An. darlingi* is the primary malaria vector. Additionally, the areas of broken forest and the mosaic of cropland and vegetation that fall within the Amazon Basin, in the state of Pará, Brazil, define zones of major anthropogenic change. A comparison of Plates 4-1 and 4-5 further defines these relationships.

Climatic Zones

No single regional classification fully encapsulates the spatial and temporal diversity of malaria and malaria transmission (for example, the predominance of falciparum malaria in some areas and vivax malaria in others). Similarly, there is no explanation of temporal variability of one type of malaria over the other in a single locality.

Investigators have defined broad regions by descriptions of climate—for example, Gabaldón's (1949b) climatic zones of malaria. The boundaries of these zones were defined by precise ranges of temperature, humidity, and rainfall. Yet, even using Gabaldón's strict definitions, we were unable to reproduce his climatic zones from satellite and ground measurement data derived from the National Centers for Environmental Prediction (NCEP). As an alternative approach, we used an unsupervised classification technique to group similar weather measurements into four classes (zones) using total precipitation, average daily temperatures, average 6:00 a.m. temperatures, and average humidity as the variables. These zones were established with a K-means unsu-

Table 4-1. Characteristics of Four Climate Zones of South America, Based on 10-Year Averages, 1990–1999

Climate region	Total precipitation	Average temperature	Average relative humidity	Average 6:00 a.m. temperature
Orange, high rainfall	4,282 (774)	24 (2.8)	90.7 (2.6)	17 (3.5)
Yellow, equatorial	2,638 (395)	23.7 (4.1)	90 (2.8)	16.3 (4.4)
Blue, paraequatorial	1,470 (337)	22.3 (6.4)	88 (4.9)	15 (6)
Green, subtropical	159 (197)	13.8 (14.4)	90.6 (10.9)	8.7 (14.8)

Note: Numbers in parentheses are the standard deviations of average values.

pervised classification algorithm for four output classes. The classification was run for 16 iterations. Using these methods with different groupings of variables and seasons, we characterized a set of climate zones based on average values and standard deviations (see Plate 4-6).

The top left section of Plate 4-6 is a classification of annual average values for all parameters listed above (we have attempted to preserve the terminology of Gabaldon's climatic zones of malaria). Actual values for the classes are presented in Table 4-1. Except for the subtropical zone (green), the discriminating variable for all other classes is rainfall. The variables of average annual temperature, minimum temperature, and relative humidity do not discriminate between the equatorial and paraequatorial zones. However, these zones are distinctly different in total amounts of precipitation.

The equatorial zone (yellow) also includes areas of very high rainfall (orange), encompassing Colombia, southern Venezuela, and much of the Amazon Basin in Brazil. A small isolated area on the eastern side of the Andes in Peru and Bolivia also falls into the equatorial zone. The northern paraequatorial zone (blue, north of the equator) includes northern Venezuela and most of Guyana and Suriname. The southern paraequatorial zone (blue, south of the equator) borders the equatorial zone and extends into a large area of southeastern Brazil. The southern subtropical zone (green) covers most of the southern part of South America to include areas of Peru and Ecuador on the Pacific coast. The small area classified as paraequatorial in southern South America is due to a classification error that resulted from very high annual precipitation and wide standard deviations for daily and minimum temperatures.

Average temperatures increase as one moves from southern South America northward. Average daily and 6:00 a.m. temperatures for the paraequatorial zone are higher than for the subtropical zone. Standard deviations of average temperatures for the paraequatorial zone are much lower than for the subtropical zone. The same relationship holds as one moves from the paraequatorial to the equatorial zone and from the equatorial zone to the high rainfall areas. Although differences in average temperatures are not large (except for in the subtropical zone), variation in temperature decreases greatly (as defined by standard deviations) with warmer and wetter climates.

We attempted several classifications of seasonal data. Unfortunately, variability in months of peak precipitation did not yield a fully acceptable classification of climatic zones. Data in Tables 4-2 and 4-3 contrast climatic conditions between midsummer and midwinter months. The wet season for much of the Amazon Basin occurs during the summer months, from January to March. In contrast, the wet midsummer months north of the equator occur from July to September. As illustrated in the top middle and top right sections of Plate 4-6, warm, wet conditions extend south of the equator during January–March and extend north of the equator during July–September.

Table 4-2. Characteristics of Four Climate Zones of South America, Based on 10-Year Averages for January–March, 1990–1999

Climate region	Total precipitation (mm/year)	Average temperature (°C)	Average relative humidity (%)	Average 6:00 a.m. temperature (°C)
Orange, high rainfall	1,318 (203)	26 (6.2)	91 (3.2)	15 (7.5)
Yellow, equatorial	843 (121)	28 (4.3)	90.2 (2.8)	16 (4.5)
Blue, paraequatorial	378 (110)	27 (8.1)	92 (3.1)	16.3 (7.8)
Green, subtropical	35 (53)	17.5 (16.6)	92 (10)	9.3 (164)

Note: Numbers in parentheses are the standard deviations of average values.

Table 4-3. Characteristics of Four Climate Zones of South America, Based on 10-Year Averages for July–September, 1990–1999

Climate region	Total precipitation (mm/year)	Average temperature (°C)	Average relative humidity (%)	Average 6:00 a.m. temperature (°C)
Orange, high rainfall	1,509 (197)	26 (2.6)	92 (3.5)	22 (2.8)
Yellow, equatorial	803 (146)	25 (2.5)	90 (3.4)	21.9 (3.4)
Blue, paraequatorial	444 (104)	24 (5.7)	91.6 (3.1)	21.2 (6.2)
Green, subtropical	31.6 (60)	16 (12)	88 (14)	13 (13)

Note: Numbers in parentheses are the standard deviations of average values.

Malaria in the Americas

Distribution

Malaria is endemic in countries of the Americas from Brazil, Paraguay, and Bolivia north to Mexico. Haiti and countries of the Guiana shield are characterized by a predominance of falciparum malaria. In other South American countries (i.e., excluding the Guiana shield), vivax malaria is more often reported than falciparum malaria. In Central America today, *P. vivax* infections clearly predominate.

Climate influences seasonal patterns of malaria transmission. Gabaldon (1949b) described the pattern of malaria far south of the equator, at Tucumán, Argentina (26° south and 65° west, at an altitude of 1,218 meters). There, malaria was governed by the seasonality of both precipitation and temperature. As a result, there was a high frequency of cases during March and April when temperatures and precipitation were higher. Vivax malaria was the cause of most cases during cooler months, whereas cases of both *P. vivax* and *P. falciparum* occurred during summer months.

The coastal region of Guyana is mostly within the northern paraequatorial zone. Data for Guyana before 1943 documented relatively high rates of malaria throughout the year, with the greatest number of cases between June and September. Hot, wet, and humid conditions occur in Guyana from July to September.

Manaus, Brazil, is located in the center of the Amazon Basin, just south of the equator and within the equatorial zone (3° south, 60° west). Malaria now occurs within the city of Manaus throughout the year, with the greatest number of cases occurring between July and October .

Farther north of the equator and west of Manaus, at Barcelona, Venezuela (10.13° north, 64.13° west), the highs and lows of malaria are more accentuated, but rates are more stable than in Tucumán, Argentina. In Barcelona (before 1949), the peak number of cases was reported from July to November. This pattern probably was a result of distinct wet and dry seasons, with most cases occurring during wet, humid months (Gabaldon 1949b).

Patterns of malaria are similar in locations closer to the equator (on both sides), but peaks and valleys in the number of cases are variable. The reversal in timing of the peak number of cases from Tucumán, Argentina, to Barcelona, Venezuela, reflects the reversal in winter and summer seasons south and north of the equator.

Environmental Capacity for Malaria

History shows that beginning in 1945, spraying DDT on house walls miraculously reduced the geographical boundaries of endemic disease and the overall number of cases (Brown, Haworth, and Zahar 1976; Mouchet et al. 1998). Today, the opposite trends of an increasing number of cases and expanding distributions of endemic disease are occurring (Roberts et al. 1997; Guarda, Asayag, and Witzig 1999; Mouchet et al. 1998; Roberts 1999; Roberts, Manguin, and Mouchet 2000). The end point of these trends is not yet in sight. For malaria, we can get a measure of where these trends could potentially lead by examining the burden of uncontrolled malaria before 1945.

Even before 1945, the level of malaria endemicity in the Americas never seemed to equal the levels of disease burden in other parts of the world. Working with statistics from the years before DDT, Gabaldon made the following assessment:

> Although some spleen indices of 100 have been reported in South America, these are exceptional, and for this reason the areas of high endemicity are here of lower intensity than those of Equatorial Africa, India and Dutch East Indies. (Gabaldon 1949b)

Both Hackett (1949) and Gabaldon (1949b) noted that proportions of falciparum malaria cases relative to *P. vivax* infections increased in a gradient from southern to northern South America and the West Indies. That old pattern of case distribution, with few exceptions, persists to the present (PAHO 1992).

Although there was less malaria in the Americas than in places such as Africa, the disease was still a devastating public health problem. Before 1945, epidemics were common within malaria-endemic areas of the Americas.

> The highest general death rate for a month, observed in a municipality of Venezuela, has been 104.3 per 1,000, which nevertheless is a very high death rate indeed. In this respect it should be pointed out that in several states of Venezuela afflicted by epidemic malaria the annual general death rates have been higher than those reached in the same states as a consequence of the influenza epidemic of 1918. (Gabaldon 1949b)

Even without epidemics, malaria death rates were a major public health problem. The nonepidemic burden of malaria deaths (number per 100,000 population) was described as follows:

> Few data are available on exact figures in South America, but it may be said that with the exception of Uruguay, where malaria is not present, and of Argentina and Chile, where the incidence is very restricted, the malaria death rate in the other countries is above 100, which is a high death rate for any disease. (Gabaldon 1949b)

Before DDT use, malaria was widely distributed, and moderate to high spleen indexes and parasite rates (slide examination data) were common. In 1932, the League of Nations Malaria Commission estimated a need for 70,000 kilograms of quinine to treat 3.5 million cases of malaria in Colombia. An estimated 817,115 malaria cases were treated in Venezuela in 1943 (Gabaldon 1949b). Other examples of malaria burden during the pre-DDT years can be drawn from Bolivia, Brazil, Chile, and Guyana in South America; Belize in Central America; and the United States in North America. Data from Guyana illustrate pre-DDT malaria rates and the impact of DDT spraying on maternal and infant mortality; data from Belize show the severe burden of malaria in northern Central America.

Bolivia. In lowland areas of Bolivia, infection rates as high as 100 were reported. In high-elevation valleys, spleen rates of 21 were recorded. In one valley at 2,770 meters, a spleen index of 21.5 was documented, and in another valley at 2,440 meters, an index of 95 was reported (Gabaldon 1949b).

Brazil. The Amazon or northern region had spleen indexes of 25–50. Falciparum malaria was more prevalent than *P. vivax* infections in areas of higher parasite rates. In the northeastern region, spleen indexes were between 10 and 50. In the eastern region, spleen indexes were between 10 and 30, and parasite rates were up to 68%; in Espirito Santo and the Valley of the Rio Doce, parasite rates of 20–50% were reported. In the southern region, the spleen index was up to 66, even in the state of São Paulo. The west central region, which includes part of the *planalto* (the great Brazilian plateau), was characterized by low prevalence and spleen indexes of 16 (Gabaldon 1949b).

Chile. Historically, the largest reported malaria-endemic sector was 360 square kilometers. A spleen index of 61 and parasite rate of 50 were recorded. Vivax malaria was most common; falciparum malaria represented about 25% of the cases (Gabaldon 1949b).

Guyana. To provide some perspective, we present data on malaria before DDT use (data and observations in this section are from Giglioli 1951) and then show how remarkable the decline in malaria was and how these results were achieved. Events in British Guiana (now Guyana), beginning in 1944, illustrate how rates were rapidly and decisively reduced by DDT-sprayed house walls.

The first test of DDT spraying in Guyana was initiated in February 1945. In that test, 80 dormitory rooms in a sugar plantation were sprayed, and 94 were left unsprayed. During the first five months after spraying, the average catch of *An. darlingi* in unsprayed rooms was 194 times greater than in sprayed rooms; 21 and 22 months after spraying, an average of 10 times more mosquitoes were captured in control rooms than in sprayed rooms. This test showed the power of DDT in reducing malaria vector activity inside houses and also showed its remarkably long residual action.

In the early 1940s, Guyana was an intensely malarious country despite functional programs of case detection and treatment. The Malaria Research Unit of the Medical Department of British Guiana—funded by the government, the Rockefeller Foundation, and the British Guiana Sugar Producers' Association—was inaugurated in 1939. The research unit compiled malariometric data for 54,500 residents of malarious sugar estates. Malaria attack rates on the sugar estates remained high through mid-1946. Again, these high rates were sustained despite programs for case detection and treatment. Six sugar plantations with an aggregate population of 10,491 people reported 15,043 hospitalization person-days as a result of malaria from July 1945 to June 1946.

Table 4-4. Effects on Malaria of DDT House-Spraying in Guyana

| | Parasite and (spleen) indexes | | |
Population surveyed	Before spraying 1943–1945	After countrywide spraying 1949–1950	Reduction (%)
Rural (pop. ~250,000)	37.7 (33.3)	0.22 (7.1)	99
Urban (pop. ~85,000)	26.8 (16)	1.1 (0.75)	96

Source: Giglioli 1951.

Table 4-5. Effects on Infant and Maternal Mortality of DDT House-Spraying in Guyana

| | Mortality per 1,000 live births | | |
Population group	Before spraying, 1943–1945 (pop. 368,498)	After countrywide spraying, 1948–1949 (pop. 408,331)	Reduction (%)
Infants	126	77.5	39
Mothers	12.67	5.5	56

Source: Giglioli 1951.

Beginning in July 1946, however, houses were sprayed with DDT. The same plantations reported only 2,932 malaria-related hospitalization person-days through June 1947, an 84% reduction in 12 months.

Systematic DDT control of malaria was begun in Guyana in January 1947, and by March 31, 1948, malaria in the whole of the coastal area was controlled. By 1954, Guyana, Puerto Rico, the United States, and Venezuela were recognized as having eradicated malaria from large geographical areas.

Table 4-4 lists statistics on parasite rates and spleen indexes in Guyana from 1943 to 1945 and from 1949 to 1950. Before the use of DDT, parasite rates were high in both rural (37.7%) and urban (26.8%) environments. In just three to four years, DDT spraying of house walls had reduced parasite rates in rural areas by 99% and in urban areas by 96%. These reductions also affected infant and maternal mortality rates (Table 4-5), which were reduced by 39% and 56%, respectively, by 1948–1949.

Belize. Formerly known as British Honduras, Belize is located in northeastern Central America. In the 1930s, malaria accounted for more than 10% of hospital/dispensary deaths and 40% of all hospitalizations in Belize (Scott 1932; Faust 1949). As much as 50% of rural populations was sick with malaria. DDT spraying was initiated in 1950, and malaria rates were reduced by 80% during the 1950s (British Honduras Health Department 1956). Only 23 cases were detected in 1961 (PAHO 1992). The spraying program was particularly effective in preventing cases of falciparum malaria. In 1959, *P. falciparum* infections were still threefold more prevalent than *P. vivax* infections. From 1963 to 1977, no cases of falciparum malaria occurred during 11 of 16 years (PAHO 1992).

United States. The first tests of DDT residues on house walls were initiated in the United States in 1943. Those initial tests showed a remarkable drop in the number of malaria vector mosquitoes in DDT-sprayed buildings and served as the first demonstration of how DDT could function to prevent malaria (Gahan et al. 1945). The United States had a preexisting malaria control program, so draining and larviciding were retained as methods of choice in towns of 2,500 or more people. However, malaria was a rural disease, and before DDT, there had been no economically feasible method of malaria control for individual households (U.S. Public Health Service 1944–1945).

The DDT-spraying program in the United States was inaugurated at the beginning of the mosquito season of 1945. In that year, a total of 18,860 cases of malaria were reported in Mississippi alone. By the end of 1945, 300,000 houses had been sprayed. Malaria essentially disappeared from the United States over the next two to three years. However, even before DDT was used in the United States, the number of malaria cases was declining (U.S. Public Health Service 1944–1945). Therefore, it seems that DDT contributed to a complex set of factors (for example, increased wealth, improved standards of living, and organized malaria control programs at the state level) that quickly led to malaria eradication. This was not the case in Guyana, where the dramatic reductions of malaria are more clearly attributable to spraying houses with DDT.

Malaria Control

Influence of Anthropogenic Environmental Changes

Concerns about human-made environmental changes and increasing malaria are not new. There should be little doubt that human-made environmental change and capacity for inducing environmental change is much greater today than in the past. Human mobility is also much greater than ever before. Nevertheless, it is instructive to examine the concerns about the effects of human-made environmental changes on malaria from an earlier time.

Hackett, working on data and observations from intervals of time before 1945, made the following insightful assessments about relationships between anthropogenic changes and malaria.

> The movements and activities of man and his increasing ability to modify his natural environment have had remarkable effects on the map of malaria ....
>
> Up to about 1850 the area subject to malaria was on the increase as the infection gradually penetrated to every corner of the world. Since then, malaria has receded from great areas in North America and western Europe, and minor gains have been registered throughout the world ....
>
> Not infrequently, however, settlement and development of land have had the effect of increasing anopheline breeding and malaria ....
>
> [Malaria increased] in Malaya when the jungle was cleared for rubber plantations letting in the sun-loving *A[nopheles]. maculatus*. It has occurred in relation to impounded water the world over. Covell, in lecture, lists the causes of malaria in New Delhi, the capital of India, as "irrigation, interference with natural drainage by railway, road and canal embankments, the backing up of water in drainage channels by high river levels, vast numbers of excavations, borrow-pits, brick-pits and quarries, artificial water collections such as hydrant-fed ornamental waters, cisterns and wells. It is evident that in most cases these factors owe their origin not so much to the forces of nature as to the mis-directed activities of man. It is not an exaggeration to say that more than half the malaria in many developed areas in the tropics is of similar origin.
>
> The migratory movements of man whether they be of nonimmunes into infected areas (e.g., armies, laborers or displaced populations), or of carriers into malaria-free zones (e.g., demobilized soldiers, nomads or migratory labor), usually provoke only transitory epidemic manifestations since the tendency is

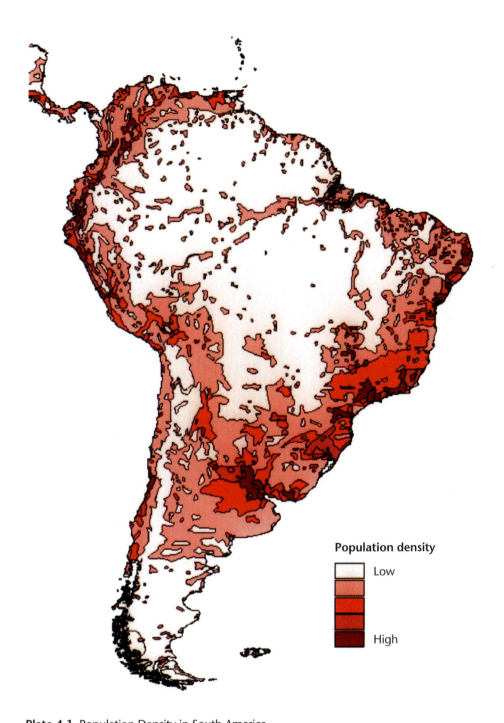

Population density

Low

High

Plate 4-1. Population Density in South America

Source: Map derived from data provided by ArcData from Environmental Systems Research Institute (ESRI).

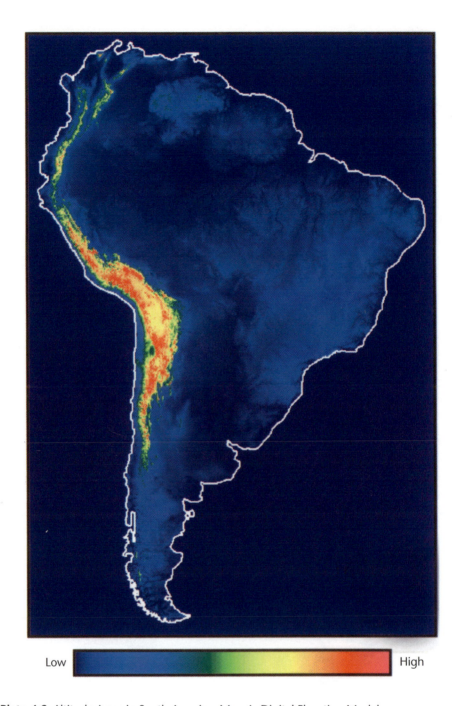

Low High

Plate 4-2. Altitude Areas in South America: Map A, Digital Elevation Model

continued on next page

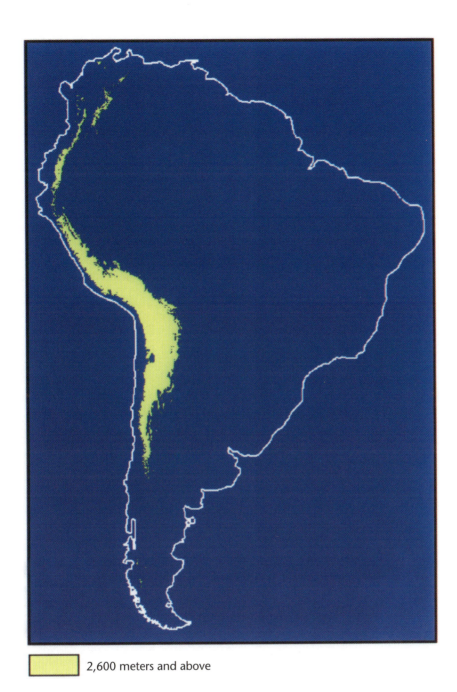

2,600 meters and above

Plate 4-2 (continued). Altitude Areas in South America: Map B, Areas Where Malaria Does Not Occur Due to High Altitude

Note: Map B (areas above 2,600 meters) is derived from Map A (digital elevation model); the highlighted areas of Map B represent high-altitude areas where malaria will not occur.

Source: Digital elevation model is from http://edcdaac.usgs.gov/glcc/glcc.html (accessed April 2000).

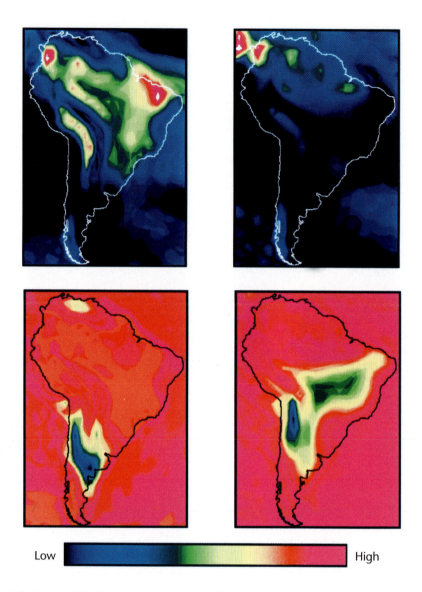

Plate 4-3. Maps of Weather Measurements for South America

Top: Total precipitation, January–March (left) and July–September (right). *Bottom:* Average relative humidity, January–March (left) and July–September (right).

continued on next page

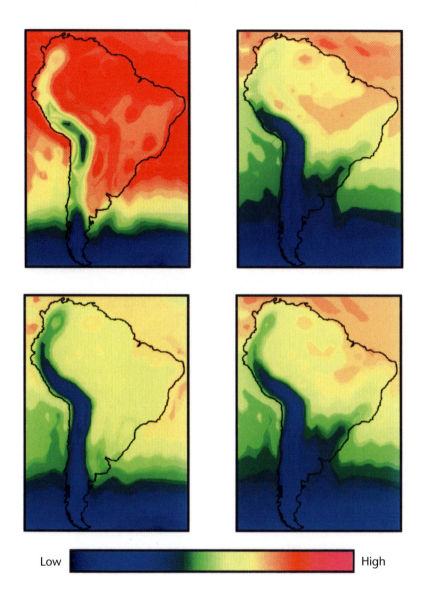

Low High

Plate 4-3 (continued). Maps of Weather Measurements for South America

Top: Average temperature, January–March (left) and July–September (right). *Bottom:* Average 6:00 a.m. temperature, January–March (left) and July–September (right).

Notes: Total precipitation is the total of the averages for three months; other maps show averages for three months. Precipitation, humidity, and temperature monthly averages were calculated from 10 years of National Centers for Environmental Prediction (NCEP) data, 1990–1999. Interactive data language programs were used to calculate the monthly averages and create the raster maps. Temperature monthly averages derived from NCEP data used measurements taken throughout the entire day. Approximate minimum daily temperature is represented by the average of the 6 a.m. measurements.

Source: Precipitation and temperature data were derived from a combination of satellite and ground measurements by NCEP.

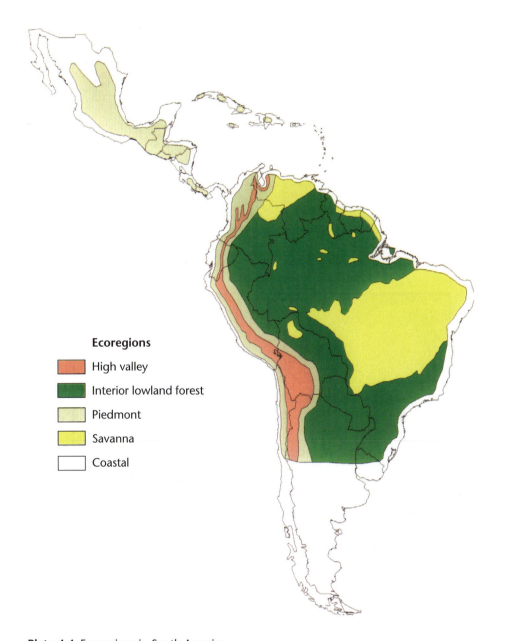

Plate 4-4. Ecoregions in South America

Ecoregions
- High valley
- Interior lowland forest
- Piedmont
- Savanna
- Coastal

Sources: Ecoregions are described in Rubio-Palis and Zimmerman 1997. Land cover data were derived by the EROS (Earth Resources Observations Systems) Data Center from advanced very high resolution radiometer images taken between April 1992 and March 1993. Data were retrieved from the EROS Data Center Distributed Active Archive System, http://edcdaac.usgs.gov/glcc/glcc.html (accessed April 2000).

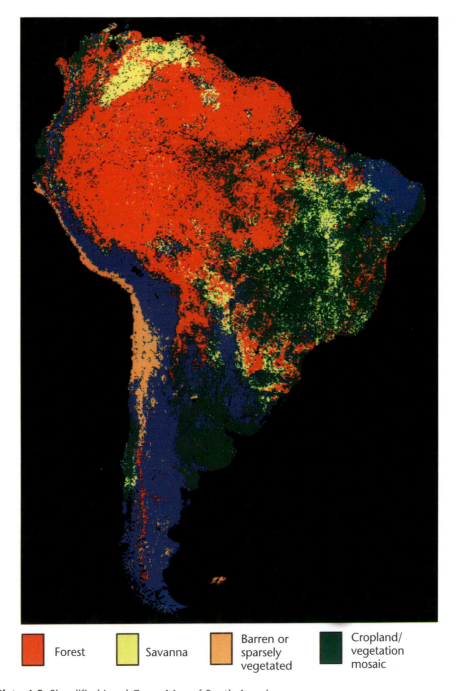

| | Forest | | Savanna | | Barren or sparsely vegetated | | Cropland/ vegetation mosaic |

Plate 4-5. Simplified Land Cover Map of South America

Note: Blue areas indicate a composite of shrublands, some grasslands, permanent wetlands, urban areas, snow and ice, and inland water bodies.

Source: South America Land Cover Characteristics Data Base in the EROS Data Center Distributed Active Archive System, http://edcdaac.usgs.gov/glcc/glcc.html (accessed April 2000).

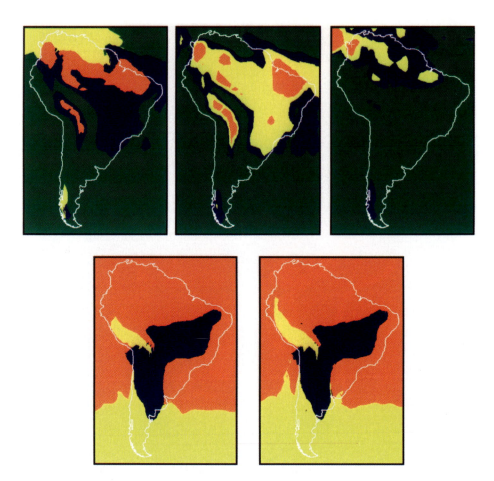

Plate 4-6. Climate Zones of South America Based on K-Means Classification Results

Notes: Orange, high rainfall areas; yellow, equatorial zones; blue, paraequatorial zones; green, subtropical zones. All classifications based on four output classes run for a maximum of 16 iterations: precipitation total and average daily temperature for January–March and July–September (*top left*); precipitation total, average daily temperature, average 6 a.m. temperature, and average relative humidity for January–March (*top middle*); precipitation total, average daily temperature, average 6 a.m. temperature, and average relative humidity for July–September (*top right*); average daily temperature and average relative humidity for January–March and July–September (*bottom left*); and average 6 a.m. temperature and average relative humidity for January–March and July–September (*bottom right*).

for conditions to return rapidly to normal. The factors which have led to the automatic suppression of malaria in a community are linked with the economic and cultural progress of the people and have great permanence, although they may be profoundly disturbed by natural or social disasters which affect the standard of living and stability of the population. (Hackett 1949)

Although one might argue with Hackett's assessment about the amount of malaria due to human-made environmental changes, his statement shows that anthropogenic environmental changes were contributing to malaria problems long before DDT appeared on the scene. Despite human-made environmental changes, residual spraying successfully eliminated or greatly reduced incidence of malaria, and it sustained control of malaria in most tropical countries. Today, health workers are confronted by an even larger scale of human-made environmental changes, but many countries no longer have the benefit of programs or even organizational structures for house spraying. Under these conditions, the malaria burden is rapidly expanding to fill a dynamic, changing environmental capacity that, in some areas, favors the proliferation of malaria vectors and disease transmission.

DDT: Mode of Action

There are critically important issues and misunderstandings about the way DDT has functioned to control malaria. DDT house-spraying programs successfully eliminated or controlled malaria in most tropical countries. Yet DDT, compared with modern insecticides, is weakly toxic. DDT opponents claim that many new chemicals are superior insecticides (WWF 1998; Physicians for Social Responsibility 1999). If we were to judge only insect-killing capabilities, we would concede that these claims are true.

How toxic is DDT? In one study, 24 human volunteers consumed 35 milligrams of DDT daily for 21.5 months without harm; 8 were clinically monitored for an additional 25.5 months and 16 for an additional five years, with no adverse health impact (Hayes 1971). As a comparison, consider that nicotine is 170 times more toxic to mammals than is DDT (Brown 1951). Nicotine is even more toxic to insects; the nicotine in a puff of cigarette smoke can be used in the field to almost instantaneously kill live mosquitoes in small, enclosed cages (Roberts, unpublished observation). DDT would have no effect under similar conditions. Certainly, many modern insecticides are hundreds to thousands of times more toxic to mosquitoes than is DDT. Thus, one would think that if toxicity were the key to successful malaria control, then newer compounds would be much more effective. On the contrary, patterns of reemerging malaria after the use of alternative insecticides suggest that the newer insecticides are inferior chemicals for malaria control—and many times more expensive.

The strong repellent and irritant actions of DDT elicit powerful avoidance behaviors in malaria vectors. These chemical actions have been repeatedly documented in 55 years of literature on malaria control (Kennedy 1945; Muirhead-Thomson 1960; de Zulueta 1960). Yet no quantitative framework describes how these behaviors contribute to malaria control. Consequently, DDT is always evaluated on the basis of its weak toxic actions. To correct this, Roberts and colleagues (2000) developed a probability model that defines, for the first time, the dominant role of DDT repellency in malaria control.

We can better understand how DDT controls malaria by first understanding the primary means of malaria transmission. A mosquito species that normally feeds outdoors has multiple host options (e.g., dogs, horses, and cows). A mosquito first must bite an infected human to acquire malaria parasites and then, following an extrinsic incubation period, must bite another human to transmit malaria. An exophagic mosquito, which normally feeds outside, probably will not bite a human and is even less likely to bite a human on two separate occasions. Alternatively, an endophagic mosquito species, which tends to enter houses to feed, will feed on humans much more frequently because humans are the only hosts available indoors. These relationships explain why the tendency to enter houses is a dangerous behavior in a potential vector species.

DDT residues induce both repellent and irritant behaviors. *Repellency* is defined as oriented movement away from a chemical without physical contact, whereas *irritancy* is movement away from the chemical after physical contact (Roberts et al. 2000). In experimental hut studies, repellency is expressed by the reduction in the number of mosquitoes that physically enter a sprayed house compared with the number of mosquitoes that enter a control (unsprayed) hut. Irritancy is expressed as the relative number of mosquitoes that exit the sprayed house without feeding on human blood, adjusted for the number of mosquitoes that exit unfed from the control hut. Mortality is defined as the percentage of blood-fed females caught exiting the sprayed house that die during a 24-hour holding period. This estimate of mortality also is adjusted by the level of mortality of females that exit the control hut and also can include the number of mosquitoes found dead inside each hut (Roberts et al. 2000).

The acts of entering, biting, escaping, and surviving are sequential acts and can be treated as conditional probabilities (Roberts et al. 2000). The main components of the model are illustrated in Figure 4-1, which illustrates examples of the total effect of DDT, assuming equal levels of effect from repellency, irritancy and repellency, and toxicity. For the calculations illustrated in the first DDT-sprayed house (Figure 4-1, top) we assume a 35% level of repellency, irritancy/repellency, and toxicity. Of the 100 females, 35 will be repelled and will not enter the DDT-sprayed house; of the 65 that enter, 23 (35%) will be irritated or repelled and exit the house without biting; of the 42 that bite indoors, 15 will exit and not survive. The remaining 27 that fed on human blood will escape and survive. The marginal values of 35 repelled, 23 forced to leave without biting, and 15 that die, show that total threat from 100 mosquitoes was reduced by 73%. Almost 80% {[(35 + 23)/73] × 100} of this reduction is due to DDT-induced avoidance behaviors.

By comparison, the second DDT-sprayed house (Figure 4-1, bottom) shows the effect of an assumed 70% repellency, irritancy/repellency, and toxicity. Of 100 mosquitoes, 70 will be repelled and never enter, 21 will enter but exit the house without biting, and 6 will die after biting. The total effect is a 97% reduction in threat. In this example, fully 93.8% of this action is due to vector avoidance of DDT residues.

When tested in the field, this model indicated that the repellent action of DDT residues can function at a level of 95% and higher (Roberts and Alecrim 1991). Data and historical literature that support this model have been reviewed and published (Roberts et al. 2000). Experimental hut studies in Belize have further confirmed the essential elements of the probability model (Grieco et al. 2000). The Belize studies also compared the effects of DDT to those of deltamethrin. *Anopheles vestitipennis*, a major malaria vector in southern Belize, aggressively enters houses during the first half of the night and continues to bite throughout the night. The repellent action of DDT residues decreased the number of mosquitoes entering houses by 97%. In the deltamethrin-sprayed house, the mosquitoes continued a normal pattern of entering and biting during the first half of the night, with only a small reduction in the number that entered. The irritant actions of deltamethrin caused most mosquitoes to exit the sprayed house before mid-

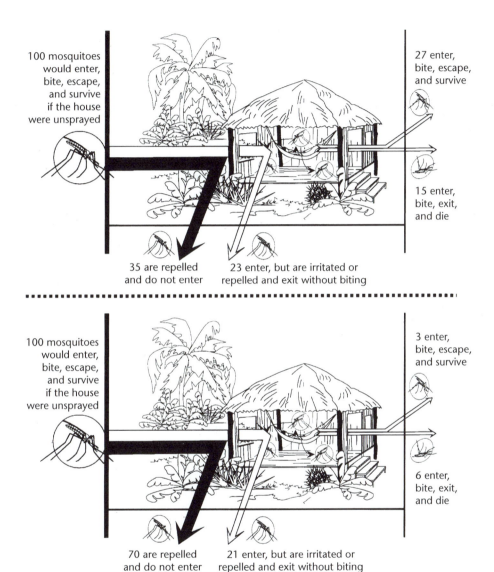

Figure 4-1. Repellent, Irritant/Repellent, and Toxic Actions of DDT

Notes: Each example assumes that 100 female mosquitoes would (if the house were not sprayed with DDT) enter, bite a human indoors, and subsequently escape the house and survive (100%). The result for each DDT-elicited behavior is listed at the bottom of each example, and the output for toxic action (death or survival) is listed on the right. *Top:* 35% level of repellency, irritancy/ repellency, and toxicity. *Bottom:* 70% repellency, irritancy/repellency and toxicity.

night, so biting after midnight was prevented. Regardless, the high number of mosquitoes entering the house and biting during the first half of night in the deltamethrin-sprayed house provided ample opportunity for the acquisition and transmission of malaria parasites (Grieco et al. 2000).

Challenge to Understanding Malaria Control and Epidemiology

The probability model poses several challenges to understanding vector behavior, interpreting epidemiological data, assessing insecticide effectiveness, and evaluating insecticide resistance. The most obvious challenge is to properly account for repellent and irritant actions of chemicals in malaria control. Mosquitoes not entering a house because of chemical residues are forced to seek hosts outside. This behavior should be recognized as chemically induced exophagy. Additionally, when houses are sprayed, paired indoor/outdoor collections of malaria vectors show that the mosquitoes are biting mostly outdoors. If epidemiological data are consistent with this action of DDT residues, then they also show a comparatively low number of malaria cases, and most cases reflect an age–sex distribution that is indicative of outdoor transmission. (*Note:* A low number of cases reflects the inefficiency of outdoor malaria transmission.) If it is assumed that malaria is controlled by killing mosquitoes, then the natural interpretation for both sets of observations is that the house-spraying program is not very effective because mosquitoes are primarily biting outdoors and malaria is being transmitted outdoors. However, if mosquitoes are outdoors only because DDT repels them from entering houses, once spraying is stopped, the vectors will begin entering houses again, malaria transmission will become much more efficient, and malaria cases will increase.

Unless one knows whether a chemical functions as a repellent, an irritant, or a toxin, it is impossible to properly interpret entomological or epidemiological data on the effectiveness of control programs. The many claims that DDT is not effective because vectors are biting outdoors should be reevaluated with the understanding that DDT actually functions as a repellent, not a killing agent. This implies that an evaluation of vector control should include repellency and irritancy as well as toxicity.

Role of Insecticide Resistance in Malaria Control

The importance of insecticide resistance in the Americas is not well understood. The work by Georghiou (1990) indicates that resistance is primarily a result of agricultural use of insecticides. The classic studies by Rachou and colleagues (1966) in El Salvador suggest that resistance of *An. albimanus* to DDT had almost no adverse impact on effectiveness of the house-spraying program. This series of studies also documents the effectiveness of the powerful excito-repellency of DDT residues in reducing resting and biting of *An. albimanus* inside houses. Rachou and others reported that *An. albimanus* is generally an outdoor biter. Exophagic behavior of *An. albimanus* was recognized even before DDT was used in malaria control (that is, it is not chemically induced exophagy) (Gabaldon 1949a,b; Hackett 1949). When house-spraying programs failed to bring malaria rates below certain levels in areas of Central America, it was almost certainly because of outdoor transmission that resulted from the natural exophagy of *An. albimanus*. The failures were also attributable to the tendencies of local people to be outside during the early evening, which coincides with the peak biting time of *An. albimanus*. Nevertheless, as demonstrated with data from Belize, house-spraying programs did reduce overall malaria burdens in Central America and greatly reduced the attack rates of falciparum malaria in particular.

The claims that DDT resistance has neutralized the usefulness of DDT for malaria control in the Americas must be balanced against the understanding that there is no clear correlation in distributions of DDT-resistant vector populations and the distributions of resurgent malaria. In Brazil, there is no DDT resistance in important vectors, yet malaria has rapidly increased (Roberts et al. 1997). In Belize, there is no significant DDT resistance in vector populations, yet malaria increased when the DDT-spraying program was stopped; rates quickly dropped when DDT spraying was resumed in 1995 (PAHO 1992). In Mexico, extensive and intensive levels of resistance occur in vector populations, yet DDT was used to effectively control malaria from 1988 onward (PAHO 1992; Roberts and Andre 1994).

Options for Malaria Control

Rapid technological advances may eventually allow for much greater success in our efforts to control arthropod-borne diseases. In the meantime, however, researchers and public health professionals continue to struggle against an established set of obstacles. Gabaldon's assessment of these obstacles (1949a) is as accurate and instructive today as it was 50 years ago.

> Malaria-control measures may be divided into three groups: (1) those directed against the parasite in man, (2) those aimed at the anopheline vector, and (3) those pointed towards the susceptible individual. The problems found in the application of these different measures are mainly due to the human element living in the afflicted areas, and to the peculiar habits and ecology of the responsible mosquitoes. The difficulties involved were so great that until recently [with advent of DDT] most authorities agreed there was no known means of eradicating malaria from the large rural areas of the neotropic region.
>
> The inhabitants of the malaria sections concerned unfortunately are people lacking education and low in economic resources. Owing to these handicaps there is little collaboration to be expected, either financial or otherwise. This is an important limiting factor in malaria control, which must be taken into consideration at all times by the organizations devoted to these activities in the neotropic region. (Gabaldon 1949a)

Gabaldon also provided a list of options for malaria control, including vector control with both natural and human-made chemicals. He placed special emphasis on screens and improved house construction. He also believed that bed nets were effective against some malaria vector species and expressed the opinion that the nets might decrease the level of *An. darlingi*–transmitted malaria in some environmental settings. He stated that some vectors feed before people go to bed, so bed nets would be less effective against those mosquitoes. He further suggested that effectiveness might be improved by spraying net material with residual insecticides.

Today, the problems of malaria are so great that no promising method should be ignored. If a method works to reduce disease and is affordable, it should be used. Unfortunately, the large number of potential methods for vector control has led some to the oversimplified view that house-spraying programs should be replaced with integrated vector management (e.g., WWF 1998; Physicians for Social Responsibility 1999). The idea is that various methods can be applied to bring about the same result that might be achieved by spraying houses. There are advantages and disadvantages with different methods and approaches to malaria control. However, if the discussion focuses on the advantages of controlling larvae or residual spraying to reduce human–vector contact, then the matter of scale should be considered.

To illustrate this point, we developed a geographical information system (GIS) for an area of southern Belize. We then selected a house site and created a 500-meter buffer zone around it, within the GIS. We mapped aquatic habitats (some were seasonal) that could serve as larval habitats for one of three important vector species that were present at the study site: *An. vestitipennis, An. darlingi,* and *An. albimanus.* The objective of this exercise was to determine surface area that would need to be controlled if we were to control malaria by eliminating populations of mosquito larvae. We used GIS functions to calculate actual surface area of the aquatic habitats that were detected with ground reconnaissance. We would need to exert control over a total of 140,000 square meters of larval habitat. Because some habitats are seasonal and most larval control measures are short-lived, multiple applications would be required each year. Unfortunately, in the real world, mosquitoes can travel over much greater distances than 500 meters; in other words, our example vastly underestimates the magnitude of the problem in such sparsely inhabited areas. By contrast, we would need to spray only 250 square meters of internal wall surface to break critical indoor contact between humans and vectors. As noted above, malaria in the Americas is basically a disease of rural populations. The matter of scale argues forcefully for spraying houses as opposed to interfering with natural aquatic habitats.

Current Status

Published reports attest to the rapid growth of malaria rates throughout malaria-endemic regions of South America (Roberts et al. 1997; Guarda, Asayag, and Witzig 1999). Relationships between the declining number of houses sprayed with DDT and the increased number of cases over what would have been expected if spraying programs had been maintained are illustrated in Figure 4-2. Global efforts to deemphasize spraying houses for malaria control began in 1979. However, no effective alternative approach to malaria control was in place. As a result, the number of houses sprayed with DDT declined, and the number of malaria cases increased. By 1995, there were an estimated 10.4 million excess cases of malaria, and almost no houses were sprayed with DDT.

Over the past few years, the slowest rates of growth in malaria burden occurred in South American countries that continued some DDT use, such as Venezuela and Ecuador (Roberts 1999). Although we focus on what is happening in South America, malaria is also reemerging in Central America. Using published methods (Roberts et al. 1997), we standardized the annual parasite indexes (APIs; annual number of cases per 1,000 people) in Guatemala, Honduras, and Nicaragua to the annual blood examination rates for 1965. Once standardized, the average APIs for those three countries were 4.25, 10.4, 9.2, and 19.5 for the years 1965, 1975, 1985, and 1995, respectively, indicating a steady increase.

Urbanization of Malaria: Amazon Basin

Although the trend of the increasing number of cases is alarming, worse still is the urbanization of malaria in the Amazon Basin. As revealed by numerous reports at the XXXVI Congresso da Sociedade Brasileira de Medicina Tropical in February 2000,

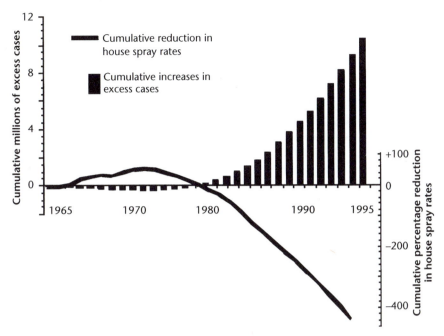

Figure 4-2. Relationships between Number of Houses Sprayed with DDT and Estimated Number of Excess Malaria Cases: Combined Data from Brazil, Colombia, and Peru

Notes: Excess cases represent the number of cases that were estimated to occur above those expected to occur (151,456 cases per year) if the DDT house-spraying program had been maintained at the 1965 to 1979 levels of spray coverage. *Reduced house spraying rates* represent reductions in spraying rates below those expected (46.2 houses per 1,000 people) to occur if DDT spraying had been maintained at levels of house spraying in the 1960s and 1970s.

Note that 1992 was the first year that 1 million estimated excess cases occurred in a single year. The actual estimate was 1,029,352 cases. Numbers were adjusted for variations in slide examination rates across years.

malaria is now well established in many urban areas that previously were relatively free of autochthonous malaria, for example, Belém (Libonati et al. 2000) and Manaus (Sandoval et al. 2000). This urbanization process is illustrated below with data from Manaus (personal communication from José J.F. Sandoval, Director of Epidemiology, Fundação de Medicina Tropical, Manaus, Amazonas, Brazil).

Between 1897 and 1906, 41.8% of 18,681 deaths in Manaus were due to malaria. And until 1939, almost all neighborhoods were infested with malaria. Surveys conducted from 1939 to 1943 revealed the presence of *An. darlingi* and seven other *Anopheles* species in Manaus. From 1950 onward, a malaria control program (which went through many organizational changes) operated within the Amazon Basin, but organized control was not initiated in Manaus until 1962. The economic opportunities offered at the free port of Manaus attracted waves of settlement that were accompanied by epidemics in 1966–1968 and in 1971–1973. During the latter interval, DDT spraying had been restricted to only 19 of 44 neighborhoods because of personnel shortages in the malaria control program. As a result of the epidemic, the spraying program was expanded with personnel from outlying areas. Spraying was resumed, and the drainage system and sanitation throughout the city were improved. The number of cases dropped in 1974, and no autochthonous malaria was recorded in 1975. *An. darlingi* completely disappeared from Manaus in 1975 and did not reappear until June 1988. The first cases of autochthonous malaria occurred in Manaus in the same year, and the number of cases per year continues to increase even now.

The Reemergence of Malaria: Belize

An example drawn from Central America illustrates how malaria can be reduced far below environmental capacity and then reemerge when the house-spraying program ends. As described earlier, Belize had a serious malaria problem before the advent of DDT spraying (Scott 1932; Faust 1949). In 1940, Komp discovered the presence of *An. darlingi* in southern Belize (Komp 1994). Soon after, in dissections of specimens caught in the wild, Kumm and Ram (1941) found sporozoites in specimens of *An. darlingi* and *An. vestitipennis* but none in *An. albimanus*. The last report of *An. darlingi* found in Belize was three years after the DDT-spraying program was initiated, in 1950 (British Honduras Health Department 1956).

An. darlingi was not represented in extensive surveys conducted in Belize in the 1970s (Bertram 1971), nor from 1990 to 1992 (Roberts et al. 1993; Harbach, Roberts, and Manguin 1993). Then, in 1993, roughly two years after countrywide DDT house spraying was stopped, Harbach, Roberts, and Manguin (1993) found *An. darlingi* along rivers in central Belize. In subsequent surveys, Manguin and colleagues (1996) found *An. darlingi* in association with every major drainage system in Belize; they also found the highest minimum field infection rates, based on the presence of malaria sporozoite antigen, in *An. darlingi* and *An. vestitipennis* (both species are strongly endophagic). Much lower minimum field infection rates were found in *An. albimanus*, which is strongly exophagic and zoophilic (Achee et al. 2000).

These observations suggest that before DDT was used, the two endophagic species were responsible for much of the malaria in Belize. For decades, the house-spraying program controlled indoor transmission by these two vectors, and malaria was almost eradicated from Belize. Simultaneously, deprived of the option to enter houses and bite humans indoors, *An. darlingi* became relatively uncommon in Belize. With the cessation of house spraying, vector populations increased, as did indoor transmission. The number of malaria cases peaked in Belize in 1994–1995. House spraying was restarted in 1995, and the number of cases quickly decreased (Roberts et al. forthcoming).

The point of these observations is that the environmental conditions were still supportive of the major vectors and of malaria transmission. Once restraints imposed by DDT-sprayed houses were removed by stopping the house-spraying program, the problem of malaria and malaria vectors started to expand within the broader constraints of environmental capacity.

Policy Recommendations

Options for the Future

Today, national and international environmental advocacy has forced many malaria-endemic countries of the Americas to stop applying insecticides (particularly DDT) for public health use. It is perfectly reasonable and desirable to use nonchemical means of malaria control. Indeed, malaria is such a devastating disease that it is reasonable to use any safe and practicable method of control. However, as a civil act, a powerfully effective public health program should not be stopped unless an equally affordable, broadly applicable, safe, and effective alternative method of control is functioning in its stead. When this criterion is met, program changes can occur with no increase in human disease. However, eliminating a highly effective program when no efficacious alternative is in place is simply unthinkable. Yet, the unthinkable has occurred.

Many modern malaria control issues require objective study and change. Global strategies for malaria control allow uncontrolled growth in malaria rates, and these strategies must be revised. Countries should be allowed to use DDT in areas where it will reduce disease, even if it means centralizing and restructuring malaria control programs. Regulations that block financial assistance to programs in countries that use DDT for malaria control are destructive and should be eliminated.

Need for Malaria Control Research

The technical issues of vector control require renewed research support. The modern specification for spraying two grams of DDT per square meter of wall surface every six months is the same method that was used during the eradication era. Funds are needed for applied research to define frequencies and methodologies of spraying that are more appropriate for long-term malaria control, as opposed to eradication.

Past research suggests that malaria might be controlled by spraying homes just once a year, given the long residual action of DDT. Research conducted by the Malaria Research Center in Tapachula, Mexico, suggests that adequate control might be achieved by partial treatments of houses with DDT (Cases et al. 1998). In addition, remote sensing and GIS technologies, in combination with historical data on malaria cases, might be used for precise definitions of malaria risk for individual households (Roberts et al. 1999; Roberts et al. forthcoming).

Risk assessments can be used to identify smaller populations of houses to be sprayed. Taken together, modified house-spraying programs could focus on small populations of high-risk households for partial spraying once a year. The net effect could be improved cost-effectiveness of time-tested malaria control methods and great reductions in the amount of insecticide used. This approach might still provide a level of control comparable to conventional house-spraying programs. In any case, these approaches to malaria control are unproven and must be evaluated through additional research and large-scale field trials. Today, unfortunately, funding policies militate against funding for such applied research in general and against funding for the public health use of insecticides in particular.

Conclusion

The environmental capacity for malaria and malaria transmission is high in the equatorial, paraequatorial, and subtropical regions of the Americas. In some regions, human-made environmental changes have, without a doubt, increased environmental capacity for malaria and malaria transmission. However, human activities can work for or against disease occurrence.

Through the application of preventive measures, we can exert powerful control over malaria and other arthropod-borne diseases and maintain malaria burden far below environmental capacity. Because national and international policies have curtailed DDT use, house-spraying programs no longer restrain malaria. The number of malaria cases is growing rapidly. The urbanization of malaria in cities of the Amazon Basin is the latest indication of this growing public health disaster. In our opinion, DDT is still needed for malaria control in the Americas.

References

Achee, N.L., C.T. Korves, M.J. Bangs, E. Rejmankova, M. Lege, D. Curtin, H. Lenares, Y. Alonzo, R.G. Andre, and D.R. Roberts. 2000. *Plasmodium vivax* Polymorphs and *Plasmodium falciparum* Circumsporozoite Proteins in *Anopheles* (Diptera: Culicidae) from Belize, Central America. *Journal of Vector Ecology* 25(2): 203–11.

ASI Global. 1997. *South America's Demographica*. http://www.asiglobal.com/vision/sa4.html (accessed April 2000).

Bertram, D.S. 1971. Mosquitoes of British Honduras, with Some Comments on Malaria, and on Arbovirus Antibodies in Man and Equines. *Transactions of the Royal Society of Tropical Medicine and Hygiene* 65: 742–62.

British Honduras Health Department. 1956. *Plan of Operation for the Malaria Eradication Programme in British Honduras*. Belize City, British Honduras: British Honduras Health Department.

Brown, A.W.A. 1951. *Insect Control by Chemicals*. New York: Wiley.

Brown, A.W.A., J. Haworth, and A.R. Zahar. 1976. Malaria Eradication and Control from a Global Standpoint. *Journal of Medical Entomology* 13(1): 1–25.

Cases, M., J.L. Torres, D.N. Bown, M.H. Rodriguez, and J.I. Arredondo-Jimenez. 1998. Selective and Conventional House-Spraying of DDT and Bendiocarb against *Anopheles pseudopunctipennis* in Southern Mexico. *Journal of American Mosquito Control Association* 14(4): 410–14.

Charlwood, J.D., and W.A. Alecrim. 1989. Capture-Recapture Studies with the South American Malaria Vector *Anopheles darlingi* Root. *Annals of Tropical Medicine and Parasitology* 83(6): 569–76.

Coetzee, M., J.G. Estrada-Franco, C.A. Wunderlich, and R.H. Hunt. 1999. Cytogenetic Evidence for a Species Complex within *Anopheles pseudopunctipennis* Theobald (Diptera: Culicidae). *American Journal of Tropical Medicine and Hygiene* 60(4): 649–53.

Davies, C.R., A. Llanos-Cuentas, J. Canales, E. Leon, E. Alvarez, J. Monge, E. Tolentino, Q. Gomero, S. Pyke, and C. Dye. 1994. The Fall and Rise of Andean Cutaneous Leishmaniasis: Transient Impact of the DDT Campaign in Peru. *Transactions of the Royal Society of Tropical Medicine and Hygiene* 88: 389–93.

de Zulueta, J. 1960. The Irritability of Mosquitoes to DDT and Its Importance in Malaria Eradication. *Rivista di Malariologia* 41(4–6): 169–78.

Faust, E.C. 1949. Malaria Incidence in North America. In *Malariology*, edited by M.F. Boyd. Philadelphia, PA: Saunders, 749–63.

Forattini, O.P. 1962. *Entomologia Medica*, Volume 1. São Paulo, Brazil: Faculdade de Higiene e Saude Publica.

Gabaldón, A. 1949a. Malaria Control in the Neotropic Region. In *Malariology*, edited by M.F. Boyd. Philadelphia, PA: Saunders, 1400–15.

———. 1949b. Malaria Incidence in the West Indies and South America. In *Malariology*, edited by M.F. Boyd. Philadelphia, PA: Saunders, 764–87.

Gahan, J.B., B.V. Travis, F.A. Morton, and A.W. Lindquist. 1945. DDT as a Residual-Type Treatment to Control *Anopheles quadrimaculatus*, Practical Tests. *Journal of Economic Entomology* 38: 223–35.

Georghiou, G.P. 1990. The Effect of Agrochemicals on Vector Populations. In *Pesticide Resistance in Arthropods*, edited by R.T. Roush, and B.E. Tabashnik. New York: Chapman and Hall, 183–202.

Giglioli, G., III. 1951. Eradication of *Anopheles darlingi* from the Inhabited Areas of British Guiana by DDT Residual Spraying. *Journal of the National Malaria Society* 10: 142–61.

Grieco, J.P., N.L. Achee, R.G. Andre, and D.R. Roberts. 2000. A Comparison Study of House Entering and Exiting Behavior of *Anopheles vestitipennis* (Diptera: Culicidae) Using Experimental Huts Sprayed with DDT or Deltamethrin in the Southern District of Toledo, Belize. *Journal of Vector Ecology* 25(1): 62–73.

Guarda, J.A., C.R. Asayag, and R. Witzig. 1999. Malaria Reemergence in the Peruvian Amazon Region. *Emerging Infectious Diseases* 5(2): 209–15.

Gubler, D.J. 1998. Resurgent Vector-Borne Diseases as a Global Health Problem. *Emerging Infectious Diseases* 4(3): 442–50.

Hackett, L.W. 1949. Distribution of Malaria. In *Malariology,* edited by M.F. Boyd. Philadelphia, PA: Saunders, 722–35.

Harbach, R.E., D.R. Roberts, and S. Manguin. 1993. Variation in the Hindtarsal Markings of *Anopheles darlingi* (Diptera: Culicidae) in Belize. *Mosquito Systematics* 25(3): 192–97.

Hayes, W.J. 1971. Evidence of Safety of Long-Term, High, Oral Doses of DDT for Man. *Archives of Environmental Health* 22 (January): 119–35.

Kennedy, J.S. 1945. The Excitant and Repellent Effects on Mosquitoes of Sub-lethal Contacts with DDT. *Bulletin of Entomological Research* 37: 593–607.

Komp, W.H.W. 1994. The Occurrence of *Anopheles darlingi* Root in British Honduras and Guatemala. *Science* 91: 522–23.

Kumm, H.W., and L.M. Ram. 1941. Observations on the *Anopheles* of British Honduras. *American Journal of Tropical Medicine and Hygiene* 21: 559–66.

Libonati, R.M.F., M.V.N. Dos Santos, A.Y.N. Pinto, V.S. Calvosa, A.M. Ventura, P.H.M. Figueiredo, J.M. Bezerra, C.H.M. Azevedo, M.P. Brito, R.S. Santos Jr., and J.M. De Souza. 2000. Malaria Autoctone na Grande Belém: Panorama Atual e Prevalencia no Ultimos Seis Anos. *Revista da Sociedad Brasileira de Medicina Tropical* 33(Suppl. 1): 347.

Manguin, S., D.R. Roberts, E.L. Peyton, I. Fernandez-Salas, M. Barreto, R.F. Loayza, F.E. Spinola, R.M. Granaou, and M.H. Rodriguez. 1995. Biochemical Systematics and Population Genetic Structure of *Anopheles pseudopunctipennis*, Vector of Malaria in Central and South America. *American Journal of Tropical Medicine and Hygiene* 53(4): 362–77.

Manguin, S., D.R. Roberts, R.G. Andre, E. Rejmankova, and S. Hakre. 1996. Characterization of *Anopheles darlingi* (Diptera: Culicidae) Larval Habitats in Belize, Central America. *Journal of Medical Entomology* 33(2): 205–11.

Manguin, S., R.C. Wilkerson, J.E. Conn, Y. Rubio-Palis, J.A. Danoff-Burg, and D.R. Roberts. 1999. Population Structure of the Primary Malaria Vector in South America, *Anopheles darlingi*, Using Isozyme, Random Amplified Polymorphic DNA, Internal Transcribed Spacer 2, and Morphologic Markers. *American Journal of Tropical Medicine and Hygiene* 60(3): 364–76.

Martin, P.H., and M.G. Lefebvre. 1995. Malaria and Climate: Sensitivity of Malaria Potential Transmission to Climate. *Ambio* 24(4): 200–7.

Mouchet, J., S. Manguin, J. Sircoulon, S. Laventure, O. Faye, A.W. Onapa, P. Carnevale, J. Julvez, and D. Fontenille. 1998. Evolution of Malaria in Africa for the Past 40 Years: Impact of Climatic and Human Factors. *Journal of the American Mosquito Control Association* 12(2): 121–30.

Muirhead-Thomson, R.C. 1960. The Significance of Irritability, Behavouristic Avoidance and Allied Phenomena in Malaria Eradication. *Bulletin of the World Health Organization* 22: 721–34.

PAHO (Pan American Health Organization). 1992. Status of Malaria Programs in the Americas. XL Report. Washington, DC: PAHO.

Physicians for Social Responsibility. 1999. *The Modern Malaria Handbook*. Washington, DC: Physicians for Social Responsibility.

Pimentel, D., M. Tort, L. D'Anna, A. Krawic, J. Berger, J. Rossman, F. Mugo, N. Doon, M. Shriberg, E. Howard, S. Lee, and J. Talbot. 1998. Ecology of Increasing Disease. Population Growth and Environmental Degradation. *BioScience* 48: 817–26.

Rachou, R.G., L.A. Schinazi, and M. Moura-Lima. 1966. Preliminary Note on the Epidemiological Studies Made in El Salvador to Determine the Causes of the Failure of Residual Spraying to Interrupt the Transmission of Malaria. *Revista Brasileira de Malariologia e Doencas Tropicais* 18(3/4): 763–79.

Roberts, D.R. 1999. DDT and the Global Threat of Re-emerging Malaria. *Pesticide Safety News* 2(4): 4–5.

Roberts, D.R., and W.D. Alecrim. 1991. Behavioral Response of *Anopheles darlingi* to DDT-Sprayed House Walls in Amazonia. *Bulletin of Pan American Health Organization* 25: 210–7.

Roberts, D.R., and R.G. Andre. 1994. Insecticide Resistance Issues in Vector-Borne Disease Control. *American Journal of Tropical Medicine and Hygiene* 50: 21–43.

Roberts, D.R., S. Manguin, and J. Mouchet. 2000. Re-emerging Malaria: A Result of Abandoning DDT House Spraying. *Lancet* 356(July 22): 330–2.

Roberts, D.R., O. Chan, J. Pecor, E. Rejmankova, S. Manguin, J. Polanco, and L.J. Legters. 1993. Preliminary Observations on the Changing Roles of Malaria Vectors in Southern Belize. *Journal of the American Mosquito Control Association* 9(4): 456–9.

Roberts, D.R., L.L. Laughlin, P. Hshieh, and L.J. Legters. 1997. DDT, Global Strategies, and a Malaria Control Crisis in South America. *Emerging Infectious Diseases* 3(3): 295–302.

Roberts, D.R., E. Vanzie, E. Rejmankova, P. Masuoka, and R. Andre. 1999. Use of Remote Sensing and Geographic Information Systems to Target Malaria Control Measures in Belize, Central America. SCOPE Malaria Research and Policy Forum. http://www.scope.educ.washington.edu/malaria/ (commentary posted December 15, 1999; accessed July 29, 2001).

Roberts, D.R., W.D. Alecrim, P. Hshieh, J.P. Grieco, M. Bangs, R.G. Andre, and T. Chareonviriphap. 2000. A Probability Model of Vector Behavior: Effects of DDT Repellency, Irritancy, and Toxicity in Malaria Control. *Journal of Vector Ecology* 25(1): 48–61.

Roberts, D.R., E. Vanzie, M. Bangs, J.P. Grieco, H. Lenares, P. Hsheih, E. Rejmankova, S. Manguin, R.G. Andre, and J. Polanco. Forthcoming. Role of Residual Spraying for Malaria Control in Belize, Central America: A Case Study. Accepted for publication in *Journal of Vector Ecology.*

Rozendaal, A. 1992. Relations between *Anopheles darlingi* Breeding Habitats, Rainfall, River Level and Malaria Transmission Rates in the Rain Forest of Suriname. *Medical and Veterinary Entomology* 6: 16–22.

Rubio-Palis, Y., and R.H. Zimmerman. 1997. Ecoregional Classification of Malaria Vectors in the Neotropics. *Journal of Medical Entomology* 34(5): 499–510.

Sandoval, J.J.F, M.G.G. Saraiva, R.D.S. Amorim, M.V.F. Guerra, B.C. Albuquerque, and W.D. Alecrim. 2000. Malaria na cidade de Manaus: Vulnerabilidade e Receptividade. *Revista da Sociedad Brasileira de Medicina Tropical* 33(Suppl. 1): 67.

Scott, H.H. 1932. Medical and Sanitary Reports from British Colonies, Protectorates and Dependencies for the Year 1930. *Tropical Diseases Bulletin* 29: 127–29.

Severo, O.P. 1955. Eradication of the *Aedes aegypti* Mosquito from the Americas. In *Yellow Fever: A Symposium in Commemoration of Carlos Juan Finlay,* Volume 105. Philadelphia, PA: Jefferson Medical College of Philadelphia, 39–59.

Tren, R. 2000. *The Economic Costs of Malaria in South Africa.* IEA Publications. http://www.iea.org.uk/env/malaria.htm (accessed April 2000).

U.S. Bureau of the Census. 1996. *Total Midyear Population for the World: 1950–2050.* http://www.census.gov/ipc/www/worldpop.html (accessed April 2000).

U.S. DOE (Department of Energy). 2000. *The Americas in a World Context.* http://www.eia.doe.gov/emeu/cabs/theamericas.html (accessed April 2000).

U.S. Public Health Service. 1944–1945. *Malaria Control in War Areas.* Report of the Federal Security Agency, U.S. Public Health Service.

WWF (World Wildlife Fund). 1998. *Resolving the DDT Dilemma: Protecting Biodiversity and Human Health.* Washington, DC: WWF.

Chapter 5

The Control of
Malaria in Brazil

Renato d'A. Gusmão

In this chapter, I review the malaria control experiences of Brazil, a country with a complex and changeable malaria situation. Brazil has coped with the decentralization of its malaria control program and a paradigm shift from eradication to disease management strategies in the face of economic constraints by prioritizing control activities. Epidemiological classification of geographic regions into malaria risk categories allowed for resources to be concentrated on the highest-priority groups and increased the ability to focus more precisely on the highest-risk population in every locality.

Malaria has been endemic in Brazil for the past three centuries. Early in the twentieth century, control activities were instituted to accommodate the classical urban demographic growth caused by the industrial revolution. Investment was concentrated on reducing mosquito breeding sites in and around human settlements and on distributing *cinchona* (bark extract) to feverish people. In the mid-twentieth century, to support the expansion of agricultural production, a national program was launched to eradicate malaria transmission from the population in rural as well as isolated areas. These activities took advantage of the newly available DDT as an indoor insecticide and synthetic chloroquine for effective treatment.

This program achieved a significant level of control. The total population almost doubled between 1959 and 1974, whereas the number of malaria cases was halved. Starting in the mid-1970s, house spraying with insecticides and active case detection for supervised treatment began to show less favorable results. The number of malaria cases increased from 66,481 in 1974 to almost 10 times as many by 1991, when the number of registered cases reached 614,431.

The Problem

Brazil had already begun searching for alternative methodologies to cope with this high increase of malaria morbidity in the early 1980s. The country tried a strategy called "zonification" that was based on the permanent presence in each highly endemic area of a national program worker, who was responsible for massive treatment and house spraying activities. The high maintenance costs of this operation could not be sustained, and its results were limited insofar as malaria incidence continued to rise. However, a great deal of epidemiological information for the planning and launching of zonification was gathered, recorded, and analyzed.

By 1989, the Brazilian Ministry of Health had procured and signed a World Bank loan to support a project designed to strengthen its malaria eradication campaign, based on a categorical campaign approach by a single institution, the Brazilian National Health Foundation. Its emphasis was on vector control (by means of intramural spraying of residual insecticides) and active case detection (house-to-house search for febrile individuals). By 1992, these activities had proven ineffective for two main reasons: the greater proportion of extradomiciliary occurrence of the malaria transmission and the logistical difficulties of reaching the population at risk due to the limited coverage of the health services delivery system.

These factors were compounded by continuous and increasing migratory and circulatory movements to and within the forested areas of the Amazon Basin, greatly reducing the potential effectiveness of the active case detection system and house-spraying activities. Moreover, rapid decentralization of the technical and administrative structure of federal institutions in 1990 led to a vacuum of control activities at the periphery of the health sector, which had been completely dependent on the centralized infrastructure for its operation. Thus, the attempt to curb malaria transmission by means of traditional eradication methods was deemed of limited success up to 1992, despite the available financial resources.

The Strategic Shift

In 1992, the Global Malaria Control Strategy (GMCS) was adopted by the Ministerial Conference on Malaria held in Amsterdam, the Netherlands (WHO 1992a, b). The Brazilian National Health Foundation requested that the Pan American Health Organization reinforce its technical cooperation for GMCS implementation and that Brazil become the first country to implement the new strategy in the Americas.

This strategy called for a radical reorientation of the malaria control program from its traditional objective (eradicating malaria transmission) to controlling the disease. It required changing the emphasis from controlling vectors to preventing mortality and reducing the social and economic burden of the disease in the at-risk population. These objectives were to be pursued through the rapid improvement of the local health services.

Efforts were focused on the individual groups of the population at risk, through

- widespread expansion of capabilities for early diagnosis and immediate treatment;
- the introduction of preventive and protective measures for individuals, families, and communities, including vector control;
- increased capability for early detection and containment of malaria epidemics; and
- analysis of the ecological, social, and economic determinants of the disease for the development of selective and sustainable control measures.

Epidemiological Intelligence at the Local Level

To define the magnitude of the malaria problem, initial project implementation efforts were directed toward practical epidemiological risk stratification by municipality (the smallest geopolitical unit of the country). This method contrasted with the traditional malaria eradication approach, which considered a malarious area as any geographical

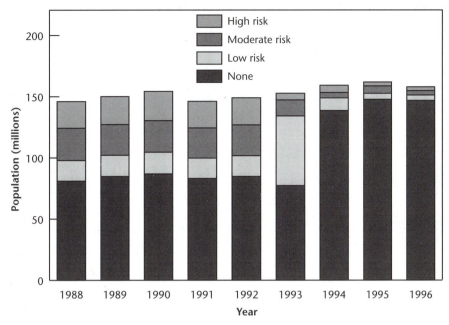

Figure 5-1. Population Exposed to Malaria Risk in Brazil, 1988–1996

Source: Brazilian Ministry of Health.

site with the ecological characteristics capable of supporting the mosquito vector. As a result of the new effort, areas with levels of malaria transmission risk (high, moderate, and low) and a large no-risk area were identified.

The accurate definition of each transmission area with a precise, spatially distributed population at risk provided a better idea of what was needed to expand services coverage for improved access to prompt diagnosis and treatment. This single analytical measure indicated that 6 million inhabitants, in several dispersed groups, were at high risk of transmission. The previous generalized analysis had identified 20 million people at high risk (Figure 5-1).

Measurable Inputs

This analysis led to a massive program of human resources development for program implementation at local and regional health education institutions so as to quickly reach the affected risk groups, such as mining prospectors, lumber workers, and newly settled agricultural families. Priority was given to educating trainers who could expand coverage and strengthen the capacity of the local and community health workers to diagnose and immediately treat suspected cases.

The strategic location of these diagnostic and treatment centers was also a direct result of the epidemiological stratification. In line with the national policy for infrastructure decentralization, the control program financed, trained, and supported the establishment of 618 new diagnostic and treatment centers during this initial phase of rapid expansion. Between 1992 and 1996, a total of 1,038 centers were completely integrated and run by the municipalities in the transmission risk areas.

Sustainability was also promoted by means of a two-pronged continuous investment:

- expanding the process for early diagnosis and immediate treatment by introducing a rapid field test for *Plasmodium falciparum* detection, which further simplified the use of multiple-drug-resistant treatments and the consolidation of GMCS implementation, and
- providing additional training and ensuring the supply of general health services facilities for prompt diagnosis and immediate antimalaria treatment, from 1,038 up to 35,000 facilities in the Amazon region.

Results of the Strategic Shift

Epidemiological stratification allowed resources to be concentrated on the populations most at risk. The expansion in early diagnosis coverage was achieved at all three levels of transmission risk. Between 1992 and 1995, the coverage of diagnosis and treatment services increased from 11% to 34% for the high-risk populations, from 1.6% to 8.0% for the moderate-risk populations, and from 0.2% to 2.2% for the low-risk populations (Figure 5-2).

With epidemiological mapping and the ability to target precisely the population at highest risk in every locality, the efficiency of the surveillance system also increased (Figure 5-3). The slide positivity rate (number of positives per number of slides taken) increased from 24% in 1992 to 42% in 1995 for the high-risk population. This improvement in the efficiency of the surveillance efforts also was observed for the areas at moderate risk (from 0.6% to 21.6% positive slides) and low risk (from 3.2% to 8.3% positive slides).

While concentrated efforts strikingly improved services in the areas of active transmission (i.e., Amazon Basin), surveillance in no-risk areas was not forgotten. In 1992, 84.8 million people were living in areas with no risk of malaria; 20,200 slides were taken

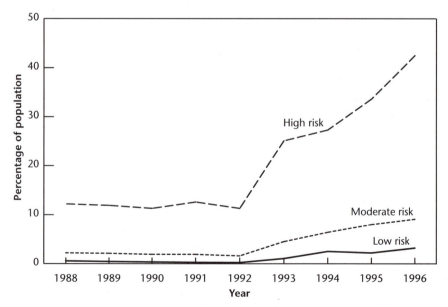

Figure 5-2. Population Covered by Case Detection Services (Annual Blood Slide Rate) in Brazil, 1988–1996

Source: Brazilian Ministry of Health.

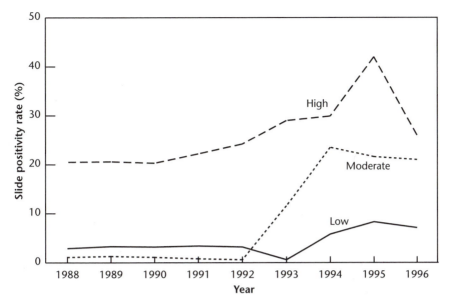

Figure 5-3. Malaria Slide Positivity Rate by Population at Risk in Brazil, 1988–1996

Source: Brazilian Ministry of Health.

that indicated a positivity rate of 17.2%. In 1995, from a population of 147.6 million, 925,191 slides were collected to diagnose 6,089 (0.6%) malaria cases outside the areas of active transmission.

Measurable Benefits

The availability of prompt diagnosis and immediate treatment was essential for the continuous reduction of *P. falciparum* circulation in the Amazon Basin. The results of this strategic shift is shown by the following statistics:

- an increase of medical attention to malaria disease (measured by hospitalization), which was available to 25% more of the *P. falciparum* cases in 1995 than in 1992;
- a reduction in the *P. falciparum* case fatality rate by 20.8% (from 0.48% to 0.38%) during the same period; and
- a reduction of the *P. falciparum* incidence rate from 13 per 1,000 people exposed to transmission to 8 per 1,000 people exposed between 1992 and 1996.

An economic evaluation of this program was carried out by the Brazilian Ministry of Health (Akhavan 1999). The evaluation was based on disability-adjusted life-years (DALYs) saved and on all expenditures from the three sources of funds disbursed for malaria-related activities between 1989 and 1996: the National Malaria Program, the World Bank loan, and the hospital and ambulatory care provided by the Unified Health Care System. These expenditures invested in malaria control have saved 8.57 million DALYs compared with the expected mortality and morbidity in the absence of any control program. The great majority of DALYs saved came from preventing death due to untreated or late-treated *P. falciparum* infections. Preventive measures such as controlling vectors and reducing the number of individuals infective to vectors accounted for a savings of 3.82 million DALYs, and prompt diagnosis and immediate treatment accounted for a savings of 4.74 million DALYs. The cost of the control program was US$616 million (adjusted to 1996 value). Based on the epidemiological trend observed between 1977 and 1988, the program prevented an estimated 1.83 million cases of malaria and 100,687 deaths for the period from 1989 to 1996.

This reduced incidence rate resulted in an estimated savings in treatment of approximately US$42.7 million; program cost-effectiveness is US$60–65 per DALY saved by the program. These results clearly support the effectiveness of the GMCS in demographic and ecologically unstable areas of development such as the Amazon region of Brazil. Table 5-1 shows the cost effectiveness of results for the categorical campaign of 1989 to 1992 with the GMCS strategy for the period from 1993 to 1996.

Conclusion

Malaria control efforts in Brazil have evolved over the last century, in response to varying levels of funding and organization, to changes in the parameters of disease transmission, the antimalaria drug and pesticide arsenal, vector and parasite resistance status, and characteristics of the human population at risk. Before the advent of the organic chemical pesticides, control activities focused on the reduction of mosquito breeding sites in and around human settlement and the distribution of *cinchona* to malaria patients.

The malaria eradication campaigns of the 1960s, which took advantage of the newly available DDT for intramural spraying and the synthetic drug chloroquine, made significant inroads initially but began to falter in the 1970s. Brazil decentralized its malaria control program over several decades and, in response to economic constraints and new and complicated malaria control demands in the expanding settlements of the Amazon Basin, shifted its emphasis from eradication to disease management. Its current strategy is to concentrate malaria control resources among the highest-risk groups, attempting to prevent mortality and reduce the social and economic burden of the disease. Although not yet fully implemented, this strategy has already shown positive results, for example, in the *P. falciparum* case fatality rate.

Disclaimer

Opinions expressed in this chapter are the author's only and do not necessarily reflect the policies and views of the World Health Organization or the Pan American Health Organization.

References

Akhavan, D. 1996. *Análise de Custo-Efetividade do Projeto de Controle da Malária na Bacia Amazônica: Relatório Final.* Brasilia, Brazil: Pan American Health Organization.

Akhavan, D., P. Musgrove, A. Abrantes, R. d'A. Gusmao. 1999. Cost-Effective Malaria Control in Brazil. Cost-effectiveness of a Malaria Control Program in the Amazon Basin of Brazil, 1988–1996. *Social Science & Medicine* 49: 1385–1399

WHO (World Health Organization). 1992a. *The Global Malaria Control Strategy.* Geneva, Switzerland: WHO.

———. 1992b. Malaria: Disease of Poverty and Underdevelopment. Press release, Ministerial Conference on Malaria, 26–27 October.

Table 5-1. Cost-Effectiveness of Malaria Control Strategies in Brazil, 1989–1996

Concept	Old strategy, 1989–1992			New strategy, 1993–1996			Entire period, 1989–1996		
	Prevention	Treatment	Total	Prevention	Treatment	Total	Prevention	Treatment	Total
Cost (millions of US$)	340.51	471.49	387.66	185.11	43.39	228.50	525.62	90.53	616.16
Expenditures prevented (millions of US$)	10.01	—	10.01	31.50	—	31.50	41.52	—	41.52
Net cost (millions of US$)	330.50	47.15	377.64	153.61	43.39	197.00	484.11	90.53	574.64
Falciparum cases prevented	257.50	—	257.50	749.37	—	749.37	1,006.87	—	1,006.87
Falciparum cases treated	—	813.53	813.53	—	595.34	595.34	—	1,408.87	1,408.87
Lives saved	25.75	75.01	100.76	74.94	54.90	129.83	100.69	129.90	230.58
Cost per life saved (US$)									
Based on total cost	13,224	629	3,847	2,470	790	1,760	5,220	697	2,672
Based on net cost	12,835	629	3,748	2,050	790	1,517	4,808	697	2,492

Note: See source for more specific information about methodology.
Source: Akhavan and others 1999.

Chapter 6

Determinants of Malaria in WHO European Region

Guido Sabatinelli

The World Health Organization (WHO) European Region consists of 51 countries located in an area that roughly corresponds geographically to Europe, Anatolia (the part of Turkey that comprises the peninsula of Asia Minor), the Caucasus (Armenia, Azerbaijan, and Georgia), Siberia, and Central Asia (Kazakhstan, Kyrgyzstan, Tajikistan, and Uzbekistan). According to Macdonald (1957), this area corresponds to the North Eurasian and Mediterranean epidemiological areas and is located entirely within the Palearctic zoogeographic region (described in detail in Chapter 9). Since 1990, malaria has reemerged—in different aspects and for different reasons—in Europe, Turkey, the Caucasus, and Central Asia.

In Central Asia and the Caucasus, political and economic instability followed the dissolution of the Soviet Union. The consequent decrease in the quality of health services, massive population movement, and environmental modifications appear to be the main determinants of this resurgence of malaria. The expansion of irrigation networks for agricultural activity is the basis of the recent epidemic in southeastern Turkey. The increased movement of international immigrants and tourists from tropical areas has resulted in a continuous rise in the importation of malaria cases in Europe, with associated high fatality rates.

A campaign launched at the end of the 1950s eradicated malaria in Europe and in almost all of the countries of the Soviet Union (reviewed in Bruce-Chwatt and de Zulueta 1980). Residual foci remained active in the Asian part of Turkey and in Azerbaijan. By the end of the 1980s, malaria was nearly forgotten in the WHO European Region (Gramiccia and Beales 1988); however, since 1993, the disease has dramatically reemerged (Majori, Sabatinelli, and Kondrachine 1999; Sabatinelli 1999).

The malaria situation in the WHO European Region presents a complex epidemiological picture characterized by autochthonous cases (transmitted and contracted locally) and cases imported from malaria-endemic countries. At present, four countries—Armenia, Azerbaijan, Tajikistan, and Turkey—are experiencing malaria epidemics. The highest number of cases was registered in 1997, when 75,685 autochthonous cases of malaria were officially reported. In occidental Europe, the malaria situation is characterized by the continuous increase in the importation of malaria cases from endemic tropical countries, mainly malaria caused by the *Plasmodium falciparum* parasite, with associated high fatality rates.

In this chapter, I describe the epidemiological situation in the countries of the WHO European Region and attempt to identify the main determinants of the epidemiological changes.

Overview of the Malaria Situation

Turkey

Turkey is a mountainous country with a diversity of climates. It encompasses areas that differ widely both in their endemicity and in their receptivity to malaria reintroduction. *Anopheles sacharovi* is the important vector, but other species—notably, *Anopheles superpictus* and *Anopheles hyrcanus*—may play roles in transmission (Giglioli 1979).

In 1945, one-third of the population under threat of malaria risk received treatment for malaria, and in 1946, a countrywide survey revealed a 25% prevalence of enlarged spleens; that same year, residual spraying of houses using DDT was introduced. A National Malaria Eradication Programme was launched in 1957, and by 1968, malaria had almost disappeared. By 1970, a total of 1,293 cases of malaria were reported, mainly from southeastern Anatolia. Before control activities began, *P. falciparum* was the predominant parasite. However, since the early 1970s, only malaria caused by the *Plasmodium vivax* parasite has been found in indigenous cases. From 1971 onward, the number of malaria cases in the Chukurova and Amikova plains (which form the provinces of Adana, Hatay, and İçel) continued to increase, reaching alarming proportions with a *P. vivax* epidemic in 1976 and 1977, when 37,320 and 115,512 cases were reported, respectively (Figure 6-1).

Several factors contributed to this deterioration of the epidemiological situation in the 1970s, including insufficient coverage by the surveillance system and the rapid agricultural development of the Chukurova plain. The situation was exacerbated by the extension of agriculture through the construction of a dam on the Seyan River and the introduction of industries along with rapid, uncontrolled urbanization (Giglioli 1979). Added to the resident population of the region of about 2.8 million (1.16 million urban,

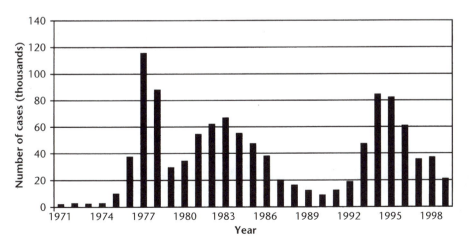

Figure 6-1. Incidence of Vivax Malaria in Turkey, 1971–1999

0.36 million suburban, and 1.31 million rural) was a large "floating" population of some 750,000 seasonal workers (Chakraverti and Uner 1975) who lived mostly in temporary dwellings such as tented encampments in grain, cotton, and rice fields during the harvest season. Laborers migrated mainly from malarious southeastern Anatolia, bringing malaria and other parasites with them. The malaria in the Chukurova area thus became the origin of disease dissemination.

Through concentrated efforts and at considerable cost, disease incidence began to recede in this area in 1978, subsequent to the reintroduction of large-scale malaria control operations (Ramsdale and Haas 1978). By 1979, the total number of reported cases had dropped to 29,323 and the epidemic was contained. During 1981, however, the situation deteriorated again, and the number of malaria cases reached more than 56,000; this growth continued until 1983 (66,681 cases).

The situation was exacerbated in the early 1980s by the appearance of *An. sacharovi* populations that were resistant to organochlorine compounds and, soon after, to several of the carbamate and pyrethroid compounds that were subsequently used. This resistance was attributable largely to the uncontrolled use of several types of insecticides for crop protection and for the pyrethroids' cross-resistance with DDT. At the same time, indoor residual spraying for malaria control decreased because of the bad smell of the organophosphate insecticides (malathion) used.

Since 1990, when only 8,680 malaria cases were reported, the malaria situation has deteriorated markedly throughout the country, with a steady increase in the number of cases from 12,218 to 84,345 between 1991 and 1994. This increase in the incidence of malaria was observed mainly in southeastern Anatolia, where the Güneydogu Anadolu Projesi (GAP) hydroagricultural project was developed.

The epidemic that developed around the GAP areas should be attributed mainly, but not only, to the impact of the expansion of irrigation networks. In fact, GAP introduced large changes in the environment, bringing water to a fertile but arid region and permitting an unprecedented expansion of agricultural production. GAP is the largest integrated project in Turkey's history. It covers 9.7% of the nation's total area and is inhabited by 10% of Turkey's population. Within an area of 75,358 square kilometers, 22 dams, 19 hydroelectric plants, and 2 irrigation tunnels are being constructed on the Euphrates and Tigris Rivers as well as their tributaries. This construction has resulted in an enormous increase in malaria vectors; a rise in malaria incidence also occurred in areas where development projects had not yet started, as a result of the importation of migrant workers infected with malaria.

Despite a significant reduction in the reported incidence of malaria cases from 60,884 to 20,963 during 1996–1999, the amount of malaria in the country is thought to be much greater and cannot be reliably assessed based on available data. Malaria transmission is concentrated in a part of the country where access to health services is poor. Underequipped and understaffed health facilities and undertrained health personnel, particularly in far-away areas, result in poor-quality disease management and prevention. Late diagnosis and delayed treatment are common. Furthermore, malaria patients usually are treated as outpatients, and many do not complete the full course of antirelapse treatment. Low awareness and knowledge of malaria result in the inadequate use of personal protective measures. In addition, some malaria patients are never seen by the public health sector or are self-treated, and these cases are not reported to the surveillance system.

The resistance of *An. sacharovi* (the principal malaria vector) to insecticides, the shortage of insecticides and spraying equipment, the limited use of antilarval measures, and the low usage rate of community-based preventive measures (including insecticide-treated mosquito nets) have resulted in present vector control operations having but limited impact. Finally, the resources invested by the government and international donors are insufficient, resulting in a diminished ability (and lack of the continuity required) to cope with the present malaria situation.

In terms of its impact on population health, development, and tourism, the malaria situation in Turkey continues to be serious. At present, more than 25% of the total population in Turkey lives at risk of contracting malaria. The malaria burden is a major obstacle to Turkey's development (Sabatinelli, Gokcinar, et al. 2000).

Armenia

Malaria has been endemic in Armenia since ancient times. Transmission occurs from June to October, and the main malaria vector is *Anopheles maculipennis*. In the 1920s and 1930s, thousands of people were affected by malaria in Armenia; 17 regions (Ararat, Armavir, Artashat, Ashaterak, Bagramian, Echmiadzin, Ekhegnadzor, Goris, Idgevan, Masis, Meghry, Kapan, Kotaik, Noemberian, Sisian, Tavush, and Vaik) and 3 towns (Diligan, Gumry, and Yerevan) were considered malarious. In 1934, as many as 200,000 malaria cases had been registered. From the 1930s to the 1960s, with the rapid development of health services and specialized malaria control institutions and with improved socioeconomic conditions, the malaria situation in the country improved. The number of malaria cases decreased to 60,000 by 1946, and to 14,500 by 1950 (Pirumov, Kazanchan, and Balasanian 1983).

During the period of malaria eradication (the 1950s and 1960s), comprehensive measures were undertaken, including indoor spraying with residual insecticides and wide-scale hydrotechnical environmental management. The number and size of *Anopheles* breeding places shrank dramatically, as did mosquito densities. By 1953, *P. falciparum* was eradicated, and only 68 vivax malaria cases occurred that year. Since 1963, no *P. falciparum*-infected vectors have been found in resting places, and only a few larvae have been detected in residual stagnant waters. *P. vivax*, too, was eradicated.

Once malaria was eradicated, however, vector control measures were progressively reduced; anopheline mosquitoes began to reappear in breeding places, and the densities of potential vectors grew. A difficult economic situation in 1990 led to even greater cuts in vector control measures. But despite sporadic cases of malaria imported from abroad, Armenia maintained its malaria-free status through 1993 as a result of a well-developed network of public health–oriented institutions. In 1994, 195 imported cases of vivax malaria were recorded (of which 91% were imported by military personnel stationed along the border with Azerbaijan), and 1 autochthonous case occurred (Davidiants et al. 1998) (Figure 6-2). In 1995, 502 cases were recorded, all imported. In 1996, the epidemiological situation worsened dramatically: 347 cases were recorded, of which 149 were autochthonous. In 1997, of 841 registered cases, 567 were autochthonous. Although 30 of 81 districts recorded malaria cases, 89% of the indigenous cases were registered in the Ararat valley in the Masis district, bordering Turkey. In addition, *An. sacharovi*, which was considered to be eradicated in the 1970s, was found again in some of the malaria foci in the valley (Boccolini et al. 2000).

In 1998, with the assistance of WHO, UNICEF, the International Federation of Red Cross, and the Red Crescent Societies, the Roll Back Malaria program was developed to eliminate the recently established foci of malaria infection and to prevent the resurgence of malaria in Armenia. In 1998, although the total number of cases increased to

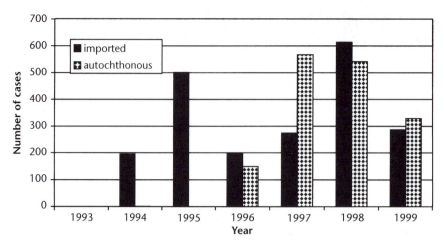

Figure 6-2. Incidence of Imported and Autochthonous Vivax Malaria in Armenia, 1993–1999

1,156, the epidemic was successfully contained; only 542 autochthonous cases were registered. In 1999, 616 cases were registered, 329 autochthonous and 287 imported (Sabatinelli, Grigorian, et al. 2000).

Azerbaijan

Malaria was practically eradicated in Azerbaijan in the 1960s; in 1967, only three indigenous cases were recorded, as compared with some 600,000 cases in 1934 (Dzhavadov, Kasimov, and Mamedov 1978). However, as a result of relaxing the surveillance activities, two large-scale malaria epidemics were reported, in 1969–1973 (Kasimov, Mamedov, and Vahabov 1979) and in 1979–1983. These epidemics were brought under control by activating the health services' existing powerful mechanisms.

The malaria situation began to deteriorate after 1990, when 24 cases were reported (Figure 6-3). The number of malaria cases increased rapidly from 667 in 1994, to 2,840 in 1995, to 13,135 in 1996. The main reason for this increase was a sharp decline in socioeconomic conditions, the displacement of nearly 1 million people from war-stricken zones (who have settled in 17 refugee camps since 1993), and the high mobility of the population living in the southern part of the country (an estimated 40% of which migrates during the agricultural season). In the absence of means to reduce malaria transmission through vector control, the specialized health services have focused their activities mainly on mass chemoprophylaxis (with chloroquine), case detection, and health education. About half the malaria cases were reported from seven districts: Imishli (14.6%), Nachishivan (10.4%), Fizuli (8.1%), Sabirabad (6.8%), Saatly (6%), Bejlagan (5.6%), and Bilasuvar (4.8%).

With international assistance, the Azerbaijan Ministry of Health resumed limited malaria control activities. In 1997, 9,911 cases of malaria were officially reported. Case detection has been actively pursued throughout the country; as a result, 75% of laboratory-confirmed malaria cases have been detected and about 600,000 people screened. A selective indoor residual spraying campaign was carried out in the refugee camps and high-risk areas. In 1998, the number of cases decreased to 5,175 (Sabatinelli, Velibekov, et al. 2000). In 1999, ENI (the Italian oil company) decided to fully finance a three-year

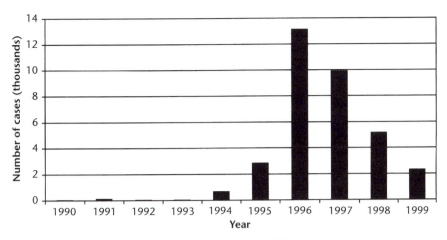

Figure 6-3. Incidence of Vivax Malaria in Azerbaijan, 1990–1999

malaria control program in Azerbaijan, through the WHO European Regional Office. That same year, a strong Roll Back Malaria partnership was established with UNICEF, the International Federation of Red Cross, the Red Crescent Societies, and Médecins sans Frontières (Doctors without Borders) Belgium. As a result of the activities carried out so far, the number of reported cases had fallen to 2,311 in 1999.

Malaria transmission occurs from June to October in two-thirds of the territory of Azerbaijan, and the main malaria vector is *An. sacharovi* (Kasimov, Mehtiev, and Mamedov 1981).

Georgia

Because of its ecological conditions, Georgia has a high potential for malaria. Between 1924 and 1928, malaria was one of the most important causes of mortality (6%) after respiratory infections, tuberculosis, and intestinal infections. To combat the malaria scourge, the Institute of Parasitology and Tropical Medicine was established in Tbilisi in 1924. Complex measures against malaria were undertaken at that time. The institute, through its specialized network, brought about a sharp decrease in morbidity by 1954, and malaria was practically eliminated in the country by 1961. Eradication was achieved by 1970 (Bakradze 1974).

However, malaria-free territories remain potentially at risk because their mosquito vectors and climatic conditions favor malaria transmission. Moreover, cases of malaria are imported into Georgia every year: 139 cases between 1970 and 1995. The conditions favorable to malaria transmission exist in 51.6% of the country (e.g., altitudes below 1,200 meters on the southern slopes of the Caucasus; between 1,300 and 1,500 meters on the northern slopes of the south Georgian uplands). About 80% of the settlements and 93% of the population are located in potentially malariogenic areas. The western and eastern parts of the country have the highest potential for malaria epidemics. Seven species of potential malaria vectors have been recorded, but the most important are *An. maculipennis,* spread in the whole territory up to an altitude of 200 meters above sea level; *An. sacharovi,* spread in the Lagodekhi, Signaghi, and Kareli regions; *Anopheles plumbeus,* spread almost everywhere there are leafy forests; and *An. superpictus,* spread mostly within eastern Georgia, on the banks of mountainous rivers.

Recent social and economic events in Georgia have negatively affected the malaria prevention system. In eastern Georgia, the situation is aggravated by the possibility of parasite introduction from bordering malarious areas of Azerbaijan. Three indigenous cases of vivax malaria were registered in districts bordering Azerbaijan (in Lagodekhi) in 1996, and 14 cases were registered in 1998 (four in Gardabani, four in Signaghi, two in Marneuli, two in Bolnisi, and two in Tbilisi) among people who worked near the Azerbaijan border. In 1999, 35 indigenous cases of vivax malaria were registered (19 in Signaghi, 4 in Marneuli, 8 in Gardabani, 3 in Dedoplistskaro, and 1 in Sagarejo) (Sabatinelli, Imnadze, et al. 2000).

Kazakhstan

Malaria was eradicated in Kazakhstan in 1960. From 1992 to 1998, about 100 malaria cases were imported from Tajikistan and Azerbaijan each year. In 1992, 1994, and 1996, only a few isolated autochthonous cases were reported; in 1998, four autochthonous cases occurred: two in the Almaty region, one in the Jambyl region, and one in the West Kazakhstan region. Of 84 imported cases observed in 1998, 51.8% were among troops demobilized from service in Tajikistan. Malaria cases were imported to all the administrative territories of Kazakhstan except the Kostanaj and Aktjubinsk regions (93.2% among adults and 6.8% among children; 19.3% among laborers and office workers, 47.4% among unemployed people). *P. vivax* was found in 89% of cases, *P. falciparum* in 3%, *Plasmodium malariae* in 1%, and mixed infections in 7%. Of people with symptoms, 52% consulted physicians within one to three days of the appearance of symptoms, and 58% of patients were diagnosed within one to three days (Sabatinelli, Spataev, et al. 2000). In 1999, 1 autochthonous case and 52 imported malaria cases were registered.

The Health Committee and the Republican Sanitary and Epidemiological Office, with the assistance of WHO, supervise the implementation of malaria prevention and control measures. Maintaining a malaria-free status requires continually screening travelers from malaria-endemic countries and local people with persistent fevers. In coordination with the Ministry of Defense and the Ministry of Internal Affairs, the Ministry of Health is organizing the preventive treatment of members of the peacekeeping forces serving in Tajikistan.

The main potential malaria vectors present in Kazakhstan are *Anopheles messeae*, *An. hyrcanus, An. superpictus,* and *Anopheles pulcherrimus.* The phenology and seasonal fluctuations in density of anophelines are systematically monitored at 117 observation points covering all the ecological regions of the country. Every year, masses of mosquitoes are collected at 400–500 selected stations. Until 1997, the vector densities were on the decrease, but in 1998, they increased in most of the country.

Kyrgyzstan

Kyrgyzstan has a mountainous terrain, and only some zones have a high malariogenic potential. Malaria epidemics occurred between 1930 and 1950; the largest epidemic was in 1944, when 60,152 cases were reported. By the end of the 1950s, malaria incidence had been reduced and was no longer a public health problem; the last indigenous case was registered in 1959. Malaria was eradicated through the development of complex measures, including vast bioenvironmental measures, through a network of specialized institutions (malaria control stations).

In the early 1980s, the malaria situation changed radically. The number of malaria cases imported from Afghanistan increased sharply, leading to the establishment of secondary foci in Tajikistan on the southern border of Kyrgyzstan. Fourteen cases of malaria were reported in Kyrgyzstan in 1986, and 10 in 1987. In 1988, 21 people contracted the disease, 11 of them local residents of the Batken district. Demobilized troops from Afghanistan were held responsible for establishing this malaria focus. Over the next several years, a few cases continued to be imported, but over the past 10 years, only one case of indigenous malaria has been reported (Chuj region in 1996). In 1997, 12 imported cases and 1 indigenous case were reported. In 1998, six cases were imported, and five were indigenous among residents of the Panfilov district. Immigrants from Tajikistan were the origin of this focus (Sabatinelli and Abdikarimov 2000).

The wave of immigration from Tajikistan, where the disease was widespread, could have led to the disease spreading in Kyrgyzstan. Kyrgyzstan has a well-developed irrigation network and many reservoirs, ponds, lakes, springs, and marshy areas around rivers. According to the specialized services of the Ministry of Health, the country has 3,861 water bodies, covering 4,605 hectares, that can serve as anopheline breeding places. According to the Ministry of Agriculture and Water Management, Kyrgyzstan has 5,440 kilometers of drainage canals, of which 1,605 kilometers have to be cleaned mechanically and 36 kilometers have to be cleaned by flushing. Hectares of potential breeding places for *Anopheles* mosquitoes need land reclamation. However, the high cost of carrying out many water sanitation projects prevents national authorities from doing so.

In the south, the climate is warm, with a long, hot season. The many ponds that form as a result of high groundwater make excellent breeding grounds for mosquitoes. The Osh and Jalal-Abad regions have a high malariogenic potential because of the immense rice-growing area (more than 2,000 hectares). Around 80% of their population are at risk of contracting malaria if the parasite were to become reestablished. The main potential malaria vectors are *An. superpictus*, *An. maculipennis*, and *An. messeae*.

Because malaria has not been a problem for more than 30 years, the present difficult economic conditions have led to a sharp drop in the number of malaria control specialists. In almost every region, the numbers of parasitologists, entomologists, and their assistants have fallen by 50–60%. There is a shortage of personnel with a thorough knowledge of the disease, experience in malaria control, and the ability to define priorities and appropriate and effective prevention measures.

The Russian Federation

During the first quarter of the twentieth century, malaria was one of the most important endemic diseases in Russia. The disease existed across the country but was particularly prevalent along the Volga River. During World War I, at least 3.5 million people in Russia suffered from malaria every year. As a result of the huge population movement and the general lowering of economic and social standards in the wake of the war, the early years (1922–1923) after the Russian Revolution saw the greatest European malaria epidemic of modern times along the middle Volga basin. According to a report by the USSR Ministry of Health, the malaria pandemic in Russia involved not fewer than 12 million cases (Bruce-Chwatt 1959).

By 1930, the situation improved greatly because of widely executed public health measures in general and malaria control measures in particular. The concept of elimination of malaria as a mass disease was adopted in the USSR in 1952, and three years later, it became obvious that total malaria eradication was possible. By 1960, malaria was eradicated in the territory corresponding to the Russian Federation, and only imported cases were registered. During the Soviet military presence in Afghanistan (1979–1989), the number of imported cases increased greatly. In 1980, 365 cases of malaria were imported by Soviet citizens and foreigners, and in 1985, at the peak of the importation of cases from Afghanistan, 1,981 cases were imported. Between 1981 and 1989, a total of 7,683 cases were diagnosed among demobilized Soviet military personnel who had been stationed in Afghanistan (Sergiev et al. 1993). The majority of these cases were vivax malaria, and isolated cases of falciparum malaria also were observed.

Another sharp rise in the number of cases of imported malaria, particularly from Azerbaijan and Tajikistan, has been observed since 1994. In 1995, for the first time in the Russian Federation, the number of cases imported from the newly independent states (NIS) exceeded the number of cases imported from the rest of the world. In 1998, a total of 1,081 cases were registered. In 1999, 789 cases were registered, of which 713 were imported. Because of high vulnerability and receptivity in large areas of the Russian Federation, local transmission began in 1996, when 10 autochthonous cases were registered. This total increased to 31 in 1997, 63 in 1998, and 77 in 1999.

In 1998, one outbreak of vivax malaria occurred in the town of Izberbash in the state of Daghestan. Subsequent to introduced cases, locally contracted cases were detected in Krasnodar (one case), Samara (one case), Tolyaty (one case), and Cherkessk (seven cases) in 1998–1999. In 1998, one case each of falciparum and vivax malaria were detected in Moscow. These infections were caused accidentally by blood transfusion.

Because of problems in procuring primaquine from abroad, not all cases of vivax malaria receive radical treatment. As a result, cases of relapsed malaria are registered every year: 20 in 1993, 37 in 1994, 45 in 1995, 59 in 1996, 99 in 1997, and 214 in 1998 (Baranova 1998; Sabatinelli, Sergiev, et al. 2000). Because of the late referral of patients with falciparum malaria, subsequent late diagnosis, and late and (in some cases) inappropriate treatment, several fatal cases occur every year; 12 fatal cases were reported during 1994–1997 and 9 in 1998–1999.

An analysis of imported cases of vivax malaria shows that of all imported cases, 83% occurred in cities (where receptivity is limited) and only 17% in rural areas (where receptivity is high). However, one-half of the cases registered in rural areas occurred during the cold (i.e., unfavorable) season for malaria transmission. Of 1,018 imported cases registered in 1998, only 200 appeared at the right time and place for prime transmission.

Tajikistan

Malaria was eradicated in Tajikistan by 1960 (Lysenko and Kalmykov 1969). However, subsequent to changes in the political structure of Afghanistan and the departure of Soviet troops in 1989, an increased incidence of malaria was observed in the country's border districts (Darvaz, Kulyab, Moscovsk, Parkhar, and Pyandzh). These outbreaks were brought under control by a major malaria control effort that included aerial spraying and mass prophylaxis.

The incidence of malaria until 1992 was about 200–300 cases a year, and on average, 40–77% of all registered cases occurred in the border districts. Most of these cases were due to *P. vivax*, but lately, cases due to *P. falciparum* have increased (Pitt et al. 1998). Between 1992 and 1998, no malaria control measures were carried out in Tajikistan because of civil war. In addition, almost all of the refugees returning from northern Afghanistan to their home region of Khatlon carried malaria parasites, which led to the rapid spread of the dis-

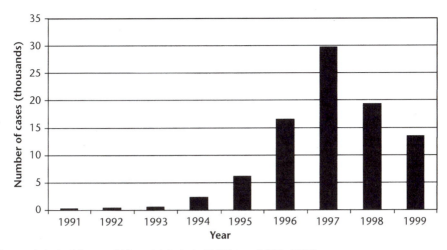

Figure 6-4. Incidence of Vivax Malaria in Tajikistan, 1991–1999

ease in Tajikistan. In 1997, the number of officially registered vivax malaria cases reached nearly 30,000, mainly in areas with refugee populations (Figure 6-4). Most of the cases (25,364) occurred in the Khatlon region (85.2%); the remaining cases occurred in the Gorno-Badakhshan Autonomous Region (3.7%), in the Centrally Administered Districts (6.6%), in Dushanbe city (4.0%), and in the Leninabad region (0.5%).

Only three species of *Anopheles* have proved to be epidemiologically important as vectors of *P. vivax* parasites in Tajikistan: *An. superpictus, An. pulcherrimus,* and *An. hyrcanus. An. superpictus,* the main vector, is highly endophagic and anthropophilic (that is, prefers to feed indoors on humans). *An. pulcherrimus* and *An. hyrcanus,* secondary vectors, are exophagic and zoophilic (that is, prefer to feed outdoors on animals).

A major international assistance program to control the malaria epidemic was launched in late 1997 in a joint effort among WHO, other international agencies, and the Tajikistan Ministry of Health. The foci complex located in southwestern Tajikistan forms a unique epidemiological entity with the settlements of northern Afghanistan (WHO 1998). In this area, military action along the border makes effective malaria control very difficult. Nevertheless, after the implementation of prevention and control measures, the number of malaria cases officially registered in 1999 dropped to nearly 13,500 (a 70% reduction compared to 1997) (Sabatinelli, Aliev, et al. 2000).

Turkmenistan

Malaria was eradicated in Turkmenistan in 1960. However, between 1965 and 1980, 23 indigenous cases of malaria were reported, all in the Maryj and Ahal districts. Nine species of potential malaria vectors are present in Turkmenistan, the most important of which are *An. superpictus, An. pulcherrimus,* and *An. hyrcanus.* Turkmenistan has large arid territories, and major changes made to the country's water system have affected anopheline distribution. The malaria-receptive territories are the Tedjen and Murgab flood plains, an area with an abundant network of water bodies fed by the Murgab and Tedjen Rivers, and the Hauz-Han Reservoir, which is fed by the Karakum Canal. A chain of 17 major reservoirs has been constructed along the Karakum Canal and river basin area, and the enormous seepage ponds that have formed around them have become anopheline breeding places (Ponirovskij, Mamednijazov, and Morozova 1988).

In recent years, because of the deteriorating malaria situation in some southern countries of the Commonwealth of Independent States (CIS; includes the former constituent republics of the USSR: Azerbaijan, Armenia, Belarus, Georgia, Kazakhstan, Kyrgyzstan, Moldova, Russia, Tajikistan, Turkmenisten, Uzbekistan, and Ukraine) and in Afghanistan, the number of malaria cases imported into Turkmenistan has risen sharply. Most of the malaria cases imported in the 1980s were among soldiers returning from Afghanistan. Despite the massive movement of population between Afghanistan and Turkmenistan from 1979 to 1989, only 204 cases were reported. Of these, 25 were indigenous and occurred in 10 villages of the Maryj region. From 1990 to 1997, the number of imported cases of malaria decreased (79 cases in total) and 27 isolated cases (acquired through blood transfusions) were reported, but no local outbreaks or secondary cases were observed.

In 1998, the epidemiological situation in the country deteriorated with the resumption of local transmission. The first autochthonous case occurred in the town of Kushka in June, and seven cases occurred in August in a nearby village. Four more cases were observed in the Dashovuz and Lebap districts among former frontier guards returning from duty in Kushka. In August, active screening for malaria was organized in Kushka and two neighboring villages. Finally in 1998, 115 autochthonous cases were registered in five foci in an area inhabited by about 10,000 people (Sabatinelli and Amangaldiev 2000). The main reasons for this outbreak were late diagnosis and treatment because of a lack of awareness, drugs, and laboratory equipment; an increased number of vectors because of a disregard for the rules of the construction and use of water installations; and late and poor-quality malaria control measures because of a lack of insecticides, equipment and vehicles, and qualified personnel (parasitologists and entomologists).

Uzbekistan

An increase in the importation of malaria into Uzbekistan has been observed as a result of the deteriorating malaria situations in neighboring countries. The epidemiological situation has become particularly tense in the cities and districts of eight provinces of Uzbekistan along the frontier with Tajikistan, where 5.6 million people live. Some 25% of the population lives in the 67 cities and districts that border Afghanistan, Kazakhstan, Kyrgyzstan, Tajikistan, and Turkmenistan. The epidemiological situation is exacerbated by migratory movements of large population groups between the countries, especially of people resettled from Tajikistan.

Imported cases of malaria are registered in all regions of the country except in the Republic of Karakalpakstan and the province of Khorezm. Between 1991 and 1998, the number of localities into which malaria has been imported increased; between 65% and 80% of cases of malaria are registered in cities. However, in recent years, the importation of cases into rural areas (where risk of malaria transmission is high because of the high density of potential malaria vectors) has increased. For example, 43% of malaria cases in the Surkhandarya region were imported into rural areas in 1996, 56% in 1997, and 100% in 1998.

In 1998, 74 cases of malaria were registered in Uzbekistan, including 17 (23%) among children up to 14 years old. All of these cases were reported as imported, and 93% were from Tajikistan. As in previous years, *P. vivax* was responsible for the majority of cases (70 cases [95%]) and *P. falciparum* for only a few (four total: three cases imported from Tajikistan, and one case from Guinea) (Sabatinelli, Majori, et al. 2000). Since 1998, the WHO Regional Office for Europe and the Istituto Superiore di Sanità in Rome, Italy, have provided technical assistance in carrying out anti-epidemic measures in foci and strengthening the technological base of the Republican Sanitary and Epidemiological Centre and the Isaev Institute of Medical Parasitology.

The environment and climate in Uzbekistan favor the development of malaria vectors. The presence of many bodies of water of differing types facilitates the simultaneous occurrence in a given locality of all the epidemiologically dangerous species: *An. maculipennis, An. pulcherrimus,* and *An. superpictus.* The temperature ensures the rapid reproduction of vectors (up to five generations) and parasites (up to eight cycles) and transmission of the disease within five months. At present, seven potential malaria vector species have been observed. The most receptive areas for malaria are the districts named after the main rivers: Amy-Darya, Chirchik, Naryn, Surkhan, and Syr-Darya (Jusupova, Pershin, and Musatova 1975; Sergiev and Gozodova 1979).

Imported Malaria in Europe

Almost all of the 51 countries in the WHO European Region maintain a national malaria surveillance system with mandatory notification of all malaria cases. The only country that has adopted a different system is France, where only indigenous cases are statutorily notifiable; the total number of imported cases is estimated by using data collected by a sentinel reporting network of selected laboratories. Diagnosis of malaria cases is confirmed by microscopic examination of blood in about 80% of the European countries.

Since the early 1970s, the number of imported malaria cases has been increasing (Figure 6-5). From 1983 to 1986, the number of cases nearly doubled (from 5,167 to 10,046 cases, respectively), and this explosive growth continued until 1989 (11,882 cases). After 1989, the number of malaria cases declined until 1992 (8,292 cases) but then increased by 50% by 1997 (12,860 cases). Malaria cases were imported mainly into the western part of the WHO European Region, particularly into countries of the Euro-

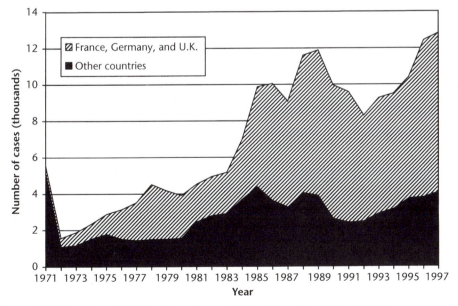

Figure 6-5. Number of Malaria Cases Imported into Countries of the WHO European Region, 1971–1997

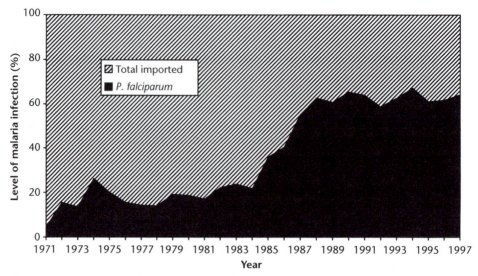

Figure 6-6. Percentage of Imported Cases of Falciparum Malaria in the WHO European Region, 1971–1997

pean Union. The highest numbers of cases were recorded in 1997: 5,377 in France, 2,364 in the United Kingdom, and 1,017 in Germany. In 1997, these three countries accounted for almost 70% of all the imported malaria cases in the WHO European Region.

From 1971 to 1997, the ratio between infections with *P. falciparum* and other *Plasmodium* species changed (Figure 6-6). From the late 1970s to the mid-1980s, *P. falciparum* was responsible for only about 20–30% of cases. The percentage of *P. falciparum* infections increased dramatically between 1984 and 1988, when *P. falciparum* became responsible for 60% of infections. Since 1988, this level has remained fairly stable. In 1997, the countries with the highest prevalence of imported cases of *P. falciparum* were France (80%), Italy (77%), and Germany (72%).

Information about fatal cases of malaria (due to *P. falciparum*) is available for only a few countries. For 1987–1997, 578 fatal cases were reported in the WHO European Region. Germany reported 25 fatal cases in 1995 and 19 in 1996; France reported 21 in 1996; the United Kingdom reported 13 in 1997; and Italy reported 10 in 1997. The countries that reported the most malaria cases also experienced the highest fatality rates. The fatality rate in Germany for the period 1987–1996 was 3.6%, one of the highest in Europe.

"Airport Malaria"

A relatively recent phenomenon has been cases of autochthonous malaria occurring in people who travel by airplane but have not visited a malarious country and people who live near airports. Since 1977, when the phenomenon was first documented, 75 cases of so-called airport malaria have been observed in Western Europe; 28 of the cases occurred in France (Mouchet 2000). Airport malaria also has been reported in Belgium, Italy, Luxembourg, Switzerland, and the United Kingdom.

Two people apparently were infected while traveling from London to Rome on an aircraft that had originated in Africa. People also have become infected during a stopover. Other autochthonous cases have been attributed to the arrival of infected tropical anophelines on airplanes; the anophelines later escaped into the adjacent countryside. Epidemiological investigations also suggest transmission through the passive transport of tropical infected mosquitoes in containers or personal belongings that arrive from tropical areas. Such cases are currently referred to as *luggage malaria*.

The highest risk of airport malaria in Europe comes from western and central Africa, because most of the air traffic from these countries includes stopovers in western Europe. Numerous *Anopheles* species can be found in all these airports, especially *Anopheles gambiae*, whose breeding season (the rainy season) takes place in West Africa during the summer (July–August), when conditions favor the survival of imported specimens (Mouchet 2000).

Analysis of Determinants

Thus far, I have outlined the malaria epidemiological situation in the WHO European Region, which is typified by autochthonous malaria and imported malaria. Next, I analyze the factors that influence both epidemiological aspects.

Malariogenic Potential

The changes in malaria incidence observed in a given area are the result of changes in the malariogenic potential. *Malariogenic potential* is the result of the interaction of two factors: receptivity, which takes into account vectors and climatic conditions in a territory, and vulnerability, which takes into account the occurrence of parasite carriers in a territory.

Receptivity. Receptivity is the tendency of an area to establish malaria transmission after the introduction of parasite carriers as a result of the presence of vectors and favorable climatic conditions. Because of the diversity of prevailing ecological conditions in the WHO European Region, several anopheline species are present in the region, and 11 have been recognized as malaria vectors: *Anopheles atroparvus, Anopheles claviger, Anopheles hispaniola, An. hyrcanus, Anopheles labranchiae, An. maculipennis, An. messeae, An. plumbeus, An. pulcherrimus, An. sacharovi,* and *An. superpictus* (WHO 1989; Ramsdale and Snow 2000). However, only a few of these species are principal vectors that generally maintain transmission; the others are secondary vectors that augment the amount of transmission but would not sustain the disease cycle efficiently without the principal vectors.

Considering the climatic factors and the distribution of principal vector species, the WHO European Region can be divided into five areas:

- northern Europe (*An. atroparvus* and *An. messeae*);
- southern Europe (*An. labranchiae, An. atroparvus, An. superpictus,* and *An. sacharovi*);
- Anatolia and the Caucasus (*An. sacharovi, An. superpictus,* and *An. maculipennis*);
- northern central Asia and Siberia (*An. messeae, An. maculipennis,* and *An. superpictus*); and
- southern central Asia (*An. superpictus* and *An. pulcherrimus*).

An. superpictus and potential malaria vectors of the *An. maculipennis* complex (*An. maculipennis sensu stricto* [*s.s.*], *An. messeae, An. labranchiae, An. atroparvus,* and *An. sacharovi*) overwinter as adults in cold natural shelters or in buildings. Where climatic conditions permit, hibernation is only partial; occasional blood meals (which do not lead to ovarian development) may be taken through the winter (Ramsdale and Haas 1978). In the areas of the WHO European Region where malaria transmission currently occurs, hibernating adults probably start to appear in August or early September. Most mosquitoes that overwinter in buildings do so in stables, where the cool, humid environment is more favorable to survival than the often dry conditions of heated human dwellings and where continued feeding on animals leads to a wastage of any sporozoites. Although the possibility obviously exists, winter transmission has little epidemiological importance. Reactivation of hibernating mosquitoes in the spring occurs at temperatures below the threshold for parasite development or under conditions in which their extrinsic cycles are greatly extended. Therefore, although newly reactivated mosquitoes are improbable vectors of malaria during the spring, they may acquire an infection at this time. Some can survive long enough to become infective (Detinova 1962).

Most of the anophelines present in the WHO European Region, including those of known or possible epidemiological importance, are markedly zoophilic and readily feed outdoors. *An. hyrcanus* will not enter buildings and is never found biting humans in the presence of cattle, but it feeds readily on humans if animals are not available. It is a crepuscular feeder, and its attacks cease entirely within about one hour of sunset. *An. pulcherrimus,* an important vector in Tajikistan, is also markedly exophilic. *An. maculipennis* s.s. and *Anopheles melanoon*, domestic mosquitoes that sometimes occur in enormous densities, are so strongly zoophilic that they probably could not maintain malaria transmission on their own. *An. superpictus* is endophilic and has a marked preference for animals but feeds on humans in the absence or relative rarity of animals. Even *An. sacharovi*, the most dangerous vector in Turkey and Azerbaijan, feeds on animals to a greater extent than it does on humans. Like *An. hyrcanus,* all these mosquitoes are active at or shortly after dusk but continue feeding, to varying degrees, throughout the night. The absence of animals is an important factor in contributing to conditions conducive to malaria transmission.

With few exceptions, vector breeding places in most of the originally rural malarious areas underwent little change during malaria eradication; as a result, vector densities returned to their original levels after vector control measures ceased. In some countries (e.g., Turkey), the surfaces for breeding places increased enormously as a result of hydro-agricultural projects, and in others (e.g., Turkmenistan), some desert areas are now receptive to malaria.

Nevertheless, the high density of *Anopheles* populations reported in some areas does not necessarily translate into a serious malaria threat. Several entomological factors influence risk of transmission. First, only some species of *Anopheles* are able to transmit malaria. It has been proven that members of the same *Anopheles* species can have different degrees of susceptibility to *Plasmodium* species from different geographic areas and different degrees of ability to transmit infection. In areas where malaria parasites have long been eradicated, it is important to determine whether the mosquitoes are still susceptible to infection with *Plasmodium* species from areas where malaria is still endemic. A few tests of susceptibility carried out with some of the *An. maculipennis* complex in the Palearctic region showed a near-complete refractoriness to African strains of *P. falciparum* (James, Nicol, and Shute 1932; Shute 1940; Ramsdale and Coluzzi 1975; de Zulueta et al. 1975). Under experimental conditions, only *An. plumbeus* was able to nurture *P. falciparum* at least to the oocyst stage, and the intensity of infection did not differ significantly from that of known vectors of *P. falciparum* (Marchant et al. 1998). However, most of species of the *An. maculipennis* complex, as well as *An. superpictus* and *An. hyrcanus*, are able to transmit *P. vivax* from different malaria-endemic areas.

Three main climatic factors govern malaria transmission: temperature, humidity, and rainfall. In the human host, the malaria parasite finds a more or less stable environment that is insulated from external conditions. However, the development of *Plasmodium* species within a mosquito is directly related to external temperature. Thus, the length of the transmission season is limited by the duration of the period during which temperatures are above the threshold necessary for completion of the parasite's extrinsic cycle.

Previously, *P. falciparum* occurred in the southern countries of the WHO European Region because its requirements of relatively high temperatures for development limited its distribution in the north. *P. vivax*, which is able to develop at lower temperatures, has been observed in the northern part of the WHO European Region, and in especially favorable years, it even has been transmitted within the Arctic Circle (Russell 1952; Bruce-Chwatt and de Zulueta 1980). The temperatures below which development in the mosquito is indefinitely retarded lie between 14.5 °C and 16 °C for *P. vivax* and between 16 °C and 19 °C for *P. falciparum* (Macdonald 1957; Moshkovsky 1946; Pampana 1963). Even so, Macdonald maintains that in regions with marked winters, the risk of *P. vivax* transmission remains slight until mean daily temperatures reach 21 °C. Similarly, because of the higher temperature requirements of *P. falciparum*, the risk of its transmission is slight until temperatures 3–4 °C higher (i.e., 24–25 °C) are reached. Some transmission at lower temperatures may be possible, but in considering the current epidemiological importance of reintroduced malaria, Macdonald's contentions are reasonably accurate. In the WHO European Region, malaria receptivity is generally nil from November to May; no malaria occurs in areas on the colder side of the 15 °C summer isotherm, and no falciparum malaria occurs on the colder side of the 21 °C summer isotherm. During the first quarter of the twentieth century, in Soviet Union territories, malaria reached 61°30′N along the Dvina River in the west and 45°N in the east (Haworth 1988).

The length of the sporogonic cycle can be estimated by using air temperatures recorded by meteorological stations; however, a more accurate estimate can be obtained by recording the temperatures of the actual mosquito resting places. Unfortunately, in most situations, mosquitoes use many different resting sites. Indoor temperatures are higher than outdoor temperatures only at night, when mosquitoes are active. Whether they spend the daylight hours inside or outside, resting mosquitoes choose the most favorable microclimate, which might be cooler or hotter than the air temperature.

A warmer climate could increase the reproductive potential of mosquitoes and their biting rates. It also could reduce the pathogen incubation period. All these changes could be conducive to increased the transmission of *Plasmodium* species. In addition, milder winters might prolong the malaria transmission season. Changes in humidity probably would affect the survival rate of adult mosquitoes (higher humidity is generally associated with higher survival), thus affecting the likelihood of transmission. Higher rainfall could increase the availability of breeding sites in some areas but have a flushing effect in others. However, such changes would not necessarily lead to a change in the distribution of the vectors, whose presence is limited by the availability of suitable breeding places and other nonclimatic factors. In addition to latitude, temperature is affected by altitude, and within the tropics, the limits of transmission have often been considered to coincide with a particular topographic contour (Hackett 1945; Wilson

1949). However, isotherms do not always follow contours in subtropical and temperate regions, and climatic conditions, even at sea level, are far from uniform. For instance, in Turkey, some locations at altitudes of more than 600 meters experience longer and hotter summers than other areas at sea level (Ramsdale and Haas 1978).

Mosquito densities depend on breeding conditions. After hibernation—a period of reduced metabolic activity that enables female anophelines to survive the cold season—mosquitoes begin to lay eggs. This reactivation takes place during the spring thaw, a time in temperate climates when rainstorms are frequent, contributing to runoff, flushing, and fluctuating water levels. Surface water is cold, so the aquatic developmental stages are extended, with a corresponding increase in the hazards to which the immature mosquitoes are exposed. Because of adverse conditions, early eggs laid by reactivated mosquitoes rarely give rise to a dramatic increase in adult densities. This comes later, with the amelioration of climatic conditions.

Densities of *An. superpictus,* whose eggs are laid in clear, sunlit eddies at the edges of streams or in residual pools in stream beds, often fluctuate in response to rainfall in the mountain catchment areas. This species is vulnerable to flushing and in general tends to increase in number as streams pool during the hot, dry summer; however, high densities can occur early in some situations, according to rainfall and the local morphology of streambeds and riverbeds.

An. sacharovi, An. maculipennis sensu lato (*s.l.*), and *An. hyrcanus* all favor marshy habitats. Their breeding grounds, which vary by location, may be either natural or human-made from an epidemiological standpoint. Many of the natural sites (e.g., marshes, swampy edges of streams or ponds, or inundated grassy depressions) that are important early in the spring tend to dry out progressively during the summer; to a certain extent, they regulate mosquito distribution and density. The importance of human-made breeding places, usually associated with irrigation systems, depends on water usage. Where water is scarce, intermittent irrigation in accordance with water rationing might (but usually does not) limit mosquito breeding in potential breeding sites that dry out every few days. Where water is plentiful, as in the rich agricultural areas of hot regions, single cash crops (principally cotton or rice) are cultivated under flood irrigation. Most of the currently malarious or high-risk parts of the WHO European Region are areas of intensive cultivation. The installation of irrigation systems modifies the ecology of large areas (such as Chukurova, Turkey), often allowing *An. sacharovi* to extend its range, and invariably provides extensive, long-lasting breeding areas.

Together, relative humidity and temperature have a great influence on the geographical distribution and longevity of *Anopheles* (Vinogradskaya 1969). The longevity of *Anopheles* is important for its effectiveness as a malaria vector; the mosquito must survive longer than the days necessary to complete sporogony to be able to transmit the disease (Gillies 1988; Detinova 1962). For most vector species, a temperature range of 20–30 °C and a minimum relative humidity of 60% are optimal (Bruce-Chwatt 1980). The life span of the mosquito decreases with rising temperatures and increases with increasing relative humidity. In general, the longevity of *Anopheles* shortens drastically with a combination of prolonged high temperature (more than 35 °C) and low humidity (less than 50%) and when niches with suitable microclimates are unavailable (Horsfall 1955; Bruce-Chwatt 1980).

Even so, optimal average daytime temperature and relative humidity differ considerably by species. For instance, *An. pulcherrimus* and *An. superpictus* show resistance to dehydration, and the density of *An. pulcherrimus* is high when humidity is low (provided that the relative humidity does not drop below 20%) (Vinogradskaya 1969). In addition, *An. pulcherrimus* is active at 16–33 °C and can resist temperatures of 38 °C. Under favorable climatic conditions, the average mosquito lifetime can be more than three to four weeks (Horsfall 1955), and many species may live two months during summer periods. Longevity is increased by hibernation (at low temperatures), and mosquitoes can survive as long as seven months during the winter season (Horsfall 1955).

The vectorial capacity of a mosquito population is the measure currently used in epidemiology to estimate the malaria transmission risk in various geographic areas. It expresses the number of potentially infectious bites that originate daily from a case of malaria in a given area or, more precisely, from a carrier of gametocytes capable of infecting all the receptive mosquitoes that feed on the carrier. The vectorial capacity (VC) of local anophelines is described by the formula $VC = ma^2p^n/-\ln(p)$, where m is the density of vectors (i.e., the number of mosquitoes per person); a is the human-biting habit (i.e., number of human blood meals taken per vector per day); p is the daily survival probability; and n is the duration of sporogony (Macdonald 1957; Moulineaux 1988).

Vectorial capacity is a useful way of expressing malaria transmission risk, because most of the factors that affect the risk of malaria transmission are included in the formula. However, calculating vectorial capacity is very difficult in practice and is associated with problems of bias and error (WHO 1979). A significant problem is the estimation of the survival probability and the density of the vector (Moulineaux et al. 1988). The estimation of the feeding habit also might be problematic, especially in areas were the vector is not entirely anthropophilic. The difficulties in measuring the ecological factors related to the vector are certainly amplified if the assessment is done on a large scale.

The receptivity to malaria in the Caucasus and Central Asia can be mapped according to climatic factors. The more favorable the climate to the vector–parasite–host development cycle, the higher the receptivity to introduced cases of malaria. This receptivity can be defined according to the level of risk of an outbreak should a new case be introduced locally. These risk levels can be defined to range from: the highly receptive climate—where reintroduction of malaria can lead to explosive outbreaks—to the no-risk climate—where introduction of malaria would not lead to any further transmission of the parasite.

A comparison of a map of climate receptivity for this region to where indigenous cases of malaria have been recorded between 1997 and 1999 shows little correspondence between climate receptivity factors and actual outbreaks. Of the 10 indigenous outbreaks between 1997 and 1999, two were in the no-risk and very-low-risk region, two more were in the low-risk region, and two were in the highest-risk region. The remaining four outbreaks took place in the medium-risk regions. This evidence provides support for the notion that, although climatic factors are important, recent outbreaks are poorly predicted by climate receptivity. As maintained throughout this volume, many other contextual variables can and do govern malaria transmission.

Vulnerability. The vulnerability of an area to malaria is determined by its proximity to malarious areas or the likelihood of a frequent influx of infected people or infective mosquitoes. In addition, public awareness concerning malaria, together with the level of efficiency of the public health services, plays an important role in determining malaria vulnerability. The different types and determinants of population migration are analyzed specifically in each epidemiological context in the following sections.

Table 6-1. Malariogenic Potential According to the Interaction of Levels of Vulnerability and Receptivity in the WHO European Region

Vulnerability	Low receptivity	Medium receptivity	High receptivity
Low[a]	Low	Medium	High
High[b]	Medium	High	High

[a]Area with few, if any, imported malaria cases.

[b]Area close to malarious areas, with a regular influx of people from malarious areas, or with sporadic but large-scale movements of people from malarious areas.

Source: WHO 1979.

The elements that affect the vulnerability appear to be difficult to quantify. For practical purposes, to stratify territories, two arbitrary levels of vulnerability are distinguished: low and high. The combination with the different levels of receptivity gives three levels of malariogenic potential (Table 6-1). In general, vulnerability deals with the socioeconomic contextual determinants of malaria, whereas receptivity refers to the components of vectorial capacity.

For example, the elements of vulnerability have contributed to malaria resurgence in the NIS. On December 26, 1991, the national parliament voted the USSR out of existence, and the USSR was eventually replaced with 12 independent states and 3 Baltic states. The profound socioeconomic changes that followed the dissolution of the Soviet Union had a negative effect on the malaria situation.

Economic and Social Determinants. One cost of the transition to democracy has been an extraordinary rise in poverty. Economic output in many of the countries of the former Soviet Union decreased sharply with the breakup of the USSR; purchasing power fell, and inflation was high. In some countries, the poverty rate remains extraordinarily high. In Armenia, according to a household survey conducted by the Ministry of Statistics in 1996, about 55% of the households were poor. In Kyrgyzstan, according to the National Statistic Committee, 71% of the population had an income below the poverty level. In Azerbaijan in 1998, about 25% of the labor force was estimated to be unemployed, 68% of households were assessed to be poor, and 24% of households were assessed to be very poor. In Tajikistan, the gross domestic product is estimated to have declined by about 30% per year between 1998 and 2000.

Since December 1991, unprecedented numbers of people have been displaced throughout the countries of the former Soviet Union. Given its scope and complexity, this displacement—estimated at more than 5 million people in 1994—constitutes the most important population movement in the region since World War II.

The main categories of population on the move in the newly independent states (NIS) are refugees, internally displaced people, illegal and transitory migrants, labor migrants, and returning military personnel. Refugee flows, which first appeared in 1989, are a new phenomenon for the region. Refugees either originated in the NIS, fled areas of armed conflict (e.g., Armenia, Azerbaijan, or Tajikistan), or arrived in the CIS from other countries, seeking asylum there or elsewhere. Internally displaced people appeared in the region at the same time as refugees as a result of armed conflicts or internal strife. They did not cross internationally recognized borders in their flight for safety but remained in their own countries (e.g., Armenia, Azerbaijan, Georgia, the Russian Federation, and Tajikistan).

In 1994, Armenia harbored over 300,000 ethnic Armenians fleeing from the cities of Baku, Nagorno-Karabakh, and Sumgait in Azerbaijan. The vulnerable population of refugees and nonrefugees was estimated to be 2.5 million of a total 3.5 million. In Azerbaijan, more than 900,000 people were displaced by the conflict in Nagorno-Karabakh. In Georgia, the military conflict that began in August 1992 brought the number of refugees and displaced people to 300,000. The civil war that erupted in Tajikistan in 1992 caused the internal and external displacement of some 500,000 people, more than 60,000 of whom fled to northern Afghanistan. Spontaneous and assisted repatriation of Tajik refugees began shortly after an amnesty agreement. An estimated 13,000 refugees have returned spontaneously to Tajikistan, and 17,000 more have returned, primarily to Piandji and Gorno-Badakhshan, with the assistance of the U.N. High Commissioner for Refugees. By the beginning of 1994, only about 39,000 Tajik refugees remained on Afghan soil; repatriation was concluded in 1995.

As in Turkey, in some NIS countries, the seasonal migration of workers is a contributing factor to the malaria situation. An estimated 40% of people in the southern part of Azerbaijan migrate during the agricultural season. Population movement should be considered the main cause of malaria resurgence in the NIS. The role played by demobilized military forces as parasite carriers also was particularly important for malaria transmission in Armenia and Turkmenistan.

Breakdown of Health Services. Recent economic difficulties have led ministries of health to reduce their budgets for preventive measures. The supply of essential equipment and materials for malaria control (e.g., antimalaria drugs and insecticides) has dried up, particularly those that used to be purchased from abroad by the Ministry of Health of the former USSR (e.g., primaquine). The lack of transport, materials, and drugs has weakened malaria prevention activities.

Difficult economic conditions also have sharply reduced the number of specialized technicians working on malaria programs. To some extent, the exodus of technicians has been understated, because some workers have been put on long-term "administrative leave" (typically unpaid but still classified as employed), whereas many of the unemployed have been put into other categories, such as "early retirement" or "inactive." In almost every region, the number of parasitologists, entomologists, and their assistants has fallen by 50–60%. Today there is a shortage of personnel with a thorough knowledge of the disease, experience in malaria control, and the ability to define priorities as well as appropriate and effective prevention measures.

The level of the population's awareness of malaria and the level of the population's and the health authorities' sophistication and health education also have important bearing on vulnerability. Lack of knowledge and experience in malaria prevention and control among health service staff who have not seen malaria for 30 years is an obstacle in the planning and effective implementation of these measures. The expertise in malaria epidemiology and control that existed in several research institutes in Europe some 20–30 years ago is now limited to only a few expert centers.

Changes in Agricultural Practice. Most agricultural lands in the former Soviet Union were cultivated as collective farms. Because of the lack of cash and credit available to the state farms as well as to the small number of privately owned farms, the performance of the agricultural sector has declined steadily since 1985. In several countries, but particularly in Azerbaijan and Armenia, the maintenance of the extensive irrigation system has been neglected, giving way to rapid deterioration and providing favorable breeding places for anophelines. In addition, in some countries (e.g., Tajikistan and Uzbekistan), people started to cultivate rice in an uncontrolled way near their dwellings, thus increasing the anopheline density and the risk of contact with potential malaria vectors.

In the past, mosquito densities dropped drastically in some countries during the summer as result of crop spraying, illustrating the positive contribution of agricultural insecticides to malaria control. However, the indiscriminate use of insecticides caused early incidence of resistance to insecticides among malaria vectors in the same areas.

Imported Malaria

A complete understanding of the epidemiology of imported malaria in the WHO European Region requires an analysis of the major determinants of the trend, which include

- the number of people exposed to malaria risk (e.g., Europeans traveling to malaria-endemic areas);
- the number of people coming from malarious areas (e.g., immigrants);
- the endemicity levels in the malarious areas (determined by different factors); and
- the sensitivity of *Plasmodium* species to antimalaria drugs (for prophylaxis or treatment).

In the following sections, I analyze the first two determinants with available information.

Travelers to Malarious Areas. The growing number of intercontinental travelers certainly has contributed to the increased importation of malaria cases into European countries (Sabatinelli, Joergensen, and Majori 1999). The general trend in the total number of travelers to malaria-endemic countries (in Africa, Asia, and Central and South America) is shown in Figure 6-7. In 1997, about 12 million Europeans were estimated to have traveled to malarious countries for tourism or work.

The malaria risk varies substantially, even within a given endemic country, from low in certain urban areas to high in rural areas. It also varies with the time spent abroad and the living conditions in endemic areas. Therefore, with only generic data about the destinations of travelers, it is almost impossible to calculate the real incidence of malaria in tourists.

Immigration from Malarious Areas. Since the 1970s, some European countries have changed from being countries with high emigration to countries with high immigration. The migrants, who originate primarily in economically depressed or politically unstable areas of Africa and Asia, seek new employment opportunities and an escape from the political and social problems of their homelands.

An accurate calculation of the number of foreigners in Europe is particularly difficult because, in addition to foreigners who are legally registered, many immigrants hold expired resident permits or have entered the country illegally. However, the total number of immigrants from Africa, Asia, and South America appears to have increased twofold between 1985 and 1991. In general, the majority of immigrants during the entire period were from Asia. Figure 6-8 shows the trend of immigration from African malarious countries to the WHO European Region between 1985 and 1995. From 1985 to 1988, the number of people emigrating from malarious areas of Africa was more or less constant, averaging about 25,000 a year. By 1993, this number had increased more than threefold, reaching about 80,000 (Statistical Office of the European Community 1998).

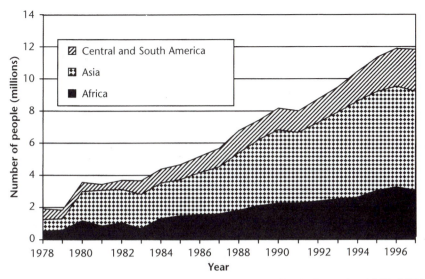

Figure 6-7. Number of Europeans Traveling to Malaria-Endemic Countries, 1978–1997

Conclusion

The malaria situation in the WHO European Region presents a complex epidemiological picture characterized by

- changes in malaria endemicity levels in Turkey;
- malaria resurgence in the NIS, specifically in the Caucasus from residual foci in Azerbaijan and in central Asia from the malaria epidemic in Afghanistan;
- imported malaria cases from tropical and subtropical endemic countries; and
- risk of malaria reestablishment in malaria-free areas.

Different determinants influence each context.

Changes in Malaria Endemicity Levels in Turkey

The explosive malaria epidemic in Turkey in recent years caused a dramatic emergency situation and affected socioeconomic development in the country. The situation is the result of many factors that arise from a historic presence of fertile but marshy soils in the Seyan plains and irrigation of arid territories in the Urfa district. No one factor was solely responsible; rather, the problem resulted from the combination of a complex ecological situation, rapid agroindustrial development that increased vector densities and attracted people from less developed and still-malarious regions, and the inability of the public health infrastructure to keep abreast of the situation. This sudden resurgence of malaria has shown that malaria epidemics can spread within the country in the future, if preparedness for malaria epidemics is lacking.

Resurgence of Malaria in the NIS

Unfortunately, the recent political, social, and economic events in the NIS have had a negative impact on the malaria situation. All the NIS countries in central Asia and the Caucasus experienced considerable problems in preventing and controlling malaria dur-

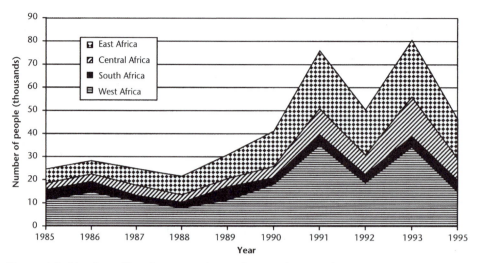

Figure 6-8. Number of Immigrants to Europe from Malarious Africa, 1985–1995

ing the 1990s. The disruption of traditional links among the former republics of the Soviet Union resulted in difficult economic conditions, massive population movement, and a sudden reduction in the quality of health care (Figure 6-9). All of these factors have resulted in a dramatic reduction in access to primary health-care systems and in an inability to respond to changes in malaria epidemiology in the southernmost areas.

The epidemic in Afghanistan (2 million estimated cases [WHO 1998]) played a particularly important role in the spread of malaria in central Asia, through the military troops used as peacekeepers along the border with Tajikistan. Massive population movement within countries as well as cross-border migrations of infected people have introduced malaria into areas that were previously malaria-free at a time when the potential breeding places for malaria vectors have increased because of poorly maintained irrigation systems.

Malaria Imported from Endemic Countries

During the past decade, the number of malaria cases imported into Europe has steadily increased, mainly as a result of two factors: the constant increase in the number of foreigners originating from countries with endemic malaria who immigrate to European countries to work or study, and the growing number of European residents who visit tropical and subtropical areas as tourists. The increase in the levels of malaria endemicity worldwide, particularly in Africa, influences the risk of travelers' contracting the disease. This increase is due mainly to the spread of drug-resistant strains of *P. falciparum* and to the spread of *Anopheles* species that are resistant to traditional insecticides, as well as to the reduction in malaria control activities as their costs escalate.

Risk of Reestablishment in Malaria-Free Areas

The possibility of resumed transmission in most of the territories where malaria has been eradicated is determined by receptivity (the residual presence in some rural areas, with favorable climatic conditions, of potential malaria vectors that have a high vectorial capacity and are susceptible to infection with malaria strains that originate in

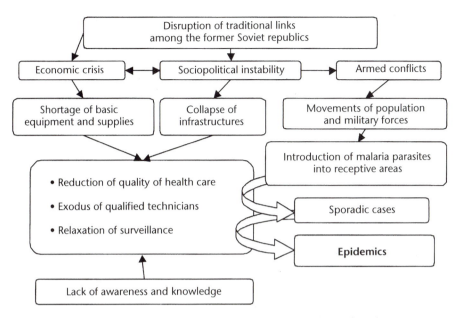

Figure 6-9. Determinants of the Malaria Situation in Newly Independent States

malaria-endemic areas) and vulnerability (the presence of parasite carriers during the seasons that are climatically favorable to transmission in receptive areas).

The malariogenic potential in most of the European Union and the Balkans appears to be very low, suggesting that the reappearance of malaria epidemics is highly improbable. Sporadic cases of autochthonous vivax malaria could, nevertheless, occur in some areas of central and southern Europe. They would not be a public health problem, however, because the health authorities would easily and quickly contain the phenomenon. The impact on a country's international image, on the other hand, would be quite serious, because malaria is a disease associated with underdevelopment. Even from an economic point of view, the occurrence of malaria cases would undoubtedly harm any country's tourist industry.

Global climate is presently in a warming phase that may be partly attributable to increased atmospheric concentrations of carbon dioxide and other greenhouse gases. Even if this warming continues, it is unlikely to have more than a limited role in the countries of the WHO European Region. Milder winters could increase the number of sporogonic cycles of *P. vivax* in a season, but they would negatively affect the geographic distribution of most of malaria vectors in the Palearctic region by reducing the extent and presence of their breeding places. An increase in temperature of a few degrees would greatly increase the probability of *P. falciparum* completing its sporogonic cycle in susceptible mosquitoes, and a climatic model suggests that global warming could allow the spread of transmission of this parasite from the tropics to Europe (Martens et al. 1995). However, in this model, no account was taken of the refractoriness to tropical *P. falciparum* strains of the well-known European potential vectors of malaria.

Acknowledgements

I am grateful to the following colleagues who provided information about the epidemiological situation of malaria in their respective countries: T. Gokcinar, C. Tabuk, and S.

Kalipci from the Ministry of Health of Turkey; G. Grigoryan and V. Davidiants from the Ministry of Health of Armenia; S.A. Velibekov, F. Huseynov, and S. Zmitrovich from the Ministry of Health of Azerbaijan; P. Imnaze and M. Iosava from the Ministry of Health of Georgia; M. Spataev, Z. Shapieva, and F. Bismildin from the Ministry of Health of Kazakhstan; S. Abdikarimov, J. Abdykadyr, and N. Usenbaev from the Ministry of Health of Kyrgyzstan; A. Branova, T. Sabgaida, G. Souleimanov, and V. Sergiev from the Martsinovskij Institute of Moscow, Russia; S. Aliev from the Ministry of Health of Tajikistan; K. Amangaldiev and S. Alieva from the Ministry of Health of Turkmenistan; and G. Shamgunova and S. Razakov from the Ministry of Health of Uzbekistan.

This chapter benefited from suggestions, comments, and various contributions from A. Kondrachine, A. Beljaev, and M. Ejov, colleagues at the World Health Organization.

Disclaimer

Opinions expressed in this chapter are the author's only and do not necessarily reflect the policies and views of the World Health Organization.

References

Bakradze, T.L. 1974. Osobennosti epidemiologii maljarii v protsesse ejo likvidatsii v Gruzinskoj SSR (Characteristics of malaria epidemiology in the Process of Its Eradication in Georgian SSR) [in Russian]. Tbilisi: Metzniereba.

Baranova, A. 1998. Malaria in Russia and CIS [in Russian]. *Meditsinkaya Parazitologiya i Parazitarnie Bolezni* 3: 58–60.

Boccolini, D., R. Romi, M. Di Luca, I. Hovanesyan, G. Grigoryan, G. Majori, and G. Sabatinelli. 2000. Entomological Investigations in the Malaria Epidemic in Armenia: Role of *Anopheles sacharovi*. *Parassitologia* 42(Suppl. 1): 124.

Bruce-Chwatt, L.J. 1959. Malaria Research and Eradication in the USSR: A Review of Soviet Achievements in the Field of Malariology. *Bulletin of the World Health Organization* 21: 737–72.

———. 1980. *Essential Malariology*. London, U.K.: William Heinemann Medical Books Ltd.

Bruce-Chwatt, L.J., and J. de Zulueta. 1980. *The Rise and Fall of Malaria in Europe. A Historico-Epidemiological Study*. Oxford, U.K.: Oxford University Press.

Chakraverti, A. and S. Uner. 1975. Demographic Factors and Provincial Immigration. Proceedings of the Second Conference on Turkish Demography. Izmir, Turkey.

Davidiants, V., M. Mannrikian, G. Sayadian, A. Parunakian, and B. Davtian. 1998. Epidemic Malaria Transmission: Armenia 1997. *Morbidity Mortality Weekly Report* 47(25): 526–8.

de Zulueta, J., C.D. Ramsdale, and M. Coluzzi. 1975. Receptivity to Malaria in Europe. *Bulletin of the World Health Organization* 52: 109–11.

Detinova, T.S. 1962. *Age-Grouping Methods in Diptera of Medical Importance*. WHO Monograph Series no. 47. Geneva, Switzerland: World Health Organization.

Dzhavadov, R.B., A.A. Kasimov, and V.I. Mamedov. 1978. To the Grouping of District Settlements of Some Landscape Zones of Azerbaijan in Accordance with Its Malaria Situations [in Russian]. *Sbornik nauchnyh trudov Nauchno Issledovatelskij Institute meditsinskoi parasitologii i tropichesko medicinyi* 10: 15–20.

Giglioli, M.E.C. 1979. Irrigation, Anophelism and Malaria in Adana, Turkey. Unpublished WHO report from a consultancy, January 17–February 8.

Gillies, M.T. 1988. Anopheline Mosquitoes: Vector Behaviour and Bionomics. In *Malaria: Principles and Practice of Malariology*, Volume 1, edited by W.H. Wernsdorfer and I. McGregor. New York: Churchill Livingstone, 453–85.

Gramiccia, G., and P.F. Beales. 1988. Recent History of Malaria Control and Eradication. In *Malaria: Principles and Practice of Malariology*, Volume 2, edited by W.H. Wernsdorfer and I. McGregor. New York: Churchill Livingstone, 1335–78.

Hackett, L.W. 1945. Malaria in the Andean Region of South America. *Revista del Instituto de Salubridad y Enfermidades Tropicales* 11: 239–52.

Haworth, J. 1988. The Global Distribution of Malaria and the Present Control Effort. In *Malaria: Principles and Practice of Malariology,* Volume 2, edited by W.H. Wernsdorfer and I. McGregor. New York: Churchill Livingstone, 1379–1413.

Horsfall, W.R. 1955. *Mosquitoes: Their Bionomics and Relation to Disease.* New York: Ronald Press.

James, S.P., W.D. Nicol, and P.G. Shute. 1932. A Study of Induced Malignant Tertian Malaria. *Proceedings of the Royal Society of Medicine* 25: 1153–86.

Jusupova, R.L., E.J. Pershin, and A.I. Musatova. 1975. Landscape Malariological Areas of Uzbek SSR [in Russian]. *Geograficheskaya Patologiya Uzbekistana, Tashkent* 190–3.

Kasimov, A.A., V.I. Mamedov, and Z.F. Vahabov. 1979. Malariological Conditions in Specific Inhabited Settlements of Kura-Araks in Lowlands and Special Arrangements for Malaria Control and Prevention: Abstract Book [in Russian]. *Research Institute for Medical Parasitology and Tropical Diseases* 11: 1119–26.

Kasimov, A.A., A.N. Mehtiev, and V.I. Mamedov 1981. Malariological Capacity of Different Physical-Geographical Areas of Azerbaijan, SSR [in Russian]. *Medical Parasitology and Tropical Medicine Baku* 1: 100–3.

Lysenko, A.J., and E.S. Kalmykov. 1969. The Basic Patterns of Malaria Eradication in Tajik, SSR [in Russian]. *Abstracts on Parasitology Dushanbe.*

Macdonald, G. 1957. *The Epidemiology and Control of Malaria.* London, U.K.: Oxford University Press.

Majori, G., G. Sabatinelli, and A.V. Kondrachine. 1999. Re-emerging Malaria in the WHO European Region: Control Priorities and Constraints. *Parassitologia* 41: 327–8.

Marchant, P., W. Eling, G.-J. van Gemert, C.J. Leake, and C.F. Curtis. 1998. Could British Mosquitoes Transmit Falciparum Malaria? *Parasitology Today* 14: 344–5.

Martens, W.J.M., L.W. Niessen, J. Rotmans, T.H. Jetten, and A.J. McMichael. 1995. Potential Impact of Global Climate Change on Malaria Risk. *Environmental Health Perspectives* 103: 458–64.

Moshkovsky, S.D. 1946. The Dependence on Temperature of the Speed of Development of Malaria *Plasmodia* in the Mosquito [in Russian]. *Meditsinkaya Parazitologiya i Parazitarnie Bolezni* 15: 19.

Mouchet, J. 2000. Airport Malaria: A Rare Disease Still Poorly Understood. *Euro Surveillance* 5: 75–6.

Moulineaux, L. 1988. The Epidemiology of Human Malaria as an Explanation of Its Distribution, Including Some Implications for Its Control. In *Malaria: Principles and Practice of Malariology,* Volume 2, edited by W.H. Wernsdorfer and I. McGregor. New York: Churchill Livingstone, 913–98.

Moulineaux, L., D.A. Muir, H.C. Spencer, and W.H. Wernsdorfer. 1988. The Epidemiology of Malaria and Its Measurement. In *Malaria: Principles and Practice of Malariology,* Volume 2, edited by W.H. Wernsdorfer and I. McGregor. New York: Churchill Livingstone, 999–1090.

Pampana, E. 1963. *A Textbook of Malaria Eradication.* London, U.K.: Oxford University Press.

Pirumov, H.I., S.M. Kazanchan, and M.A. Balasanian. 1983. On Cases of 4-Day Malaria after Blood Transfusion [in Russian]. *Meditsinkaya Parazitologiya i Parazitarnie Bolezni* 4: 7–9.

Pitt, S., B.E. Pearcy, R.H. Stevens, A. Sharipov, K. Satarov, and N. Banatvala. 1998. War In Tajikistan and Re-emergence of *Plasmodium falciparum. Lancet* 352: 1279.

Ponirovskij, E.N., O. Mamednijazov, and K.V. Morozova. 1988. Malariological Zoning of Turkmen, SSR [in Russian]. *Zdravoohr. Turkmenistana* 7: 30–6.

Ramsdale, C.D., and M. Coluzzi. 1975. Studies on the Infectivity of Tropical Strains of *Plasmodium falciparum* to Some Southern European Vectors of Malaria. *Parassitologia* 17: 39–48.

Ramsdale, C.D., and E. Haas. 1978. Some Aspects of Epidemiology of Resurgent Malaria in Turkey. *Transaction of the Royal Society of Tropical Medicine and Hygiene* 72: 570–80.

Ramsdale, C.D., and K. Snow. 2000. Distribution of the Genus *Anopheles* in Europe. *European Mosquito Bulletin* 7: 1–26.

Russell, P. 1952. *Malaria: Basic Principles Briefly Stated.* Oxford, U.K.: Blackwells.

Sabatinelli, G. 1999. Determinants in Malaria Resurgence in the Former USSR. *Giornale Italiano di Medicina Tropicale* 4: 53–62.

Sabatinelli, G., and S. Abdikarimov. 2000. The Malaria Epidemiological Situation in Kyrgyzstan. *Parassitologia* 42(Suppl. 1): 147.

Sabatinelli, G., and K. Amangaldiev. 2000. The Malaria Epidemiological Situation in Turkmenistan. *Parassitologia* 42(Suppl. 1): 149.

Sabatinelli, G., P. Joergensen, and G. Majori. 1999. Imported Malaria in the WHO European Region, 1971–1997. *Giornale Italiano di Medicina Tropicale* 4: 1–5.

Sabatinelli, G., M. Spataev, and Z. Shapieva. 2000. The Malaria Epidemiological Situation in Kazakhstan. *Parassitologia* 42(Suppl. 1): 155.

Sabatinelli, G., S. Aliev, M. Ejov, and V. Verbitsky. 2000. The Malaria Epidemiological Situation in Tajikistan. *Parassitologia* 42(Suppl. 1): 148.

Sabatinelli, G., T. Gokcinar, S. Serttas, and M. Ejov. 2000. The Malaria Epidemiological Situation in Turkey. *Parassitologia* 42(Suppl. 1): 150.

Sabatinelli, G., G. Grigorian, G. Majori, R. Romi, and A. Kondrachine. 2000. The Malaria Epidemiological Situation in Armenia. *Parassitologia* 42(Suppl. 1): 151.

Sabatinelli, G., P. Imnadze, G. Majori, and A. Kondrachine. 2000. The Malaria Epidemiological Situation in Georgia. *Parassitologia* 42(Suppl. 1): 152.

Sabatinelli, G., G. Majori, G. Shamgunova, and S. Razakov. 2000. The Malaria Epidemiological Situation in Uzbekistan. *Parassitologia* 42(Suppl. 1): 153.

Sabatinelli, G., V.P. Sergiev, T. Evgueni, A. Baranova, and G. Souleimanov. 2000. The Malaria Epidemiological Situation in the Russian Federation. *Parassitologia* 42(Suppl. 1): 154.

Sabatinelli, G., S.A. Velibekov, A. Kondrachine, and A. Madera. 2000. The Malaria Epidemiological Situation in Azerbaijan. *Parassitologia* 42(Suppl. 1): 156.

Sergiev, V.P., and G.E. Gozodova. 1979. Use of Natural Prerequisites for the Assessment of Malariogenicity of the Territory of Uzbekistan [in Russian]. *Aktuali. vopr. med. parazitol. Tashkent* 57–59.

Sergiev, V.P., A.M. Baranova, V.S. Orlov, L.G. Mihaijlov, R.L. Koustnezov, N.I. Neujmin, L.P. Arsenieva, M.A. Shahova, L.A. Glagoleva, and M.M. Osipova. 1993. Importation of Malaria into the USSR from Afghanistan, 1981–89. *Bulletin of the World Health Organization* 71(3/4): 385–8.

Shute, P.G. 1940. Failure to infect English specimens of *Anopheles maculipennis* var. *atroparvus* with certain strains of *Plasmodium falciparum* of tropical origin. *Journal of Tropical Medicine and Hygiene* 43: 175–8.

Statistical Office of the European Community. 1998. *Eurostat Database: Theme 3* [CD-ROM]. Durham, U.K.: New Cronos.

Vinogradskaya, O.N. 1969. *Geographic Distribution of Mosquitoes: Vectors of Infections on the Basis of Their Xerophily and Hygrophily* [in Russian]. Moscow, USSR: Medsina.

WHO (World Health Organization). 1979. *Receptivity to Malaria and other Parasitic Diseases*. Report of a WHO Working Group. Copenhagen, Denmark: WHO Regional Office for Europe.

———. 1989. *Geographical Distribution of Arthropod-Borne Diseases and Their Principal Vectors*. Document 967. Geneva, Switzerland: WHO Vector Biology and Control Division.

———. 1998. Occurrence of Malaria in Five Northern Provinces in Afghanistan. *Weekly Epidemiological Record* 73(March 27): 96–8.

Wilson, D.B. 1949. In *Malariology*, edited by M.F. Boyd. Philadelphia, PA: Saunders.

Chapter 7

Determinants of Malaria in Oceania and East Asia

Allan Schapira

In this chapter, I present the current and potential malaria endemic areas within Oceania and East Asia. For the purposes of this discussion, I have further divided the region into three major geographic regions: southwest Pacific and Australia, which are part of the Australasian zoogeographic region; tropical East Asia, which belongs to the Oriental zoogeographic region; and northeast Asia, which belongs to the Palearctic zoogeographic region (discussed in detail in Chapter 9).

Because contextual determinants of malaria are highly variable in space and time, a classification of malaria systems is necessary to manage the variability. Over the past two decades, the previous rigid geographical stratification has been replaced by an identification of local eco-epidemiological types of malaria as a basis for malaria control. Like any typology, such a classification is never free of some overlap and arbitrariness in its delimitations; however, the greatest usefulness of such types is in identifying different sets of social and environmental determinants of risk.

This review is based on published literature as well as databases and reports held by the World Health Organization (WHO) Regional Office for the Western Pacific. Since the 1980s, the following annual data have been consistently collected from each country by the WHO Western Pacific Regional Office:

- number of confirmed malaria cases,
- number of falciparum malaria cases, and
- number of deaths attributed to malaria.

However, several countries have also reported clinical malaria cases (Table 7-1), which are usually understood as fever cases that are suspected of being malaria (blood samples may or may not have been examined by microscopy) and treated with antimalaria drugs.

In the following discussion, the reported incidence of confirmed malaria is considered as the main indicator of transmission intensity. In general, this indicator grossly underestimates the incidence of malarial disease and, even more so, infection. The incidence of clinical malaria depends heavily on local practices; in general, the less developed a health system is, the greater the tendency to classify all fevers as "malaria." Nonetheless, even the incidence of clinical malaria is probably more often than not

Table 7-1. Summary of Reported Malaria Data from Malaria-Endemic Countries in the WHO Western Pacific Region, 1998

Indicator	Cambodia	China	Republic of Korea	Lao People's Democratic Republic	Malaysia	Papua New Guinea	Philippines	Solomon Islands	Vanuatu	Vietnam
Population at risk of malaria	2,500,000	37,100,000	1,917,635	3,659,872	2,217,970	4,400,000	10,704,786	441,840	188,185	41,939,624
Number of microscopically confirmed cases	58,874	27,090	3,992	41,623	13,491	20,900	50,709	72,808	6,181	72,091
Slide positivity rate	27%	0.31%	NA	13.60%	0.76%	10.5%	7.59%	21%	11.82%	2.61%
Number of Plasmodium falciparum cases	53,795	4,042	60[a]	39,930	6,795	NA	36,806	47,989	3,137	55,070
Number of clinical malaria cases	140,843	31,319	3,992	337,594	NA	1,414,765	374,917	NA	NA	383,341
Number of reported malaria deaths	621	24	0	485	27	651	NA	33	0	183
Estimated total malaria deaths	10,000	120	0	5,000	NA	NA	NA	NA	0	NA
Number of insecticide-treated nets in population	127,251	4,880,400	NA	NA	310,933	NA	148,633	192,711	103,970	5,432,443
Population protected by insecticide-treated nets	292,677 (estimate)	8,134,000	NA	353,010	814,572	NA	594,532	250,525	145,623	11,050,285
Population protected by indoor residual spraying	0	11,423,000	NA	NA	287,711	11,965	967,038	86,829	NA	2,637,913

Note: NA = data not available.

[a]All imported; only vivax malaria is endemic in Republic of Korea.

underestimated, because most people with malaria do not use public health services. In many situations, the slide positivity rate, although often lumped from different data sources and not an indicator of the amount of malaria in a population, is a better indicator of trends because it is relatively robust to variations in health service performance. Absolute estimates of the size of the malaria burden or transmission intensity are few and far between in Asia and Oceania because of the instability of transmission and enormous spatial variability.

Southwest Pacific and Australia

Historically, malaria has occurred in northern Australia, the island of New Guinea, the Solomon Islands, and Vanuatu (recent incidence in the latter three areas is illustrated in Figure 7-1). There has never been malaria transmission east of 170°E and south of 20°S. The genus *Anopheles* does not occur in the Pacific Island countries east of the so-called Buxton line, probably because it was never introduced there (Buxton 1926). The southernmost island of Vanuatu, Aneityum, was erroneously considered by Buxton to be nonendemic. In fact, malaria was endemic there, but it was eliminated in the 1980s (Kaneko, Taleo, and Kalkoa 1998). In all the endemic and formerly endemic countries, it is possible to make a distinction between malaria transmitted by anophelines that breed in brackish water in coastal areas and malaria transmitted in inland areas.

Coastal Areas

The dominant vector, *Anopheles farauti*, is versatile, partially exophilic, and efficient; it transmits *Plasmodium falciparum* as well as *Plasmodium vivax*. It breeds in almost any type of water and tolerates salinity in excess of 0.8%. To make matters worse, it bites relatively early in the evening; this behavior is possibly acquired, resulting from the

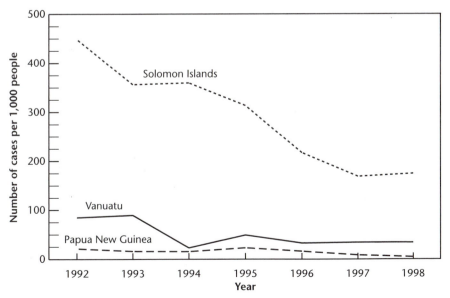

Figure 7-1. Reported Incidence of Confirmed Malaria Cases in Three Countries in the Southwest Pacific, 1992–1998

genetic selection pressure of control interventions (Taylor 1975). Coastal malaria transmitted by *An. farauti* is the main malaria type in Solomon Islands and Vanuatu and accounts for roughly 50% of the malaria in Papua New Guinea. *An. farauti* also was the malaria vector in Australia in the past.

During World War II, Guadalcanal (the main island of Solomon Islands) became a battlefield, and the human-made creation of new breeding sites for *An. farauti* on the coastal belt led to an enormous outbreak. American troops experienced a daily incidence of up to five cases per thousand people. As is often the case, it is difficult to disentangle social factors (the invasion of a large nonimmune population) from ecological factors, but the environmental disturbance was clearly important in this case. Social unrest that led to considerable population movement in the Solomon Islands in 1999 could have led to considerable increases in malaria incidence, were it not for the targeting of malaria control efforts to the populations at high risk. The continued worsening of the situation in 2000 and 2001 led to an increase in malaria transmission, although the maintenance of some control interventions seems to have prevented a major epidemic.

Chloroquine-resistant *P. vivax* has been observed in Papua New Guinea since 1989 and probably is present in the Solomon Islands now, adding to the difficulty of control of this parasite.

Australia: The Southern Fringe. *An. farauti* is the only malaria vector that is native to Australia. The epidemics in the early part of the twentieth century in the Northern Territory and Queensland north of 19°S were most often caused by gold miners returning from New Guinea (Buxton 1926). The last indigenous case in Australia was in 1962, but sporadic introduced cases have been recorded since. Cases still occur in the Torres Strait islands, which are geographically and culturally close to Papua New Guinea, but only 5% of these are due to local transmission (Walker 1998). When imported cases are detected in north Queensland, a mosquito survey is carried out and, if the density of *An. farauti* is compatible with transmission, vector control is carried out (Hanna, Brookes, and Ritchie 1998).

Climate modeling with effects of global warming, including increasing inundation of some areas, indicates that by 2030, the area receptive to malaria could extend an additional 800 kilometers south along the east coast of Queensland (Bryan, Foley, and Sutherst 1996). However, with the current surveillance-and-response system, such an increase is unlikely.

Control Experiences. Drainage was used effectively in World War II in the Milne Bay swamps of Papua New Guinea. More recently, flushing with seawater in Honiara, the capital of the Solomon Islands, has greatly reduced breeding of the vector. Gambusia fish also have been effective in the past. Although DDT residual spraying was initially successful, financial constraints and community objections rendered the program ineffective in Papua New Guinea as well as the Solomon Islands and Vanuatu.

All three countries, but most markedly the Solomon Islands, have a history of cycles of malaria control efforts followed by relaxation, severe resurgence of malaria, and new efforts. In the Solomon Islands, the recorded incidence of confirmed cases reached more than 400 cases per 1,000 people in 1991. Nowadays, the main control measure is the large-scale use of insecticide-treated nets (ITNs), which have some impact on transmission despite the tendency of local mosquitoes to bite early. The large-scale use of ITNs together with early and effective treatment has been associated with dramatic reductions of the incidence of falciparum malaria and, more slowly, vivax malaria in Vanuatu and the Solomon Islands. Subsequent developments in Honiara, Solomon Islands, provide good examples of urban malaria control interventions using a mix of control methods, including ITNs, residual house spraying, larval control, lagoon drainage, improved diagnosis and treatment, and intensive surveillance.

During the 1990s, Vanuatu made steady progress in control and may well eliminate falciparum malaria from some islands during the coming decade. In contrast, in recent years, investment in control in Papua New Guinea has been minimal but is expected to increase as a result of the Roll Back Malaria mobilization.

Inland Areas of Papua New Guinea

In Papua New Guinea, the main vector in inland areas is *Anopheles punctulatus*. In addition, in some parts of the country, *Anopheles koliensis* is an important vector in both coastal and inland areas. Before large-scale control efforts began in the 1950s, parasite rates were 35% overall and 64% in children under 10 years of age.

Repeatedly, malaria epidemics have occurred when economic development projects or military activities have led to the influx of large workforces anywhere in Papua New Guinea. The Ok Tedi Mine is a gold and copper mine in the western part of the country, located 524 meters above sea level. Malaria increased when external workforces (totaling 5,000 people) entered. Transmission peaked during construction, which provided additional breeding sites. Remarkably, there was no correlation between rainfall and malaria.

The Highland Fringe. New Guinea is located 0–10ºS; malaria generally occurs up to approximately 1,500 meters above sea level, but sporadic foci have been observed at around 2,000 meters. The highland fringe areas above 1,200 meters are the most densely populated areas in Papua New Guinea because of the low malaria risk. In the early twentieth century, practically no malaria was found in these areas, but the creation of human-made stagnant water collections and increased population movement (especially of labor forces between the highlands and the coast) led to malaria epidemics and gradually to the establishment of endemic malaria at the lower ranges (Radford, Leeuwen, and Christian 1976). Epidemics in recent years also could have been caused by increased temperatures, but the causes of these epidemics, which often are reported late, have not been rigorously evaluated. There is no evidence that the highland epidemics have become more frequent in recent years or that the average upper limits of transmission have moved upward.

Control Experiences. The vectors of inland Papua New Guinea are more amenable to insecticidal control than *An. farauti*, and the results of house spraying have generally been satisfactory. At the Ok Tedi Mine, after three years of semiannual spraying and other control measures, the infant parasite rate was reduced from 70% to less than 10% (Schuurkamp 1992). In the 1970s, malaria was thought to be so well controlled in the highlands that spraying was withdrawn (Reilly 1986). Epidemics ensued. Currently, a plan to map out the epidemic-prone highland fringe and to ensure regular house spraying is under development.

Generalizations

In the Australasian region, malaria in the coastal areas is generally stable. However, environmental changes that lead to increased stagnant water collection can cause increased vector densities, whereas drainage may have the opposite effect. Control nowadays must rely on a combination of measures, among which ITNs have a central role. Climate changes are unlikely to have any impact, except in the Australian southern fringe, where temperature is the factor that limits transmission. With the current surveillance and alert system in Australia, a malaria epidemic is very unlikely; however, prevention may become more costly.

Although population movement is an important determinant in all areas, particularly when nonimmune populations enter an endemic area, environmental changes that accompany development have been important in introducing malaria in the lower ranges of the highland fringe of Papua New Guinea during the mid-twentieth century. In the inland areas of New Guinea, residual house spraying plays a stronger role in control, especially in the highlands, where sometimes mosquitoes are so few and malaria so rare that people are not motivated to use ITNs. At the highland fringe in central Papua New Guinea, increased temperatures could seriously increase malaria risk for hundreds of thousands of people. If current efforts at improving control are developed, expanded, and well maintained, then the problem should not lead to any major increase in morbidity or mortality.

Tropical East Asia

This region includes Malaysia and the Philippines, China south of 25°N, Cambodia, Lao People's Democratic Republic (PDR), Myanmar, Thailand, Vietnam, and the Ryukyu archipelago of Japan. Internationally, attention is currently focused on the Mekong region (or Greater Mekong subregion), which includes Cambodia, the Yunnan province of China, Lao PDR, Myanmar, Thailand, and Vietnam and is home to severe multiple-drug resistance. In two areas that marginally belong to this zone, malaria has now been eradicated, namely, Japan's Ryukyu archipelago (Miyagi, Toma, and Malenganisho 1996) and Taiwan. In Brunei, malaria has been eradicated as a result of an intense control program. Recent incidence of malaria in six countries of this region is illustrated in Figure 7-2.

In tropical East Asia, the malaria vectors that breed in rice fields are inefficient. Therefore, malaria in the densely populated rural areas dominated by irrigated rice fields is rare and sporadic. Another distinctive characteristic of this subregion is the absence of urban malaria. From an ecological viewpoint, the two major disease types are coastal malaria and malaria in forested and hilly areas. The latter is divided into several subtypes, mainly determined by social and demographic factors

Coastal Malaria

In coastal areas of the Philippines (e.g., in the Sulu archipelago), *Anopheles litoralis* is an important vector that breeds in brackish water with a salinity of 1%—for example, in rock holes and on coral reefs. In Cambodia, Malaysia, Thailand, and Vietnam, *Anopheles sundaicus* (which breeds in brackish water) is found mainly in stagnant water collections, often associated with human-made disturbances of the environment. The coastal areas are generally densely populated with accessible health services. Hence, incidence of severe malaria and mortality is generally not high.

During the 1990s, the northern two-thirds of the Mekong delta in Vietnam were desalinated to increase the agricultural value of the land. Since then, malaria transmission has virtually disappeared. Malaria incidence, however, has been reduced little in

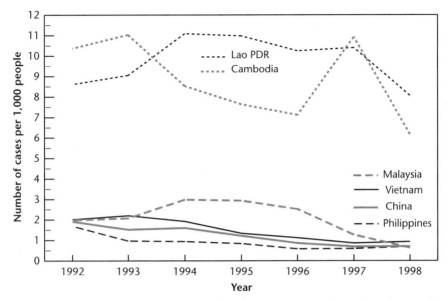

Figure 7-2. Reported Incidence of Confirmed Malaria Cases in Six Countries of Tropical East Asia, 1992–1998

the two southernmost provinces of Ca Mau and Bac Lieu, which cannot be desalinated. In these two provinces, the breeding of *An. sundaicus* is now associated with aquaculture. Shrimp ponds become diluted with rainwater during the rainy season so that the shrimp cannot breed; however, the lower salinity provides the perfect breeding conditions for *An. sundaicus*.

In coastal areas of Malaysia, drainage was introduced in 1911 to eliminate stagnant brackish water collections. Malaria has been eradicated from Singapore mainly as a result of such operations. In other areas, environmental measures probably have been underutilized. In general, the conventional insecticidal measures (ITNs or spraying) have been effective in reducing transmission, though rarely interrupting it completely.

Malaria of Forested and Hilly Areas

Vectors. *Anopheles maculatus* is the main vector in northern peninsular Malaysia. One study found that vector density and incidence of malaria was about three times higher during the dry season than during the wet season, because anopheline larvae were washed out in heavy rains and fast-flowing streams (Rahman, Adanan, and Abu Hassan 1998). In Sarawak (Malaysia), the main malaria vectors, *Anopheles leucosphyrus* and *Anopheles donaldi,* breed in shaded pools and streams, in contrast to the sun-loving *An. maculatus*. Over a period of four years—while an originally forested area was sequentially subjected to clearing, burning, and cultivation with oil palms—the human-biting rates of the two main vectors, the entomological inoculation rates, and the malaria incidence decreased by 80% (Chang, Hii, and Buttner 1997).

In the Philippines, the principal vector is *Anopheles minimus flavirostris,* which breeds along the shaded margins of clear freshwater streams in foothills and on mountain slopes. Density of this species is highly dependent on rain and thus is highest at the end of the rainy season. It is partially exophilic and exophagic and prefers cattle and buffaloes to humans. Development (i.e., clearing of steams, pollution, and semiurban-ization) tends to reduce the density of this vector.

In Sabah (Malaysia) and Palawan (the Philippines), exophagic vectors that belong to the *An. leucosphyrus* group are dominant. For this reason, malaria is more difficult to control in these areas, where drug resistance also is emerging as a major problem (Mak, Jegathosan, and Lim 1992).

Continental southeast Asia was called the Indochinese Hills zone by George Mac-donald (1957) in recognition of the dominant role of one vector, *Anopheles minimus*, which is found in foothills in slowly running streams. In hilly areas, where *An. minimus* and *An. maculatus* are the main vectors, transmission is usually relatively independent of rainfall but may be reduced temporarily after torrential rains or prolonged drought. Although this species is now relatively unimportant in Thailand, it remains the main vector in Vietnam, even in densely forested areas (Quang et al. 1997). The more typical forest vector is *Anopheles dirus*, which is also often found in plantations. It breeds mainly in shaded, stagnant water collections and often in temporary rainwater puddles. Its den-sity may therefore be rain-dependent. In Myanmar, where the forest has receded, this species now breeds in wells (Htay-Aung, Minn, and Thaung 1999). In Thailand, it is found in gem pits (Scanlon and Sandhinand 1965) and elephant footprints, especially in forests with heavy logging operations (Sharma 1991).

Multiple-drug resistance is now found in all areas of tropical East Asia where falci-parum malaria is highly endemic, with the possible exception of Lao PDR. A complete discussion of this phenomenon is beyond the scope of this chapter. However, the important point is that resistance to the generally used treatment makes malaria more transmissible. In other words, the generalized introduction of early and fully effective treatment may play an important role in reducing transmission.

Human Ecology. In this context, human ecology is understood as human interaction with the environment, especially concerning agricultural activities, population move-ment, and habitat. Within forested and hilly environments in tropical Asia, these deter-minants occur in certain combinations, making it possible to identify the following epidemiological subtypes (or epidemiological presentations) of malaria.

Subsistence Agricultural Villages in Forested Areas. Although the populations that live in forested areas and practice subsistence agriculture are small, this category possibly accounts for most of the severe disease and death in southeast Asia. Ethnic minority groups reside in villages, which often are small and isolated and have basic or no health services. This pattern is found among the Orang Asli group in central peninsular Malaysia, whose population is fewer than 1 million. It is estimated that in Cambodia, about 600,000 people live in forests. In some areas of eastern Cambodia, malaria transmission is intense; the prevalence of infection in children is more than 50%. Morbidity is high among young children, whereas adults rarely become ill from the infection. In Lao PDR, most of the Lao Theung people (population about 1.3 million), are similarly affected, although transmis-sion may be less intense (Anothay and Pongvongsa 1998). The use of bed nets is often hampered by cost, lack of knowledge of their benefits, and frequent long migrations on foot. Communication is often difficult because of cultural and language differences.

Forest Fringe and Transition Areas. The prevalence of plasmodial infection in forest fringe and transition areas (between plains and hills) is typically less than 3%, if detectable at all. The population usually is made up of ethnic majorities (Thai, Kinh, Khmer, Lao Loum) who have a relatively high level of education and better access to health services. Some village areas are close enough to the forest to have perennial transmission. However, the risk of malaria infection is higher for people who stay periodically in the forest (Vien et al. 1997a) to gather forest products or engage in agriculture (e.g., maize or rice farming); among this group, the whole family may stay for days or weeks in makeshift huts that offer no protection against mosquitoes. In foothill areas in northern Thailand, farmers who live in villages with little arable land enter forests for slash-and-burn agriculture and logging.

Remoteness has been identified as an important factor in malaria transmission (Singhanetra-Renard 1993). When access to markets is difficult, farmers have to grow or find a broader range of products in the forest. The forest activities of adult men often have been prolonged or illegal, and have led to encounters between infected and noninfected groups. In a low-endemic community in Bataan (Philippines), in areas of low malaria incidence, nightly forest activities were an important risk factor; in another area with higher incidence, however, this pattern was not identified (Lansang, Belizario, and Bustos 1997).

In some areas of the western high plateau of Vietnam, where forests are being replaced by coffee plantations, malaria incidence is highest during the dry season (April–May), when people spend more time in the forest. During the El Niño drought in central Vietnam in 1998, malaria outbreaks were observed in some provinces. Although *An. minimus* was found breeding in some pools in irrigation canals, the main reason for the outbreaks appeared to be that farmers were being forced to seek food and marketable products in the forests because the rice harvests were failing.

Temporary Migrants. Temporary migrants often come from other countries and enter forests for logging, gemstone mining, and military activities. The common risk factors are a high turnover of exposed people, a relatively short exposure time, and no immunity to malaria (Verdrager 1995). The great majority of migrants are young men. This group accounts for a major proportion of recorded mortality. The pattern is notorious in the gemstone mining areas on the Thai borders with Cambodia and with Myanmar, but it also is found in Vietnam.

Plantation Workers and Other Organized Migrants. Rubber plantations are associated with malaria risk, although whether it is because they create conditions favorable to vectors or because plantation workers are exposed to vectors by beginning work before dawn is not clear. Malaria risk is also high in fruit plantations in Thailand (accounting for a major proportion of malaria in Thai nationals) (Singhasivanon, Thimasarn, and Yimsamran 1999) and in coffee plantations (Suvannadabba 1991). In parts of peninsular Malaysia, the durian season is associated with increased malaria incidence, possibly because owners stay up at night to prevent theft (Ponnampalam 1975). Similar patterns of exposure affect road workers and many other groups of people who regularly enter malarious areas for shorter or longer periods (Xu and Liu 1997). Nowadays, people who recruit the workers usually are aware of the risk and ensure precautionary measures in the form of curative services, temporary chemoprophylaxis, ITNs, and house spraying. Mortality therefore is not high.

Dam projects often increase malaria risk; the reason appears to be the displacement of populations from areas with no or low malaria risk to areas where agriculture begins with an attack on the forest. The best-documented example of this is possibly the Nam Ngum Dam in Vientiane province, Lao PDR (Watson 2000).

Large Population Groups and Border Areas. When large groups of people who have little or no immunity to malaria settle or resettle in forested areas, the risk of epidemic is high. Major uncontrolled population movement related to changes in security has been common in western Cambodia until recently and still is important on the Thailand–Myanmar border. Inside Cambodia, the malaria situation worsened around 1998, as tens of thousands of people reclaimed land that had become accessible after the demise of the Khmer Rouge.

Border areas are characterized by high levels of transmission and mobility, high-risk human behavior, recurrent outbreaks, and variability of drug resistance patterns. National statistics indicate that migrations across borders have a major influence on malaria incidence on the Thailand–Myanmar border and on China's (Yunnan province) border with Lao PDR and Myanmar. Most of the deaths attributed to malaria in Thailand are related to cross-border movements. In the Philippines, from the 1970s to the present, civil unrest and warlike activities in Mindanao have been associated with the maintenance of malaria transmission.

Highland Fringe. According to the literature, the upper limit of transmission in the northern areas of the Lao PDR and Vietnam is about 1,000 meters, whereas in the southern Lao PDR and central Vietnam, it is about 1,500 meters. Epidemic malaria occurs when highland tribes move to lower lands. When these movements are known by the authorities (who sometimes organize them), it is easy to take precautionary measures. Otherwise, disasters may result because these people have little knowledge of malaria and move into areas with poor access to health services.

Another important factor for highland fringe malaria is increased temperature. Higher temperatures in 1998 (El Niño year) possibly caused an outbreak in a mountain area in Kontum province, Vietnam; however, as is often the case, the local temperature variations were not documented. In general, increased temperatures likely could push the limits of transmission upward in southern China, Lao PDR, Myanmar, Thailand, and Vietnam. The populations in each locality are small, and such events may remain undetected because of the remoteness.

Control Experiences. During the 1960s, malaria disappeared from most of peninsular Malaysia, except among the ethnic minority groups in the central thinly populated forested areas. The program in Malaysia now promotes ITNs as the tool of choice. Studies in Malaysia, the Philippines, and Vietnam have highlighted the problems of low ITN usage, which is particularly evident in populations that do not understand the importance of reducing mosquito exposure to prevent malaria (Miguel et al. 1999). Volunteer workers in Sabah, Malaysia, have been trained to take blood samples and prepare them on slides, dispense antimalaria drugs, and promote ITN usage; this effort has been associated with a salutary improvement in recent years.

In the Philippines, by the mid-1930s, the annual number of reported malaria cases was 2 million in a population of 13 million. During World War II, the number of cases doubled (Cabrera and Arambulo 1977). In 1955, an eradication campaign began; transmission proved intractable in certain areas, such as Palawan, northern Luzon, Mindanao, Sulu, and Tawi-Tawi. Technical and operational difficulties led to the reappearance of malaria in many provinces by the mid-1970s.

Among the Mekong countries, it is possible to draw a line between China, Thailand, and Vietnam (which have made good progress and now have low incidence of malaria) and Cambodia, Lao PDR, and Myanmar (where progress started later and has been more limited, and where both incidence and mortality are relatively high). In particular, the case fatality rate for falciparum malaria in Myanmar is much higher than that in other countries. In some areas of Myanmar, malaria mortality reaches 20–28 deaths per 100,000 people per year.

ITNs have replaced residual house spraying in several countries, and they have had an impact on malaria in some situations. Studies in Thailand indicate, however, that there may be no reduction of vectorial capacity when the vectors are highly exophilic subspecies of *An. minimus* or *An. dirus* (Somboon, Lines, and Aramattana 1995). However, there is not a constant association between patterns of mosquito behavior and ITN effectiveness. Anophelines bite mainly at night, so human nighttime behavior is at least as important a determinant of whether some effect can be obtained (Meek 1995). In fact, humans in forests are often also highly "exophilic"; housing in tropical forests is often very open and made of bamboo, providing no barriers to mosquito entrance (Linhua 1995). In a trial among migrant workers in eastern Thailand where attention was paid to health education, risk was reduced 25% by using insecticide-impregnated nets compared with nonimpregnated ones (Kamol-Ratanakul and Prasittisuk 1992). In a forest area in Vietnam, it was concluded that ITNs would reduce *An. minimus* bites by 80% and *An. dirus* bites by 60% (Vien et al. 1997b). It appears that the critical factor in relation to effectiveness of ITNs is, not surprisingly, the populations' willingness to use ITNs consistently from early evening to dawn. A longstanding habit of using nets (as among the Han Chinese, Thais, Tais, the Lao Loum majority in Lao PDR, and the Kinh majority in Vietnam) is associated with some impact (Butraporn, Kamolratanakul, and Prasittisuk 1999). Experiences with ITNs in Yunnan have not been promising so far, in contrast to areas farther north in China (Zhang and Yang 1996).

In Vietnam, malaria incidence was reduced by more than 50% in almost all parts of the country from 1991 to 1996; during the same period, coverage of ITNs increased from a few hundred thousand to more than 10 million, and coverage of house spraying reached 2 million homes. Several community-based studies indicated that ITNs were effective in most areas, but rarely in ethnic minority groups that lived in a forest environment. An evaluation of malaria control in 30 districts did not show convincingly (nor exclude) that the reduction in incidence was due to the use of insecticide-impregnated nets (Vietnam Ministry of Health 1998). It has been suggested that the reduction of malaria incidence in Vietnam was due to the widespread availability of artemisinin drugs, which have an effect on gametocytes (Price et al. 1996). The use of artemisinin derivatives, however, does not correlate with the decreasing morbidity. Thus, the widespread use of artemisinin derivatives was at most a contributing factor to the reduction of malaria transmission with other factors such as improved vector control coverage, increased access to antimalaria drugs in general, and reduced population movement as a result of economic progress.

One particular situation precludes the use of insecticides for disease vector control in parts of east Asia, namely, the breeding of silkworms that is common in parts of Cambodia, Lao PDR, and south central Vietnam. Unfortunately, there is little concrete data on the malaria burden in the silkworm farming populations, but because they are part of the modern economy and live in relatively densely populated areas, the burden is not expected to be very severe.

Generalizations

In tropical East Asia, coastal malaria is highly sensitive to environmental changes: aquaculture may increase malaria transmission, whereas desalination (undertaken for agriculture, not malaria control) and other environmental measures may decrease malaria. Population movement plays a limited role, because it rarely takes place on a large scale. Insecticidal vector control can reduce, but rarely interrupt, transmission.

In forested and hilly areas, malaria transmission closely correlates with the integrity of the forest cover, decreasing with deforestation and, in some but not all areas, reemerging with the establishment of fruit, rubber, and other plantations. Apart from forest cover changes, environmental factors play a minor role in these areas. Malaria is most prevalent in ethnic minority groups who live in forest villages and have poor access to curative and preventive services. In villages at forest fringes, malaria incidence is related to the extent of activities in the forests. Demographic pressure and poverty are the root causes of movements of nonimmune populations into forests, which lead to increased malaria incidence. Multiple-drug resistance of *P. falciparum* in this region contributes to malaria transmission. House spraying is often ineffective; ITNs may have some effect, but their effectiveness depends highly on the pattern of usage.

The hilly areas have a highland fringe where temperature increase could lead to increased transmission. The populations at risk are dispersed ethnic minority groups, so documentation of association is difficult, and some outbreaks may remain undetected.

Northeast Asia

Some areas of China always have been malaria-free: the cold, high-altitude area in the southwest; the dry desert in the northwest and north; the loess plateau in the north; and mountainous districts in the northeast. Falciparum malaria has been eliminated from central China, and only vivax malaria has ever been found in China north of 32°N and the Korean peninsula (Ho 1965). Currently, malaria incidence north of 32°N and in the zone between 25°N and 32°N, where vivax foci are found, is only sporadic. As recently as the early 1990s, vivax epidemics were still recorded in eastern Heilongjiang province, where *Anopheles messeae* is the vector. *Anopheles anthropophagus* is the main vector in hilly areas between 25°N and 32°N (Tang, Qian, and Xu 1996). In plains areas in most of China, the highly exophilic and zoophilic but rather inefficient *Anopheles sinensis* is found. It breeds in stagnant water, especially rice fields, and is also the main vector in the Korean peninsula. It is therefore possible to distinguish two malaria types in northeast Asia: malaria associated with rice fields, and malaria of hilly areas.

Malaria disappeared from the Republic of Korea (South Korea) during the 1970s. Since 1993, vivax malaria cases have been detected (Kho et al. 1999); 21 cases were diagnosed in 1993 and 1994, distributed in a narrow area along the demilitarized zone. A total of 1,724 cases were confirmed in 1997. Information from the Democratic People's Republic of Korea (North Korea) portrays almost a mirror image of South Korea. Reemergence began in 1992 from near the demilitarized zone. However, recent information indicates a substantial increase in the number of cases in 1999 to several hundred thousand. The geographical pattern of distribution and the importance of military service as a risk factor in South Korea indicate that some military activities, perhaps nightly patrols along the demilitarized zone, play a role in maintaining transmission.

Vivax malaria was indigenous in Japan, with some 20,000 cases per year in the 1930s, but the disease became extinct around 1960 (Anonymous 1997). *An. sinensis* was the sole vector (Haworth 1988).

Control Experiences

Chinese malaria control programs have historically emphasized basic elimination as their objective. Between 1985 and 1990, the emphasis shifted from spraying to insecticide treatment of mosquito nets. The reason for the success is probably the existing tradition of using nets (Xu, Xiao, and Webber 1998). In conjunction with positive economic development, these efforts helped reduce the number of reported cases from 364,000 in 1986 to 33,000 in 1996. Where the annual incidence rate is less than 0.01%, case detection, investigation, and monitoring of migrant populations and vectors are emphasized. Great attention has been paid to maintaining efficient and effective surveillance systems because vector control coverage has been gradually reduced. However, in some cases, malaria has rebounded epidemically after cessation of vector control, despite surveillance (Sleigh, Liu, and Jackson 1998).

Mass use of ITNs greatly reduced the density of the endophilic *An. anthropophagus* (Tang, Qian, and Xu 1996). In the plains areas, where the highly exophilic and zoophilic *An. sinensis* is the vector, ITNs still seem to have had some effect by diverting the mosquitoes to cattle (Ge, Cao, and Luo 1996). Intervention against this species also includes chemical and biological larviciding and source reduction.

In the past in this part of the world, temperature has determined the northern and altitude limits of transmission. As in Europe, the disappearance of first falciparum malaria and now, gradually, vivax malaria is not a result of climate change but of control efforts, access to treatment, better housing, and changed agricultural practices. Temperature increases could increase the receptive areas; however, given current economic development and capabilities of the control program, any sign of increase would be expected to be curbed early. Thus, as in Australia, climate change is not expected to lead to an increase in malaria but possibly to an increase in control expenditures.

Generalizations

In rice fields and hilly areas, changed agricultural practices may have an impact. Insecticidal control is effective in hilly areas, less so in rice field areas. The incidence of vivax malaria on the Korean peninsula is highest near the demilitarized zone and among military personnel. Increasing temperatures could increase the receptive area in central China but, as in the case of Australia, increased malaria incidence is unlikely because of the existence of a proactive and reactive control program.

Conclusion

Despite enormous variability, the determinants of malaria from Vanuatu and Australia to northern China show some interesting similarities.

Environment

Malaria parasites occur naturally under certain ecological conditions that favor the proliferation of mosquito vectors when humans are present. These conditions include tropical forests and hilly areas with streams. Certain coastal areas with anophelines that breed in brackish water are also prone to malaria, although it is a matter of conjecture whether the brackish water breeders have ever attained sufficient density in coastal areas, unless there also has been a human disturbance of the environment—such as aquaculture—that leads to the accumulation of stagnant, brackish water. What is certain is that such disturbances can greatly increase the vectorial capacity in coastal areas. Conversely, well-designed environmental management can reduce malaria transmission in coastal areas, and desalination schemes carried out to improve agriculture can have a similarly unintended beneficial side effect.

In inland areas, accidental human environmental changes can increase the risk of malaria, for example, when elephants and trucks leave depressions in forest soil or when irrigation canals in rice terrace areas create the optimal conditions for *An. minimus*. In general, such effects are of minor importance, enhancing the density of a vector that is already present. Yet some evidence shows that in the early part of the twentieth century, the opening of the inlands of Papua New Guinea to economic development led to a substantial increase of breeding sites.

In tropical Asia, deforestation is clearly the most important unintended mechanism that reduces malaria. Change in land use and reforestation, especially as certain kinds of plantations, may have an inverse effect.

Human Migrations and Population Movement

The movement of large groups of people is, without a doubt, the most important factor in causing malaria outbreaks. Problems occur when nonimmune populations venture into malaria-endemic core areas and when they return to receptive, malaria-free areas. Such migrations are often impossible to monitor. Their consequences on malaria do not follow simple models; there is some interaction with change of environment and often with climate.

Human Behavior

Human activities or behaviors that influence malaria incidence include entry into nearby forests at night, the time people go to bed, use of preventive measures such as bed nets, willingness to seek treatment, and compliance with treatment and prophylaxis regimens. To some extent, behavioral patterns are determined by knowledge, but economy and tradition may have overriding influence. Behavior interacts with migration, agriculture, health services, and specific malaria control efforts in extremely complex ways.

Housing

The quality of housing, in terms of being mosquito-proof, has implications for malaria risk that have been studied little in this part of the world. Housing interacts with climate, ecology, and vector control. Inside hot and humid tropical forests, the walls may be so incomplete that they do not provide a barrier to mosquito entry, whereas in highland areas, walls tend to be relatively complete. Small houses may be impractical for the use of bed nets but allow spraying at a low cost per capita.

Climate

Rainfall may have positive or negative effects on mosquito breeding, whereas temperature influences transmission as well as mosquito reproduction. Some evidence indicates that climate variations caused by El Niño have been associated with malaria epidemics; one example is Vietnam in 1998, when the drought forced people to enter forests more frequently. To my knowledge, there is no example of any increasing temperature trend in recent years having changed malaria transmission in East Asia or the Pacific.

Increased temperatures could cause increased malaria transmission and geographic spread of malaria in highland fringe areas such as the central highlands of Papua New Guinea and the highlands in tropical Asia. Spread of malaria also could occur southward on the Australian east coast and northward in China, but in both cases, existing control programs would be expected to curb any problem.

Improved Health Services and Malaria Control Efforts

The impact of standard vector control methods is so variable that it is impossible to project with any degree of certainty the expected reduction of malaria from a given intervention. Yet it has been observed repeatedly that the combination of good curative services with effective drugs, appropriate health education, and well-managed vector control (spraying, ITNs, or environmental) together have a substantial impact on malaria transmission. Despite uncertainties such as variation in the cost-effectiveness of standard vector control interventions and problems with drug resistance, it is likely that coverage with malaria control interventions will continue to be the most potent and predictable determinant of malaria.

General Economic Development, Social Stability, and Security

Genuine, equitable development with improvement of education, health services, and income has the potential to reduce migration due to economic hardship or political instability. It will be associated with better preventive and curative services, better knowledge about how to avoid malaria, greater certainty that needed curative care is affordable, better housing, decreased family size, and decreased acceptance of malaria risk. Conversely, economic and political degradation, warlike activities, and civil strife usually have the opposite effects. However, in some cases, insecurity may be a factor that reduces human contact with forests and other environments with high malaria risk.

Disclaimer

Opinions expressed in this chapter are the author's only and do not necessarily reflect the policies and views of the World Health Organization.

References

Anonymous. 1997. Malaria in Japan. *Infectious Agents Surveillance Report* 18(11): 1–2.

Anothay, O., and T. Pongvongsa. 1998. Childhood Malaria in the Lao People's Democratic Republic. *Bulletin of the World Health Organization* 76: 29–34.

Bryan, J.H., D.H. Foley, and R.W. Sutherst. 1996. Malaria Transmission and Climate Change in Australia. *Medical Journal of Australia* 164: 345–7.

Butraporn, P., P. Kamolratanakul, and M. Prasittisuk. 1999. Cost-Effectiveness Analysis of Lambda-Cyhalothrin-Treated Nets for Malaria Control: The Patients' Perspective. *Southeast Asian Journal of Tropical Medicine and Public Health* 30: 427–31.

Buxton, P.A. 1926. The Depopulation of the New Hebrides and Other Parts of Melanesia. *Transactions of the Royal Society of Tropical Medicine and Hygiene* 19: 420–454.

Cabrera, B.D., and P.V. Arambulo. 1977. Malaria in the Republic of the Philippines. *Acta Tropica* 34: 265–79.

Chang, M.S., J. Hii, and P. Buttner. 1997. Changes in Abundance and Behaviour of Vector Mosquitoes Induced by Land Use during the Development of an Oil Palm Plantation in Sarawak. *Transactions of the Royal Society of Tropical Medicine and Hygiene* 91: 382–6.

Ge, Y.F., R.X. Cao, and D.P. Luo. 1996. Pyrethroid Insecticide-Treated Bed Nets for Malaria Control in the People's Republic of China. *Southeast Asian Journal of Tropical Medicine and Public Health* 27: 841–3.

Hanna, J.N., D.L. Brookes, and S.A. Ritchie. 1998. Malaria and Its Implications for Public Health in Far North Queensland: A Prospective Study. *Australia and New Zealand Journal of Public Health* 22: 196–9.

Haworth, J. 1988. The Global Distribution of Malaria and the Present Control Effort. In *Malaria: Principles and Practice of Malariology*, Volume 2, edited by W.H. Wernsdorfer and I. McGregor. Edinburgh, U.K.: Churchill Livingstone, 1408.

Ho, C.I. 1965. Studies on Malaria in New China. *Chinese Medical Journal* 84: 491–97.

Htay-Aung, S., S. Minn, and S. Thaung. 1999. Well-Breeding *Anopheles dirus* and Their Role in Malaria Transmission in Myanmar. *Southeast Asian Journal of Tropical Medicine and Public Health* 30: 447–53.

Kamol-Ratanakul, P., and C. Prasittisuk. 1992. The Effectiveness of Permethrin-Impregnated Bed Nets against Migrant Workers in Eastern Thailand. *American Journal of Tropical Medicine and Hygiene* 47: 305–9.

Kaneko, A., G. Taleo, and M. Kalkoa. 1998. Malaria Epidemiology, Glucose-6-phosphate Dehydrogenase Deficiency and Human Settlement in the Vanuatu Archipelago. *Acta Tropica* 70: 285–302.

Kho, W.G., J.Y. Jang, S.T. Hong, H.W. Lee, W.J. Lee, and J.S. Lee. 1999. Border Malaria Characteristics of Reemerging Vivax Malaria in the Republic of Korea. *Korean Journal of Parasitology* 37: 71–6.

Lansang, M.A.D., V.Y. Belizario, and M.D. Bustos. 1997. Risk Factors for Infection with Malaria in a Low Endemic Community in Bataan, the Philippines. *Acta Tropica* 63: 257–65.

MacDonald, G. 1957. *The Epidemiology and Control of Malaria*. London: Oxford University Press.

Mak, J.W., M. Jegathosan, and P.K. Lim. 1992. Epidemiology and Control of Malaria in Malaysia. *Southeast Asian Journal of Tropical Medicine and Public Health* 23: 572–7.

Meek, S.R. 1995. Vector Control in Some Countries of Southeast Asia: Comparing the Vectors and the Strategies. *Annals of Tropical Medicine and Parasitology* 89: 135–47.

Miguel, C.A., V.L. Tallo, L. Manderson, and M.A. Lansang. 1999. Local Knowledge and Treatment of Malaria in Agusan del Sur, the Philippines. *Social Science and Medicine* 48: 607–18.

Miyagi, I., T. Toma, and W.L. Malenganisho. 1996. Historical Review of Mosquito Control as a Component of Malaria Eradication Program in the Ryukyu Archipelago. *Southeast Asian Journal of Tropical Medicine and Public Health* 27: 498–510.

Ponnampalam, J.T. 1975. The Durian Season in Peninsular Malaysia as a Factor in the Epidemiology of Malaria [letter]. *Transactions of the Royal Society of Tropical Medicine and Hygiene* 69: 285.

Price, R.N., F. Nosten, C. Luxemburger, et al. 1996. Effects of Artemisinin Derivatives on Malaria Transmissibility. *Lancet* 347(9016): 1654–8.

Quang, N.T., N.T. Vien, N.S. Hai, et al. 1997. The Malaria Mosquitoes in Khanh Phu Commune, Khanh Vinh District, Khanh Hoa Province, Central Viet Nam. In *The Khanh Phu Malaria Research Project*, edited by Medisch Committee Netherlands–Viet Nam and National Institute of Malariology, Parasitology and Entomology. Hanoi, Vietnam: Medical Publishing House.

Radford, A.J., H. van Leeuwen, and S.H. Christian. 1976. Social Aspects in the Changing Epidemiology of Malaria in the Highlands of Papua New Guinea. *Annals of Tropical Medicine and Parasitology* 70: 11–23.

Rahman, W.A., C.R. Adanan, and A. Abu Hassan. 1998. A Study of Some Aspects of the Epidemiology of Malaria in an Endemic District in Northern Peninsular Malaysia near Thailand Border. *Southeast Asian Journal of Tropical Medicine and Public Health* 29: 537–40.

Reilly, Q. 1986. The Control of Malaria in Papua New Guinea. *Papua New Guinea Medical Journal* 29: 3–4.

Scanlon, J.E., and U. Sandhinand. 1965. The Distribution and Biology of *An. balabacensis* in Thailand. *Journal of Medical Entomology* 2: 61–9.

Schuurkamp, G.J.T. 1992. The Epidemiology of Malaria and Filariasis in the Ok Tedi Region of Western Province, Papua New Guinea. Ph.D. dissertation. University of Papua New Guinea, Port Moresby.

Sharma, V.P. 1991. Magnitude of Forest Related Malaria in the WHO Southeast Asia Region. In *Forest Malaria in Southeast Asia,* edited by V.P. Sharma and A.V. Kondrashin. New Delhi, India: Malaria Research Centre.

Singhanetra-Renard, A. 1993. Malaria and Mobility in Thailand. *Social Science and Medicine* 9: 1147–54.

Singhasivanon, P., Thimasarn, and S. Yimsamran. 1999. Malaria in Tree Crop Plantations in Southeastern and Western Provinces of Thailand. *Southeast Asian Journal of Tropical Medicine and Public Health* 30: 399–404.

Sleigh, A.C., X.L. Liu, and S. Jackson. 1998. Resurgence of Vivax Malaria in Henan Province, China. *Bulletin of the World Health Organization* 76: 265–70.

Somboon, P., J. Lines, and A. Aramattana. 1995. Entomological Evaluation of Community-wide Use of Lambda-Cyhalothrin-Impregnated Bed Nets against Malaria in a Border Area of Northwest Thailand. *Transactions of the Royal Society of Tropical Medicine and Hygiene* 89: 248–54.

Suvannadabba, S. 1991. Deforestation for Agriculture and Its Impact on Malaria in Southern Thailand. In *Forest Malaria in Southeast Asia,* edited by V.P. Sharma and A.V. Kondrashin. New Delhi, India: Malaria Research Centre.

Tang, L.-H. 1995. Social Aspects of Malaria in Heping, Hainan. *Acta Tropica* 59: 41–53.

Tang, L.-H., H.-L. Qian, and S.-H. Xu. 1996. Malaria and Its Control in the People's Republic of China. *Southeast Asian Journal of Tropical Medicine and Public Health* 27: 367–71.

Taylor, B. 1975. Changes in the Feeding Behaviour of a Malaria Vector, *Anopheles farauti Lav,* following Use of DDT as a Residual Spray in Houses in the British Solomon Islands Protectorate. *Transactions of the Royal Entomological Society of London* 127: 277–92.

Verdrager, J. 1995. Localized Permanent Epidemics: The Genesis of Chloroquine Resistance in *Plasmodium falciparum. Southeast Asian Journal of Tropical Medicine and Public Health* 26: 23–8.

Vien, N.T., N.T. Hung, N.T. Thuy, et al. 1997a. Malaria in Three Groups of People Living in a High Transmission Focus in Vietnam. In *The Khanh Phu Malaria Research Project*, edited by Medisch Committee Netherlands–Viet Nam and National Institute of Malariology, Parasitology, and Entomology. Hanoi, Vietnam: Medical Publishing House.

Vien, N.T., N.T. Quang, N.S. Hai, et al. 1997b. The Effect of Bed Nets Impregnated with Permethrin on Bites by Malaria Vectors in Khanh Phu Commune, Khanh Hoa Province, Central Viet Nam. In *The Khanh Phu Malaria Research Project*, edited by Medisch Committee Netherlands–Viet Nam and National Institute of Malariology, Parasitology and Entomology. Hanoi, Vietnam: Medical Publishing House.

Vietnam Ministry of Health. 1998. Preliminary Evaluation of the Malaria Control Programme in Viet Nam for the Period 1992–1995: Results of Surveys in 30 Districts. Unpublished report. Hanoi, Vietnam: Vietnam Ministry of Health.

Walker, J. 1998. Malaria in a Changing World: An Australian Perspective. *International Journal for Parasitology* 2: 947–53.

Watson, L. 2000. Unpublished report on malaria in Lao PDR. Lao–EU Malaria Control Project. Vientiane, Lao PDR.

Xu, B., X. Xiao, and R.H. Webber. 1998. Comparison of the Effect of Insecticide-Treated Bed Nets and DDT Residual Spraying on the Prevalence of Malaria Transmitted by *An. anthropophagus* in China. *Transactions of the Royal Society of Tropical Medicine and Hygiene* 92: 135–6.

Xu, J., and H. Liu. 1997. Border Malaria in Yunnan, China. *Southeast Asian Journal of Tropical Medicine and Public Health* 28: 456–9.

Zhang, Z., and C. Yang. 1996. Application of Deltamethrin-Impregnated Bed Nets for Mosquito and Malaria Control in Yunnan, China. *Southeast Asian Journal of Tropical Medicine and Public Health* 27: 367–71.

Chapter 8

Determinants of Malaria in South Asia

Vinod Prakash Sharma

Malaria determinants in the World Health Organization's (WHO) South East Asia (SEA) Region are embedded in its climate, terrain, vectors, sociocultural milieu, and persistent neglect. Reemergence of malaria has established new ecotypes in areas of human activity. Even as malaria incidence increases, the Asian financial crisis and reductions in the allocation of funds for malaria control have aggravated the existing financial, technical, and operational constraints. Sustainable malaria control requires a primary attack on poverty, health system reforms, emphasis on community-based approaches, and investments in research and development.

The WHO SEA Region is made up of the countries of Bangladesh, Bhutan, Democratic People's Republic of Korea (North Korea), India, Indonesia, Maldives, Myanmar, Nepal, Sri Lanka, and Thailand; within this region, the distribution of malaria is highly uneven. An estimated 525 million people (35%) live in areas of moderate to high malaria risk. The remaining 975 million (65%) live in low-risk or malaria-free areas, which extend from the valley of the Ganges in the west to the plains of Bangladesh, to central Thailand, and to Java in the southeast. Between 1995 and 1998, reported malaria cases in the region fluctuated between 2.8 and 3.7 million per year, slide positivity rates varied from 3.0 to 3.8, *Plasmodium falciparum* percentages ranged from 37.6 to 41.7, and the number of deaths due to malaria was 5,240–8,061. During the same period, estimated incidence increased 10-fold, and malaria deaths increased 6-fold. Of an estimated 20 million cases of drug-resistant malaria in the world, 6 million (30%) cases are in the SEA Region.

Figure 8-1 shows the distribution of malaria in countries of the WHO SEA Region. Note that about 75% of malaria cases are in India, whereas about 60% of malaria deaths are in Myanmar; such a difference may reflect problems in surveillance and reporting rather than the actual situation. Exact statistics of deaths due to malaria are not available, and in both India and Myanmar, data show discrepancies between estimates based on death rates and actual deaths reported.

In this chapter, I examine the decisive roles of the major malaria determinants: vector (including distribution, biology, behavior, and insecticide resistance), parasite, host, environment and climate, ecosystem, and socioeconomics. I also present some success stories and suggest some rational approaches to malaria control.

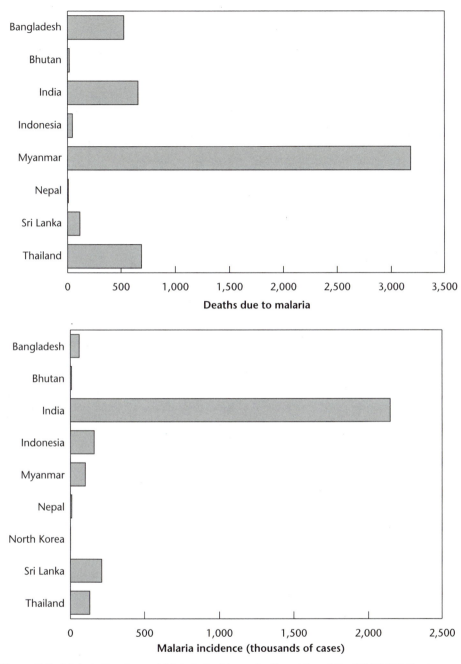

Figure 8-1. Malaria Deaths and Malaria Incidence in Countries of the WHO SEA Region

Source: WHO SEA Regional Office, New Delhi, India.

Vector Determinants

Malaria vectors—that is, carriers of *Plasmodium* parasites—are the most important deter-minants of malaria. The distribution of vectors and their biological adaptation and resi-dence in a particular environment are the determining factors in establishing malaria endemicity; for example, there has been no indigenous malaria transmission in the Republic of Maldives for more than a decade as a result of effective vector control.

Distribution of Vectors

As classified by Macdonald (1957), Asia has three epidemiological zones. Vector distribution is distinctly different in each zone, depending on the biotic and abiotic characteristics. In the Indo-Iranian region, with its arid, semiarid, and deciduous dry climates, the principal malaria vectors are *Anopheles stephensi, Anopheles culicifacies,* and *Anopheles fluviatilis.* In the Indochinese hills, with its tropical monsoon climate, the principal malaria vectors are *Anopheles dirus, Anopheles minimus,* and *An. fluviatilis.* In the Malaysian tropical monsoon climate, the principal malaria vectors are *Anopheles balabacensis, Anopheles maculatus, Anopheles umbrosus,* and *Anopheles sundaicus.*

Vector Biology

Biology of the immature and adult mosquitoes profoundly impacts malaria transmission and vector invasion. Three main groups of mosquitoes have adapted to various ecological conditions, as described next.

Group 1. *An. stephensi, An. culicifacies,* and *An. fluviatilis.* These mosquitoes transmit rural and urban malaria in India. Developments under the five-year plan to boost the national economy and eliminate poverty have provided tremendous opportunities for *An. stephensi* and *An. culicifacies* to breed in the newly created havens throughout the country. The invasion of these vectors is related to irrigation and urbanization, including the industrial growth of the country. *An. fluviatilis* is active in the foothills and transmits malaria either independently or in combination with *An. culicifacies.* Malaria is exacerbated with the onset of rains.

An. stephensi is distributed in the arid and semiarid zones from Iran, Afghanistan, and Pakistan to India. It is an important vector in urban and rural areas where the climate is dry. The female adult feeds on humans and animals, and the species is especially adapted to an urban environment. Its questing distance is three kilometers or more, which maintains high human–mosquito contact. *An. stephensi* influences malaria transmission in the western arid countries of Asia and does not occur in hilly, wet terrain. It breeds in wells, overhead tanks, cisterns, sumps, marshy lands, ponds, artificial containers, and in rainwater collections. In rural areas, *An. stephensi* breeds profusely where water harvesting is practiced, for example, in the desert of Rajasthan, India, where water is stored in underground tanks. Adult mosquitoes rest near the breeding sites and occasionally in houses on hanging objects, thus avoiding contact with sprayed walls. The National Malaria Eradication Programme in Bharatpur, Rajasthan, conducted a study to control *An. stephensi* by spraying deltamethrin at a concentration of 25 milligrams per square meter; this spraying failed to interrupt transmission mainly because of vector resting habits (i.e., on hanging objects rather than on walls) (Kalra 1991).

An. culicifacies is a monsoon-associated species that is distributed widely in the rural areas in dry and semihumid climates. It breeds in natural and human-made water bodies, banks and beds of canals, subcanals, peripheral channels, seepages, and small water collections such as hoof prints, wheel ruts, freshly dug pits, and borrow pits. Breeding accelerates with the onset of rains. Adults are zoophilic and rest indoors but readily feed on humans. Its migration is generally three kilometers or more. *An. culicifacies* originated in central India, and therefore its eradication from India is nearly an impossible task.

An. culicifacies has high polymorphism, as displayed by the presence of five sibling species. Table 8-1 shows the biological characteristics of *An. culicifacies* as investigated

Table 8-1. Biological Variations among Members of *An. culicifacies* Sibling Species Complex

Characteristic	Sibling species				
	A	B	C	D	E
Anthropophilic index[a] (%)	0–4	0–1	0–3	0–1	80
Biting activity	All night	All night	All night	Until midnight	NA
Peak biting time	22:00–23:00	22:00–23:00	18:00–21:00	18:00–21:00	NA
Vector potential[b]	Vector	Nonvector	Vector	Vector	Vector
Sporozoite rate (%)	0.51	0.04	0.3	0.4	20
Resistance					
DDT	Slow	Fast	Fast	NA	NA
BHC	Fast	Fast	Fast	NA	NA
Malathion	Slow	Intermediate	Fast	NA	NA

Notes: NA = data are not available. For resistance, Slow = 9–10 years, Intermediate = 6–7 years, and Fast = 4–5 years.

[a] Proportion of mosquitoes biting the human population.

[b] *P. vivax* and *P. falciparum* malaria.

Source: Malaria Research Center, New Delhi, India.

over a period of 30 years. Species B is a nonvector; all other species transmit malaria. Species B populations are sympatric with species A in India from north to south and with species C from west to east. Rural malaria is high in north India because of high vector densities of species A, in contrast to the south, where the prevalence of species A is low and there is little rural malaria. In areas where species B populations are allopatric—such as in eastern Uttar Pradesh and north Bihar—there is no malaria (Subbarao, Vasantha, and Sharma 1988). Malaria transmission in Rameshwaram Island was a paradox with exclusive populations of species B until the discovery of species E (Kar et al. 1999). A similar situation may be found in Sri Lanka.

In *An. culicifacies,* each sibling species has a niche to fill; they differ in biology, response to insecticides, biting rhythm, and capacity to transmit malaria. The presence of sibling species determines the malaria profile and the impact of insecticides. *An. culicifacies* is active in malaria transmission in Afghanistan, India, Iran, Pakistan, and Sri Lanka. *An. culicifacies sensu lato* has become triple resistant, and control of its populations is one of the most difficult challenges of malaria control. A rational malaria control strategy requires the selective application of residual insecticides, based on the knowledge of the sibling species and its resistance status (Sharma et al. 1986). Bioenvironmental malaria control has emerged as the most appropriate, cost-effective, and sustainable method of control for malaria transmitted by *An. culicifacies* (Sharma 1987).

An. fluviatilis species S has a wide distribution range and essentially is a vector of hills and foothills up to an altitude of 2,500 meters. True to its name ("fluviatile"—of fresh water origin), the mosquito is well adapted to breeding in the flowing water of springs, rivulets, and seepage channels of dams and irrigation channels as well as slow-running streams in the foothills and plains. The mosquito is adapted to a humid climate and rests outdoors at altitudes of 600 meters and above in Orissa, India. It frequently rests in human dwellings at the lower altitudes. *An. fluviatilis* is highly anthropophilic and maintains high degree of transmission within the dispersal range of about 1.5 kilometers. It is an efficient vector of malaria and, wherever present, joins *An. culicifacies* in transmitting malaria during the latter part of the year.

Table 8-2. Biological Characteristics of *An. fluviatilis* Sibling Species Complex

Characteristic	S	T	U
Inversion genotypes on chromosome arm2	$+ q^1 + r^1$	$q^1 + r^1$	$+ q^1 r^1$
Density (MHD)	Low (1–40)	High (up to 200)	High (up to 200)
Feeding preference	Anthropophagic	Almost totally zoophagic	Almost totally zoophagic
Sporozoite positives	Found	Not found	Not found
Preferred adult habitat	Human dwellings	Cattle sheds	Cattle sheds
Observed in Ecotype	Hilly forests and foothills	Foothills & plains	Foothills and plains
Epidemiological areas	Hyperendemic	Hypoendemic	Hypoendemic

Notes: MHD = man hour density (mosquitoes are collected by using a suction tube for 15 minutes in one room, and density is calculated as the number of mosquitoes per hour).
Source: Subbarao 1998, 36.

An. fluviatilis is a complex of three sibling species, designated as species S, T, and U (Subbarao et al. 1993). Table 8-2 shows the biological characteristics of *An. fluviatilis* in India. Studies have shown that species S is the vector, and species T and U are nonvectors. Species S prefers to inhabit undisturbed ecology; therefore, development activities lead to its disappearance, such as in Terai, Uttar Pradesh, India. Species T and U occupy newly created niches. The role of *An. fluviatilis* in malaria transmission has been minimized in some regions. Insecticide-treated mosquito nets have emerged as the most cost-effective method of controlling malaria transmitted by *An. fluviatilis* (Yadav et al. 1998).

A study of the role of malaria vectors in India (Table 8-3) discovered that *An. culicifacies* is the most important malaria vector in the region (Sharma 1998). This vector alone transmits 65% of the malaria in India and nearly 50% of the malaria in the SEA Region. In India, 80% of expenditures on malaria control are incurred in the control of *An. culicifacies*. The second vector of emerging importance, distributed as widely as *An. culicifacies,* is *An. stephensi*. This mosquito transmits about 12% of the malaria cases in urban, industrial, and desert conditions; lack of surveillance in urban areas is the main reason for its low epidemiological indices. *P. falciparum* transmission by *An. fluviatilis* is high, because *An. fluviatilis* populations increase when *P. falciparum* is the predominant parasite species (Sharma 1998).

Group 2. *An. dirus, An. minimus,* and *An. fluviatilis.* These mosquitoes maintain stable malaria, and vector control is a formidable challenge. *An. dirus* and *An. minimus* occupy inhospitable terrain in the forests and at international borders. The incidence of *P. falciparum* is high, and drug resistance has reached menacing proportions.

An. dirus is a primary vector of stable malaria in the jungles of northeast India, Chittagong Hill Tracts of Bangladesh, Myanmar, and Thailand (Rosenberg, Andre, and Somchit 1990). In areas under its influence, malaria transmission is intense and persistent. *An. dirus* breeds in water bodies with shade, such as small, shallow, temporary pools; edges of streams, springs, and gem-mining pits; bamboo stumps; elephant footprints; and wells. It enters houses for feeding and rests outdoors afterward. *An. dirus* is highly anthropophilic, and its migration is about two kilometers. Because of its exophilic behavior, *An. dirus* does not come in contact with sprayed walls; in Arunachal Pradesh,

Table 8-3. Role of Vectors in Malaria Transmission in India

Major malaria vector	Transmission potential	Malaria cases (%)	Falciparum cases (%)
Peninsular India			
An. culicifacies	+	65	55
An. stephensi	++	12	5
Regional India			
An. fluviatilis	++	15	30
An. minimus	+++	5	5
An. dirus	+++	3	5
Coastal areas			
An. sundaicus	++	0.039	0.001

Notes: for potential values, + = low, ++ = medium, and +++ = high. Percentages were calculated on the basis of 1996 malaria incidence in India.
Source: Sharma 1998.

India, for example, malaria transmission remained completely uninterrupted despite DDT spraying between 1964 and 1969 (Sen et al. 1973). During the wet season, however, *An. dirus* enters houses to feed and rest, thus indoor residual spraying has been reported to be useful in curtailing transmission in such places as Indonesia (personal communication from N.L. Kalra). Insecticide-treated mosquito nets have been effective in the control of *An. dirus* transmitted malaria in Thailand (personal communication from Malini Prasittisuk).

An. minimus is a primary vector of malaria in Bhutan, India, Myanmar, and Thailand. The clearing of jungles and the presence of streams led to invasion by *An. minimus*. It breeds in slow-moving forest hill streams with grassy margins exposed to sunlight. Dispersal is generally up to two kilometers. *An. minimus* displays pronounced exophilic behavior and thus maintains stable malaria in the forests (Dev and Sharma 1995). Together with *An. dirus, An. minimus* is active in malaria transmission in the vicinity of deep forests and, with *An. fluviatilis,* in the degraded forests. Successful malaria control has been demonstrated by the use of insecticide-treated mosquito nets in Assam, India (Jana-Kara et al. 1995)

Group 3. *An. balabacensis, An. maculatus, An. umbrosus,* **and** *An. sundaicus.* These vectors inhabit various islands in Indonesia (Figure 8-2) and maintain moderate to high transmission. They are highly efficient vectors of malaria but have limited distribution.

An. balabacensis is closely related to *An. dirus* with practically the same vector bionomics. It is one of the most efficient malaria vectors in the Kalimantan and in the Java and Bali islands of Indonesia. It breeds in various small water collections and in well-shaded areas in deep jungles. It is exophilic, exophagic, and highly anthropophilic, and it maintains almost perennial malaria. It is susceptible to insecticides but does not come in contact with sprayed walls.

An. maculatus breeds primarily in streams but also in sunlit water bodies such as ponds, tanks, and riverbed pools. It is basically zoophilic and exophagic, with low vector potential. Along with *An. minimus,* it transmits malaria in Bhutan, Nepal, and Thailand.

An. umbrosus is a vector in Kalimantan in Indonesia. It breeds in stagnant shallow waters in jungle pools and slow-running streams; it prefers shade and thick vegetation. It is a strong flier, is exophilic and exophagic, and transmits malaria in the forest. *An. umbrosus* is active throughout most of the day, with peak biting just before nightfall.

An. sundaicus is prevalent in coastal areas and in mangrove forests. The common breeding sites are the stagnant brackish water, wells, marshy low-lying areas, creeks, swampy pits, and lagoons. Heavy breeding can be found in putrefying masses. It rests both indoors and outdoors; adults rest outdoors in jungles after feeding. *An. sundaicus* is a major vector of malaria in the Andaman and Nicobar Islands, in the outer islands of Indonesia, in Sumatra and Kalimantan, and in the Java and Bali islands. In India, before the launching of the malaria control program, *An. sundaicus* was a major vector of malaria in Chilka Lake, Orissa; the east and west coasts; and in the Andaman and Nicobar Islands. DDT spraying uprooted *An. sundaicus* from the mainland, and it has not returned. The manipulation of water quality by either maintaining a high salt content or installing one-way sluice gates to prevent seawater flooding into creeks is also effective in controlling *An. sundaicus*.

Behavior of Vectors

Vector breeding behavior determines the range of colonization by a particular species. *An. stephensi* breeds in small water collections in houses and related structures in both urban and industrial townships and is the basis for "urban malaria" and "industrial malaria" in India. *An. culicifacies* is a vector of rural malaria; because of its intense breeding in irrigation systems such as dams, canals, subcanals, and seepage areas, it is known as "irrigation malaria." *An. fluviatilis, An. minimus*, and *An. maculatus* breed in running-water streams and maintain malaria in the hills and foothills, whereas *An. dirus* breeds in puddles in deep forests. These four vectors are responsible for "forest malaria" and, at international boundaries, create "border malaria" (Pattanayak et al. 1994). *An. sundaicus* breeds in brackish water and maintains perennial malaria transmission in the coastal areas.

During evolution, some malaria vectors adapted to the climatic conditions by conserving water to avoid desiccation in the dry climate. During the night, under favorable temperature conditions, these mosquitoes (e.g., *An. stephensi* and *An. culicifacies*) migrate long distances (three kilometers or more) in search of food and oviposition sites in the arid and semiarid or deciduous dry zones. These vectors are endophilic and endophagic and generate unstable malaria. In contrast, vectors belonging to the tropical monsoon humid climate have no requirement of water conservation. These vectors (e.g., *An. dirus* and *An. minimus*) display pronounced exophilic behavior, have limited dispersal, and maintain holoendemic malaria. Studies show that spiracular openings in the respiratory system of mosquitoes correlate to climate conditions (personal communication from B.N. Nagpal). In mosquitoes belonging to arid and semiarid zones, spiracular openings are small so as to conserve water; in contrast, in the tropical humid climate, spiracular openings are large. Such mosquitoes have limited dispersal and live in foci of ideal humidity and temperature conditions.

The biting rhythm of the vectors has direct consequences on the success of insecticide-treated mosquito nets. Although some mosquitoes start biting early (e.g., species C and D of *An. culicifacies*), other species (e.g., *An. minimus*) bite relatively late. Some mosquitoes (e.g., *An. stephensi*) stop biting after midnight, whereas others (e.g., *An. culicifacies sensu lato*) continue to bite all night. People who receive a significant number of bites before going to bed may reduce the impact of insecticide-treated mosquito nets (Nanda et al. 1996).

Insecticide Resistance

An. culicifacies is the most important vector of malaria in Asia. In almost all areas of its distribution, it has become resistant to DDT and, in most areas, to hexachlorocyclohexane (HCH) as well. Resistance to malathion has emerged in Gujarat, Maharashtra, and small regions in many parts of India, Sri Lanka, and Pakistan. In India, HCH has been banned, DDT is being phased out, and malathion has high refusal rates because of its pungent odor. Synthetic pyrethroids are being used increasingly in the control of *An. culicifacies*, but there are reports of resistance, and in the coming decade, widespread resistance probably will develop (Sharma and Mehrotra 1986; Raghavendra et al. 1991, 1992). Insecticide resistance then would become the most important determinant of malaria in rural India.

Table 8-1 lists the impact of three insecticides on the development of resistance in three sibling species of *An. culicifacies* in the field. Species A has high capacity to transmit malaria, but development of resistance to malathion was very slow. It took 10 years of three rounds of malathion spraying in Sonepat, Haryana, India, for species A to develop some degree of resistance (Subbarao, Vasantha, and Sharma 1988). In contrast, species C developed resistance to malathion in three years in Gujarat (Rajagopal 1977). Resistance to DDT builds up very slowly in species A but rapidly in species B. DDT spraying in *An. culicifacies sensu lato* populations produces an epidemiological impact on malaria because it selectively kills species A in the sympatric populations of species A and species B. Malaria control in species C areas by spraying DDT and malathion is unlikely to be productive in the long run, and programs should rely on alternate strategies, such as bioenvironmental methods and insecticide-treated mosquito nets.

Such information has become vital in planning malaria vector control in India. The problem of vector resistance is pronounced in the mosquitoes in arid and semiarid zones. These mosquitoes are endophilic and endophagic and rest on the walls after a blood meal. Susceptible individual vectors die on sprayed walls, resulting in the selection of resistant strains. *An. stephensi* and *An. culicifacies* belong to this group. For *An. stephensi*, the control strategy is antilarval; therefore, resistance is not the main obstacle in its control. Successful control of *An. culicifacies* in the initial stages of the malaria eradication program in Pakistan, India, and Sri Lanka resulted from endophilic and endophagic vector behavior. In contrast, in the case of malaria vectors belonging to the tropical monsoon climate (e.g., *An. dirus* and *An. minimus*), exophilic vector behavior rather than insecticide resistance continues to be a major hurdle in malaria control.

Parasite Determinants

In the SEA Region, all four of the human malaria parasites are encountered, but *Plasmodium ovale* is almost negligible. *Plasmodium malariae* has retracted but is still found in some areas in the foothills, such as in Orissa, India. *Plasmodium vivax* is the predominant species in this region, followed by *P. falciparum*. *P. vivax* causes high morbidity but rarely death. It causes relapses, which become the source of resurgence, as occurred in India in the late 1960s. Also, the Democratic People's Republic of Korea (North Korea) had enjoyed malaria-free status, but during the past four to five years, *P. vivax* has widely reemerged; about 200,000 cases are recorded annually.

During the past 20 years, *P. falciparum* incidence has increased in an unstoppable march. *P. falciparum* is the killer parasite, and its control has become the most formidable challenge in Asia because of the emergence of mono- and multiple-drug resistance. The initial epicenter of drug resistance in southeast Asia was located on the Thailand–Cambodia border (Clyde 1987). This region was particularly receptive to *P. falciparum* transmission on account of the presence of highly efficient malaria vectors such as *An. dirus* and *An. minimus*. In this region, large parasite populations produced mutants with continued superinfection in the human host. These mutants intermingled and exploded in infected children. The infected population with low-grade parasitemia provided a constant flow of gametocytes. DDT spraying failed to control *An. dirus* and *An. minimus*. Human–mosquito contact remained high because of the outdoor habits of people and work opportunities in the forests.

The epicenter of resistance by *P. falciparum* to chloroquine, and later sulfadoxine–pyrimethamine (a two-drug combination for treating malaria), was the Thailand–Cambodia border. Resistance spread rapidly and passed through the center of Myanmar and entered the Chittagong Hill Tracts of Bangladesh. High transmission in forests, population movement, gem and gold mining, and nonimmune migrant populations living in temporary settlements that lacked proper health facilities for malaria treatment were the primary reasons of the evolution of multiple-drug resistant strains and their spread to new areas (Nosten et al. 1991; Thein and Soe 1989; Singhanetra-Renard 1986). In India, drug resistance spread westward, entered the high transmission areas of Orissa, crossed central India, moved south, and reached Sri Lanka; from central India, drug resistance entered Pakistan.

In Asia, drug resistance by *P. falciparum* is now widespread and progressing toward multiple-drug resistance. Drug resistance enhances morbidity and increases mortality 5- to 15-fold, and the cost to treat drug-resistant malaria increases by a factor of 10–40 or more. In poor communities, where treatment is unaffordable, residents develop immunity and live as carriers, spreading drug-resistant malaria to new areas of their settlements. Resistance to chloroquine by *P. vivax* has been reported in Papua New Guinea, Indonesia, and India (Dua, Kar, and Sharma 1996), but it may be present in many other countries in much higher numbers. Unfortunately, reliable information on the status of chloroquine resistance by *P. vivax* is not known. The present trend of multiple-drug resistance by *P. falciparum* and the development of chloroquine resistance by *P. vivax* have emerged as a formidable challenge in malaria control and an important determinant of malaria.

Combination drug therapy is a scientific approach to eliminating the drug-resistant foci. Single- to multiple-drug resistance in *P. falciparum* has emerged as a major problem in achieving high malaria cure rates (Trape 2000). A rational approach to prolonging the therapeutic life of existing antimalaria drugs would be to combine them, as practiced in the treatment of HIV/AIDS [human immunodeficiency virus/acquired immune deficiency syndrome], tuberculosis, leprosy, and some cancers. Drug combination is likely to delay the development of resistance that arises out of independent mutations to component drugs that have different modes of action (White 1999a, 1999b).

Host Determinants

Among hosts, many factors contribute to high malaria transmission rates, including human genome diversity, living in inhospitable and often inaccessible terrain, high receptivity to malaria, socioeconomic and sociocultural milieu, nutrition, health infrastructure, and nonimmune populations (particularly children younger than five years old).

An epidemiological investigation (NAMP 1999) studied the tribal population of India, 69 million people living in 179 districts in 14 states. This population contributes more than 40% of the malaria cases, more than 65% of the *P. falciparum* cases, and more than 50% of the deaths due to malaria. Various malaria control interventions have had little impact on these statistics. It should be noted that during the height of malaria eradication, 9% of India's population lived in areas that did not respond to indoor residual spraying with DDT for 10–12 years. These areas, which largely coincide with tribal settlements, were designated as persistent malaria transmission areas (Sharma 1996a). Malaria transmission in this population is almost perennial, with a high proportion of *P. falciparum*.

Several studies in the forested and deforested areas of Madhya Pradesh state, India, show persistent malaria transmission by *An. culicifacies* and *An. fluviatilis*. For example, in Mandla district, which is predominantly tribal (80% Gond tribe), *P. falciparum* incidence was high, and chloroquine resistance by *P. falciparum* reached menacing proportions (Singh and Sharma 1989). Host immunity with low parasitemia is the characteristic feature of this population, producing asymptomatic carriers.

Hemoglobinopathies and enzymopathies are prevalent genetic traits among the tribal population settled in forests. These genetic traits provide survival advantages regarding malaria, indicating that malaria is the underlying cause of this human polymorphism. An important example is the Duffy group antigen, which is a definitive determinant of *P. vivax* malaria. The absence of the Duffy group antigen (a– b–) in the African population provides 100% protection from *P. vivax*. In Asian populations with the Duffy group antigen (a+ b+), *P. vivax* is the dominant infection (Miller 1994). Hemoglobinopathies produce carriers, thus contributing to malaria transmission, and may cause malaria outbreaks in new settlements of nonimmune populations. Malaria control in the tribal settlements continues to be a formidable challenge. Insecticide-treated mosquito nets are being introduced to reduce malaria related mortality and morbidity in predominantly tribal populations in the Asian countries.

Environmental Determinants

Temperature

For most vectors of malaria, 20–30 °C is the temperature range optimal for development. Relative humidity higher than 55% is optimal for vector longevity (enabling successful completion of sporogony). Malaria transmission requires a minimum average temperature higher than 15 °C for *P. vivax* and 19 °C for *P. falciparum*, and this temperature minimum should be exceeded over a period of time for the completion of sporogony in mosquitoes.

Altitude

Vectors can transmit malaria at various altitudes, but malaria transmission ceases at altitudes above 3,300 meters. For example, malaria transmission occurs at 3,300 meters in Kenya (vectors *Anopheles gambiae* and *Anopheles funestus*); at 2,000 meters in the Indochinese hills (vector *An. minimus*); and in rare instances, *An. fluviatilis* transmits malaria at 2,000–3,300 meters. *Anopheles sacharovi* and *Anopheles superpictus* are efficient vectors at sea level, but *An. sacharovi* can transmit malaria at altitudes up to 1,000 meters and *An. superpictus* up to 700 meters (NMEP 1986).

Rainfall

Heavy rainfall is associated with flooded rivers and canals and waterlogged conditions. Several studies have shown that enhanced vector breeding as a result of heavy rainfall has resulted in widespread malaria epidemics throughout northwest India, especially in areas within the Indo-Gangetic plains (Gill 1923; Swaroop 1946). The relationship of rainfall to malaria was investigated, and epidemic forecasting methods were developed by Swaroop (1946) for Punjab, where malaria flares up after the July and August rains. The malaria mortality figures of Punjab from 1867 to 1943 indicated that malaria peaks were separated by an eight-year interval (Yacob and Swaroop 1945). According to Christophers (1911), however, a malaria epidemic in Punjab in 1908 that caused 300,000 deaths in a population of 20 million over a period of three months as well as other deaths in the same area could be attributed to high humidity rather than rainfall.

Rainfall promotes breeding of all malaria vectors, but it has a profound impact on the breeding of *An. culicifacies*. *An. culicifacies* breeds in sunlit water collections on the ground, a condition created by the rains. Therefore, India's malaria is also a rainfall phenomenon. The impact of rainfall is more pronounced in northwest and central India because of the presence of *An. culicifacies* sibling species A and C. In southern India, with relatively low rural malaria, irrigation promotes malaria transmission by encouraging the breeding of species A in channels, seepage, and subsurface water. (For other studies connecting rainfall and malaria incidence in India, see Mathur et al. 1992; Shukla, Pandey, and Mathur 1995; and Raghavendra et al. 1992.)

In Sri Lanka, malaria is also closely associated with the pattern of rainfall. In the past (1934–1935 and 1967–1968), serious malaria epidemics in Sri Lanka have been associated with monsoon failure. On the basis of annual precipitation, Sri Lanka has been divided into three zones: dry (less than 2,000 millimeters of rainfall), intermediate (2,000–2,500 millimeters of rainfall), and wet (more than 2,500 millimeters of rainfall). *An. culicifacies*, the malaria vector, breeds in streambeds. Abundant rainfall throughout the year in the wet zone keeps the rivers flowing, thus preventing the formation of riverbed pools. Vector breeding is poor, and there is no malaria transmission in the normal years.

Failure of southwest monsoons, however, creates stagnant water pools in the rivers, an ideal breeding ground for *An. culicifacies*. Thus, malaria epidemics in Sri Lanka are associated with droughts. The dry zone gets its rainfall during the northeast monsoon, when many surface water pools are formed. When water bodies dry between monsoon storms, breeding of *An. culicifacies* increases in streams and riverbeds to maintain endemic malaria. The intermediate zone has a pattern of rainfall and malaria transmission between the two zones (van der Hoek et al. 1997). Gill (1936) analyzed the relationship between rainfall and malaria in eight districts of Sri Lanka from 1901 to 1934 and also concluded that droughts bring malaria.

Climate Change

Malaria epidemics have been linked to temporary climate changes such as abnormal rains, extended periods of humidity, and high temperatures. Epidemics also have been linked to permanent changes in the microclimate as a result of agriculture, tree plantations, developments in irrigation, and resettlements. Because of these indicators, epidemics can be predicted with a reasonable degree of precision in time for preventive interventions (Trigg and Kondrachine 1998).

Cycles of rain and drought also have a relationship with the El Niño–Southern Oscillation, a meteorological phenomenon that occurs every 2–10 years and affects the world's climate (see Chapter 11). While some areas receive excessive rainfall, others experience drought. In Sri Lanka, malaria epidemics were significantly more prevalent during El Niño years, when the southwest monsoons did not arrive. In contrast, epidemics in western Rajasthan in 1994 were related to the El Niño phenomenon of excessive rainfall and flooding (Bouma and van der Kaay 1994). In Pakistan, periods of increased falciparum transmission showed a relationship to higher late-season temperatures associated with El Niño years (Bouma, Sondorp, and van der Kaay 1994; Bouma and van der Kaay 1996).

When there is a progressive rise in surface temperature due to increased production of greenhouse gases, the increased temperature may profoundly affect the transmission of vector-borne diseases (Lindsay and Birley 1996). During the past 20 years, the average minimum temperature in northern India has increased by 2 °C, but the average maximum temperature has not increased; this climatic change may enhance malaria transmission by extending the transmission season and the transmission zones.

Ecosystem Determinants

Human-made ecological changes disturb the natural equilibrium of malaria transmission, leading to the changes in vector prevalence and the formation of new malaria ecotypes as described below.

Forests

In forests, the exploitation of natural resources, deforestation for resettlement and agriculture, additional land availability for industries and projects, and migration contribute enormously to the enhancement of malaria transmission and epidemics. Malaria vectors maintain perennial malaria transmission in the forest (Sharma and Kondrachine 1991). *An. dirus* and *An. minimus* are responsible for maintaining stable malaria and high malaria-related morbidity and mortality in children, pregnant women, and migrants who live in and near the forests. Malaria control has been difficult to eliminate in the forests because of persistent malaria transmission, difficult terrain, and poor health services. Table 8-4 shows malaria incidence in the population settled in forests. The incidence of *P. falciparum,* the parasite responsible for mortality, is high.

An. dirus is associated with the transmission of drug-resistant malaria in the WHO SEA Region. In Bangladesh, an estimated 7 million people who live in the Sylhet area in the Chittagong Hill Tract are exposed to the bites of *An. dirus* (Rosenberg and Maheswary 1982). *An. dirus* and *An. minimus* transmit intense malaria in the forests in Myanmar, on the Thailand–Myanmar and Thailand–Malaysia borders, and in India, along the borders with Bangladesh, Myanmar, and Bhutan. In forests with streams, *An. dirus* and *An. minimus* are active and produce a heavy rate of infective bites. *An. fluviatilis* combines with *An. minimus* to play a major role in the forest and foothills of northern India and to serve as the primary vector in Assam and Meghalaya in India; *An. fluviatilis* combines with *An. dirus* and *An. minimus* in the eastern region of the Myanmar border. In forest fringe and degraded forest areas, *An. minimus* and *An. fluviatilis* maintain high transmission. In Nepal, *An. fluviatilis* is a primary vector of malaria in the foothills and river valleys and joins *An. maculatus* in maintaining transmission, although

Table 8-4. Malaria Incidence in the Forests of the Countries in the WHO SEA Region, 1989

Country	No. of all malaria cases		No. of malaria cases in forests		Percentage of malaria cases in forests	
	All types	Falciparum	Total	Falciparum	Total	Falciparum
Bangladesh	50,738	35,780	44,365	35,237	87.43	98.73
Bhutan	20,585	9,660	NA	NA	NA	NA
India	2,017,823	746,219	632,721	389,980	31.35	52.26
Indonesia	22,736	NA	10,003	NA	43.99	>50
Myanmar	135,194	116,267	NA	NA	NA	NA
Nepal	22,333	2,371	11,016	1,697	49.32	71.57
Sri Lanka	258,727	66,640	NA	NA	NA	NA
Thailand	299,137	NA	125,638	NA	42.01	>50

Notes: All forests have not been included. NA = data are not available.
Source: Sharma, Prasittisuk, and Kondrashin 1991.

An. maculatus is largely a zoophilic species. In the forests of peninsular India, *An. culicifacies* and *An. fluviatilis* are a serious combination in malaria transmission.

A population of approximately 42 million tribal people in the plains of India are settled in areas with intense malaria transmission. Annually, this population contributes 33% of the malaria cases in the country and 57% of the *P. falciparum* cases. This is the most vulnerable population with varying degrees of transmission maintained by *An. culicifacies* and *An. fluviatilis,* either independently or in combination; when the two vectors are active, the transmission of *P. falciparum* is extended by *An. fluviatilis.* For this reason, although *An. fluviatilis* vectors in India are not as widely distributed as those of *An. culicifacies* or *An. stephensi,* they transmit 30% of the falciparum malaria cases, second only to *An. culicifacies* (see Table 8-3).

An. culicifacies and *An. fluviatilis* transmit malaria in the forests in central India. Both vectors can maintain high and perennial transmission. From 1987 to 1988 in Kundum, Jabalpur, Madhya Pradesh, malaria transmission remained unaffected despite four rounds of HCH spraying and chemotherapeutic measures; In these areas, a very high degree of drug resistance by *P. falciparum* was encountered. *P. falciparum* was the predominant infection in forested villages and *P. vivax* in the deforested villages in Mandla district of India (Singh, Singh, and Sharma 1996).

Gem Mining. The association of malaria and gem mining is well known in Thailand, Myanmar, and Sri Lanka, where gem mines are usually located in forest areas. *An. culicifacies* breeds in gem pits in Sri Lanka, and *An. dirus* and *An. minimus* in Myanmar and Thailand. Mining activities attract nonimmune populations to these high-risk areas, resulting in high morbidity and mortality in temporary settlements. Thus, population movement is an important determinant in the rise of malaria and in the high death rates in Myanmar. Malaria in Myanmar is almost perennial; the country's forests and forest fringes constitute a permanent reservoir, diffusing infection into the plains and resulting in a large number of epidemics. The epidemic malaria situation in the Borai border area of eastern Thailand is another such situation; thousands of gem miners entering and leaving Cambodia spread malaria.

In Sri Lanka, a malaria eradication program was initiated in 1958, and by 1963, malaria had been nearly eliminated. The discovery of new gem fields, however, reversed that progress. Miners were attracted from malaria-endemic areas, and a large number of pits were dug in search of gemstones. These pits became the locus of *An. culicifacies*, the predominant malaria vector in Sri Lanka. In 1967, new outbreaks of *P. vivax* were detected in two foci that led to an epidemic resurgence of malaria. In 1968, malaria incidence reached preeradication levels (Figure 8-2). Spraying was resumed, but the vectors had developed resistance to DDT (Rawlings, Herath, and Kelly 1985). Indoor residual spraying with malathion replaced DDT spraying, but the mosquitoes soon developed resistance to malathion, too, and malaria cases multiplied. In 1987, more than half a million cases were recorded: 502,134 cases of *P. vivax* and 184,326 cases of *P. falciparum*. The same year, a shortage of insecticide allowed for only 50–60% of houses to be sprayed (Gratz 1999). Dam construction and irrigation projects continue to provide new grounds for the breeding of *An. culicifacies* (Amerasinghe and Ariyasena 1990).

Malaria control in Sri Lanka is now based on the synthetic pyrethroids for indoor residual spraying to control *An. culicifacies*, but the malaria situation has not improved. The epidemiology of malaria in Sri Lanka is quite revealing, because although malaria may have been eliminated at one time, relapses or introduced cases seeded in the non-immune population turned back the clock.

Tribal Communities. The tribal communities are isolated and thus have access to only primitive subsistence-oriented technologies. Households tend to combine hunting and food gathering with some settled agriculture. Tribal populations migrate in groups to urban areas to look for work. Because of their specialization in agriculture, this labor population migrates to the fields in Punjab, Haryana, Uttar Pradesh, West Bengal, and Assam (India). The epidemiological role of tribal migrants in the dissemination, maintenance, and enhancement of malaria transmission once they are back in the forests is well-established.

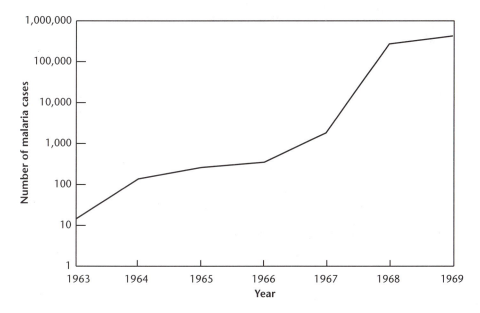

Figure 8-2. Posteradication Return of Malaria to Sri Lanka

Note: Near-eradication of malaria had left a residual focus of 17 cases. Within five years, the number of malaria cases reached about 100,000.

Source: Sharma et al. 1999.

Deforestation. Deforestation for agriculture has resulted in an ecological succession of vectors and enhanced transmission. Several examples are included here.

The Terai region in Uttar Pradesh, India, was known for hyperendemic malaria. Several attempts to colonize this area failed due to the ravages of malaria. Deforestation dislodged *An. minimus* in the early 1950s, and *An. fluviatilis* entered the area instead. In the 1960s, DDT spraying eradicated *An. minimus,* and *An. fluviatilis* assumed the role of the principal malaria vector and remained so for about a decade. Additional developments in agriculture resulted in the entry of *An. culicifacies,* and both vectors began malaria transmission. In the Cholburin province of Thailand, malaria was hyperendemic in forests, which amounted to 49% of the province's area in 1961. *An. dirus* was the main species that was breeding in rock pools, footprints, pits, and moist sand. Deforestation in subsequent years reduced forest cover to about 6% by 1985. This changed ecology reduced breeding sites for *An. dirus,* but the degraded areas were soon occupied by *An. minimus* and malaria returned in the resettled population (Suvannadabba 1991; Bunnag et al. 1979).

In the Bo Ploi district of Kanchanaburi province of Thailand, large-scale deforestation and clearing of land for sugar cane cultivation eliminated the breeding sites of *An. dirus*. However, digging for minerals and visits to the forests resulted in exposure of settlers to *An. dirus*, and malaria incidence is particularly high in this population.

In the Chantaburi district of Thailand on the Cambodian border and the Kanchanaburi district on the Myanmar border, forests were cleared from 1986 to 1995 for commercial tree crops for rubber plantations and orchards. These areas were under intense malaria transmission by *An. dirus*, but malaria declined sharply with deforestation. However *An. dirus* adapted itself to the changed environment, and malaria reemerged.

Human Migration. Population migration cuts across all types of malaria ecotypes and spreads new strains and drug-resistant malaria. In fact, several epidemics in India have been associated with population migration. Populations that settle in forests migrate to various destinations in other states for the purpose of cattle grazing, agriculture, urban construction, road projects, forest work, and industrial work. Migration is more pronounced from poorly developed areas that lack job opportunities. In such cases, labor movement is from high-transmission districts and thus spreads malaria to new places of employment.

The gender of migrants is related to migration patterns. In long-distance movement, men tend to outnumber women, but in short-distance movement, women tend to outnumber men. Migration after marriage is particularly important, because it involves nearly 25% of women of childbearing age. Such movement is within and between districts.

Malaria Control in Forests. Control of forest malaria is difficult, but a few success stories show promise in this area.

During World War II in the eastern theater, Indian troops were protected from malaria by organizing drainage in Assam. As a result, there were malaria-free roads, railway stations, and camps for the troops in the heart of a region with stable malaria. Therefore, good drainage and clearance of streams can eliminate malaria transmitted by the *An. minimus.*

A classic example of the complete disappearance of malaria without a deliberate attempt by humans to control it comes from the Malnad region in the states of Karnataka and Kerala, India, where malaria transmission ceased as a result of developments

for coffee plantations. The climate of Malnad was ideal for coffee plantations, and deforestation for coffee plantations began in the 1950s. Deforestation removed forest litter
and reduced rainwater percolation and seepage that were the principal sites of *An. fluviatilis* breeding, the only malaria vector in Malnad. Small dams were constructed for irrigation that trapped the seepage and runoff water. The new habitats were unsuitable for
An. fluviatilis breeding, and as a result, vector populations completely collapsed and
malaria disappeared from Malnad (Kalra 1991).

Irrigation

Agricultural growth was essential to sustain the growing human population of India. It
required increased irrigation, the introduction of high-yielding crops, and the use of fer-
tilizers and pesticides. Irrigation is an important determinant of malaria, particularly in
areas with *An. culicifacies*. This mosquito breeds profusely in irrigation systems. In India,
where irrigation increased from 22.6 million hectares in 1950 to more than 95 million
hectares in 1998, malaria vectors have proliferated along the irrigated land, affecting
about 200 million rural inhabitants.

Malaria transmission via irrigation begins with the aggregation of labor. Dam construction for a canal system attracts 1,000–20,000 temporary laborers, who live in camps
for several years. Conditions of these labor settlements are far from satisfactory, and
unhygienic conditions cause many diseases. After the canal system becomes operational, irrigation raises the groundwater level, which results in adjacent areas becoming
waterlogged. Vector breeding is further accelerated by the lack of "on-farm development" for drainage. For example, in Haryana and Punjab, India, transmission of malaria
has been high in waterlogged areas after the introduction of irrigation (NMEP 1986).
Other examples of irrigation increasing malaria incidence in India can be found in the
upper Krishna project, the Narmada irrigation project, and the Bagri Dam.

In Sri Lanka, malaria outbreaks are directly related to hydrological changes brought
about by major irrigation and hydroelectric schemes on the Mahaweli River. Human
migration between malaria-endemic and -nonendemic areas and resettlement near the
dam reservoir were the main factors contributing to increased malaria transmission
(Amerasinghe and Indrajith 1994; Wijesundera 1988).

Urban Centers

Urban malaria is a major problem in India; the vector of urban malaria, *An. stephensi,*
generates an estimated 12–15% of the malaria cases in India. *An. stephensi* is responsible
for the creation of urban malaria and industrial malaria because of its peculiar habits of
colonizing human-made structures built to store water. Historically, urban malaria in
India was a problem in port cities. Later, *An. stephensi* invaded towns along the rivers or
colonized wells in inland towns such as Delhi, Lucknow, and Hyderabad. Malaria
entered most Indian cities along with the introduction of piped water supplies, and the
process is leading to the invasion of *An. stephensi* in rural areas, followed by the *Aedes
aegypti*. Before the 1950s, malaria was considered a rural disease, but as malaria was
declining and disappearing in rural India, cases were multiplying in the urban areas.

Population growth and opportunities for a better life in the cities have resulted in
unprecedented growth in urban areas. People settle in undeveloped and low-lying areas
that lack proper water supplies and drainage, and their dwellings are poorly made.
Water is scarce and rationed, and water storage leads to mosquito production. *An.*

stephensi invades water storage containers and gradually establishes itself to cover an entire town. Urbanization of rural areas is providing opportunities for *An. stephensi* invasions; along with *An. stephensi* and *Ae. aegypti,* the vector of dengue fever is spreading in all towns and in the urbanized rural areas. As a result, dengue fever and dengue hemorrhagic fever are encountered with increasing intensity in the towns and villages.

To combat urban malaria, the Indian government launched the Urban Malaria Scheme (UMS) in 1971–1972 in 132 towns with populations of more than 40,000 people. Implementation was slow; it took 20 years to cover all the identified towns. The urban population had increased from 62 million in 1951 to 218 million in 1991, and by 1991, 25.7% of the total Indian population lived in towns. In the past 50 years, urbanization has swallowed 1 million hectares of agricultural land.

Urban malaria control relies on source reduction and weekly destruction of larval breeding habitats supplemented by biological control methods, minor engineering interventions, and legislative measures. As a result of failure in the detection and destruction of mosquito breeding, peri-urban and urban malaria is increasing in most towns of the country.

Malaria control requires an interruption of transmission, but because of problems in achieving vector control, excessive use of drug treatments is causing the emergence of drug-resistant malaria. Malaria control also requires indoor residual spraying and the implementation of antilarval methods, both of which are poorly implemented in urban areas. As more people migrate to cities, the number of malaria cases and the problem of drug-resistant malaria multiply. Yet of the 3,768 towns in India, malaria control is carried out only in the 132 towns with more than 40,000 inhabitants. Settlements in peri-urban areas have created a new malaria ecotype known as "peri-urban malaria," which affects 100 million people. In these areas, *An. stephensi* and *An. culicifacies* are the primary malaria vectors.

Industrial Areas

Industrial developments to improve the national economy and the quality of life have resulted in the creation of "industrial malaria." Industries require water, which becomes an ideal place for protected breeding of *An. stephensi* and *An. culicifacies*. *An. stephensi* breeds in stored waters in homes and industries, and *An. culicifacies* breeds in the stagnant water of ponds and pits.

A study in the 1980s surveyed 292 major projects under way in various sectors of the Indian economy and examined the connection between industrial development and malaria (NMEP 1986). For example, during the construction phase of the Mirzapur Thermal Power Project, the number of malaria cases suddenly increased in the district, from 2,421 cases in 1979 to 11,455 cases in 1980. At a steel plant in Vizag, 50% of the total malaria cases in the district were recorded at the steel plant. Similarly, high malaria transmission was maintained at other industrial complexes, such as Bharat Heavy Electricals Ltd. Hardwar; the oil refinery in Mathura, Uttar Pradesh; and mining areas in Orissa, Bihar, and Madhya Pradesh.

Industrial labor is concentrated in malaria-endemic areas, and about 10% of the laborers are asymptomatic carriers. A study of the labor force working on various projects in the northeastern states revealed that in seven states, 46 projects employed 253,000 workers, including 28,000 seasonal laborers. On average, the malaria prevalence rate was 11.1% (4.0% *P. vivax* and 7.1% *P. falciparum*) (NMEP 1986). In Panaji (Goa state), a malaria epidemic was the result of migrant labor imported for construction work from malaria-endemic states (Kumar, Sharma, and Thavaselvam 1991).

Bioenvironmental methods were used in malaria control at the Bharat Heavy Electricals Ltd. Hardwar. Ponds and ditches were filled with industrial fly ash; the areas were then converted to playgrounds and parks. A cost calculation showed that malaria control was highly beneficial because it reduced absenteeism as well as hospital costs; malaria had accounted for about 30% of bed occupancy in a 200-bed hospital (Dua et al. 1997).

Health impact assessment and implementation of preventive malaria control strategies should become integral parts of all industrial projects, as was done before the arrival of DDT, when a 3% project cost was mandatory for malaria prevention on industrial projects. Unfortunately, this cost was later converted to curative services and now is spent on hospital maintenance.

International Borders

Although international borders are not usually considered ecosystems, in the SEA Region, borders have characteristics that exacerbate malaria problems. Border districts have poor vector control and inadequate treatment facilities; substandard drugs are freely available; and unscrupulous medical personnel are common. Populations move freely because the international borders are highly porous, as in, for example, Bangladesh, Bhutan, India, and Nepal. Smaller countries such as Bhutan and Nepal have high percentages of their population living on the borders: 40% in Bhutan and 70% in Nepal. Among larger countries, 70.8 million Indian citizens and 11.2 million Bangladeshis are at risk of contracting border malaria (NAMP 1999).

P. vivax had been the dominant malaria parasite species in Asia, but during the past 20–30 years, *P. falciparum* has been on the rise. Chloroquine resistance in *P. falciparum* was first reported on the Thailand–Cambodia border, and from this epicenter, it spread far and wide. A precarious situation of multiple drug–resistant *P. falciparum* has been created in the eastern and southern Shan state of Myanmar in the vicinity of intensive mining activity (85% of infections are multiple-drug resistant). Malaria has declined in the previous epicenter on the Thailand–Cambodia border as a result of a halt in the cross-border population movement. The areas of eastern Shan state, Myanmar; Thailand; the People's Republic of China; and Laos have now become the epicenter of drug-resistant *P. falciparum*. This epicenter is extending south in the Kayah and Karen states of Myanmar and to the north toward Kachin state (ACTMalaria 2000).

Socioeconomic Determinants

Other important determinants of malaria are population, poverty, and political unrest. Every day, 250,000 new people come into the world. In 1995, the world population was 5.7 billion; Asia's share was 3.4 billion. By 2020, the SEA Region's population is expected to be 2 billion, more than one-quarter of the world's projected 7.9 billion people. Population growth will be accompanied by rapid urbanization. The urban population in the SEA Region is expected to reach 43% by 2020. The ceaseless flow of people into cities is likely to lead to further unhygienic living conditions in slums and to culminate in the proliferation of infectious diseases. Today, 1.3 billion people live in absolute poverty (on less than US$1 per day), 840 million people suffer from hunger, and 2 billion are malnourished; 70% of these people are Asians, and half of the developing world's poor live in southern Asia. Together, Bangladesh and eastern India have as many poor as all of sub-Saharan Africa. Malaria is restricted to the world's low- and middle-income countries.

An estimated 80% of the children in Southeast Asian countries suffer from protein-calorie malnutrition, and anemia continues to be an important factor in contributing to the high prevalence of low birth weights and high maternal mortality. In India, Nepal, and Bangladesh, as many as 48% of boys and 52% of girls weigh less than 5.5 pounds (2.5 kilograms) at birth and suffer considerable initial disadvantages (Kondrachine, Jung, and Akiyama 1991). Low birth weights have serious health consequences in malaria-endemic regions, because anemia commonly accompanies malaria and is often a life-threatening complication. Severe malaria-related anemia is more common in areas where infection is sustained throughout the year. Hemolysis is the main factor contributing to anemia of acute *falciparum* malaria (Marsh 1992). Preexisting iron deficiency significantly aggravates the severity of the anemia that accompanies malaria (Das et al. 1999).

In many instances, political disturbance has been responsible for major malaria outbreaks, and special health services were mobilized to contain the outbreaks. Examples of such disturbances include the 1959 migration of nearly 80,000 Tibetan refugees to 10 states in India and the 1971 influx of refugees from Bangladesh to Assam, West Bengal, and Tripura. Because of the civil unrest in many states in India, today there is no spraying or surveillance in areas such as northeastern India, where the problem of drug-resistant malaria is most pronounced. The Dandakaranya resettlement project in Bastar district, Madhya Pradesh, India, was established in 1958 for displaced people from East Pakistan (now Bangladesh); an estimated 35,000 families were settled there by 1986. The area was surrounded by tribal settlements with high incidence of *P. falciparum,* and in 1977 and 1978, an explosive outbreak of malaria occurred in first the Dandakaranya project and then the entire Bastar district (NMEP 1986). The problems of the Karen tribe in Myanmar and temporary settlements in Thailand are additional examples of high malaria-related morbidity and mortality in areas of political unrest.

In most tribal areas in India, frequent plastering of mud on insecticide-sprayed walls eliminates the effectiveness of insecticides. This population suffers the most from malaria because of poor health services, inaccessibility of settlements, and high receptivity for *P. falciparum* transmission. Large tribal populations settled in forested areas still believe that diseases are due to divine vengeance for wrongdoing, the effects of evil spirits, or planetary positions. Villages are near rivers or streams; houses are made of mud and thatched roofs and often are shared with cattle. The terrain is very difficult, lacking all-weather roads, and large areas remain inundated with rainfall for months during the transmission season. Deep jungles and degraded forests, along with weak health infrastructures, make the people most vulnerable to malaria and other diseases.

In eastern Thailand, socioeconomic status, the location of houses near malaria breeding sites, the presence of vegetation for resting mosquitoes, alternative hosts for feeding, and various interventions affect the exposure of humans to mosquito bites (Suvannadabba 1991). In southern Sri Lanka, the risk of malaria was found to be 2.5 times higher in residents of poorly constructed houses than those living in well-constructed houses (Gunawardena et al. 1998; Gamage-Mendis et al. 1991); living close to a stream was also a risk factor for malaria (van der Hoek et al. 1998).

A study of the economic burden of malaria in India showed that in 1991, malaria was responsible for an economic loss of half a billion to a billion U.S. dollars annually, and, because malaria receptivity is constantly increasing, this economic burden will continue to rise (Sharma 1996b). The World Bank estimated 0.9 million disability-adjusted life years (DALYs) for 1990 (World Bank 1993), and the malaria situation has considerably deteriorated since then. Treatment of malaria is expensive, particularly for people who live in poor communities. The relative cost of malaria treatment for one full course of treatment for an adult was calculated by WHO (1990) as US$0.08 for chloroquine, US$0.13 for a sulfadoxine–pyrimethamine combination, US$0.99 for intravenous quinine, $1.50 for quinine pills, US$1.92 for mefloquine, and US$5.31 for halofantrine. In terms of economic loss, a seven-day wage loss is common. The average cost of malaria treatment comes to US$5–10 and, in complicated cases, the treatment cost may go up to US$500–1,000 or more. The prevailing cost of malaria treatment is beyond the affordable limits of poor people.

A shortfall in the supply of insecticides—by roughly 50%—is another factor in malaria prevalence. When there is not enough insecticide available, partial spraying results in the rise of malaria and, eventually, epidemics. The excessive use of antimalaria drugs to combat malaria, combined with improper use, generates asymptomatic carriers and results in a rising trend of mono- and multiple-drug resistance. This situation further enhances malaria-related morbidity and mortality, and the cost of treatment of drug-resistant malaria increases by factors of 10–40 or more. In some areas, insecticides intended for public health applications are diverted to agriculture, resulting in poor malaria control and food chain contamination. A community's perception that malaria control is the sole responsibility of the government is also a major obstacle to achieving their sustained participation.

Conclusion

It is important to underscore the importance of the Roll Back Malaria initiative launched in 1998 by WHO. Roll Back Malaria envisions a partnership in malaria control and works at the community level, with a primary emphasis on malaria control for the poor and marginalized populations who have little access to health care. Sustainable malaria control requires a primary attack on poverty, health system reforms, an emphasis on community-based approaches, and investments in research and development.

In closing, I wish to quote L.W. Hackett (1937): "Everything about malaria is so molded by local conditions that it becomes a thousand epidemiological puzzles. Like chess, it is played with a few pieces but is capable of an infinite variety of situations."

Disclaimer

Opinions expressed in this chapter are the author's only and do not necessarily reflect the policies and views of the World Health Organization.

References

ACTMalaria. 2000. Malaria Situation in 1999. *ACTMalaria* 4: 1–8.

Amerasinghe, F.P., and T.G. Ariyasena. 1990. Larval Survey of Surface Water-Breeding Mosquitoes during Irrigation Development in the Mahaweli Project, Sri Lanka. *Journal of Medical Entomology* 27: 789–802.

Amerasinghe, F.P., and N.G. Indrajith. 1994. Postirrigation Breeding Patterns of Surface Water Mosquitoes in the Mahaweli Project, Sri Lanka, and Comparisons with Preceding Developmental Phases. *Journal of Medical Entomology* 34: 516–23.

Bouma, M.J., and H.J. van der Kaay. 1994. Epidemic Malaria in India and the El Niño Southern Oscillation. *Lancet* 344(8937): 1638–39.

———. 1996. The El Niño Southern Oscillation and the Historic Malaria Epidemics on the Indian Subcontinent and Sri Lanka: An Early Warning System for Future Epidemics. *Tropical Medicine and International Health* 1(1): 86–96.

Bouma, M.J., H.E. Sondorp, and H.J. van der Kaay. 1994. Climate Change and Periodic Epidemic Malaria. *Lancet* 343(8910): 1440.

Bunnag, D., S. Sornmani, S. Pinichpongse, and C. Harinasuta. 1979. Surveillance of Water-Borne Parasitic Infections and Studies on the Impact of Ecological Changes on Vector Mosquitoes of Malaria after Dam Construction. In *Proceedings of the Twenty-first SEAMEO-TROPMED Seminar, Environmental Impact on Human Health in South East and East Asia, Tokyo and Tsukuba*, edited by Mir Mulla. SEAMEO-TROPMED: Bangkok, Thailand, 656–60.

Christophers, R. 1911. *Malaria in the Punjab: Scientific Memoir, Medical and Sanitary Department, Government of India*. Calcutta, India: Government Printing Press.

Clyde, D. 1987. Variations in Response of Malaria Parasites to Drugs in Asia and Oceania. *La Medicina Tropical* 3: 3–21.

Das, B.S., N.K. Nanda, P.K. Rath, R.N. Satapathy, and D.B. Das. 1999. Anaemia in Acute, *Plasmodium falciparum* Malaria in Children from Orissa State, India. *Annals of Tropical Medicine and Parasitology* 93: 109–18.

Dev, V., and V.P. Sharma. 1995. Persistent Transmission of Malaria in Sonapur PHC Kamrup District. *Journal of Parasitic Diseases* 19: 65–68.

Dua, V.K., P.K. Kar, and V.P. Sharma. 1996. Chloroquine-Resistant *Plasmodium vivax* Malaria in India. *Tropical Medicine and International Health* 1(6): 816–19.

Dua, V.K., S.K. Sharma, A. Srivastava, and V.P. Sharma. 1997. Bioenvironmental Control of Industrial Malaria at Bharat Heavy Electricals Ltd., Hardwar, India: Results of a Nine-Year Study (1987–1995). *Journal of the American Mosquito Control Association* 13: 278–85.

Gamage-Mendis, A., R. Carter, C. Mendis, A.P.K. de Zoysa, P.R.J. Herath, and K.N. Mendis. 1991. Clustering of Malaria Infections within an Endemic Population: Risk of Malaria Associated with the Type of Housing Construction. *American Journal of Tropical Medicine and Hygiene* 45: 77–85.

Gill, C.A. 1923. The Prediction of Malaria Epidemics. *Indian Journal of Medical Research* 10: 1136–43.

———. 1936. Some Points in the Epidemiology of Malaria Arising out of the Study of the Malaria Epidemic in Ceylon in 1934–35. *Transactions of the Royal Society of Tropical Medicine and Hygiene* 5: 427–66.

Gratz, N.G. 1999. Emerging and Resurging Vector-Borne Diseases. *Annual Review of Entomology* 44: 51–75.

Gunawardena, D.M., A.R. Wickremasinghe, L.Muthuwatta, S. Weerasingha, J. Rajakaruna, T. Senanayaka, P.K. Kotta, N. Attanayake, R. Carter, and K.N. Mendis. 1998. Malaria Risk Factors in an Endemic Region of Sri Lanka, and the Impact and Cost Implications of Risk Factor-Based Interventions. *American Journal of Tropical Medicine and Hygiene* 58: 533–42.

Hackett, L.W. 1937. *Malaria in Europe*. Oxford, U.K.: Oxford University Press.

Jana-Kara, B.R., W.A. Wajihullah, B. Shahi, V. Dev, C.F. Curtis, and V.P. Sharma. 1995. Deltamethrin Impregnated Bednets against *Anopheles minimus* Transmitted Malaria in Assam, India. *Journal of Tropical Medicine and Hygiene* 98: 73–83.

Kalra, N.L. 1991. Forest Malaria Vectors in India: Ecological Characteristics and Epidemiological Implications. In *Forest Malaria in South East Asia,* edited by V.P. Sharma and A.V. Kondrachine. Delhi, India: Malaria Research Centre, 94–114.

Kar, I., S.K Subbarao, A. Eapen, J. Ravindran, T.S. Satyanarayan, K. Raghvendra, N. Nanda, and V.P. Sharma. 1999. Evidence for a New Malaria Vector Species, Species E, within the *Anopheles culicifacies* Complex (Diptera: Culicidae). *Journal of Medical Entomology* 36: 595–600.

Kondrashin, A.V., R.K. Jung, and J. Akiyama. 1991. Ecological Aspects of Forest Malaria in Southeast Asia. In *Forest Malaria in South East Asia,* edited by V.P. Sharma and A.V. Kondrachine. Delhi, India: Malaria Research Centre, 1–28.

Kumar, A., V.P. Sharma, and D. Thavaselvam. 1991. Malaria Related to Constructions in Panaji, Goa. *Indian Journal of Malariology* 28: 219–26.

Lindsay, S.W., and M.H. Birley. 1996. Climate Change and Malaria Transmission. *Annals of Tropical Medicine and Parasitology* 90: 573–88.

Macdonald, G. 1957. *The Epidemiology and Control of Malaria*. Oxford, U.K.: Oxford University Press.

Marsh, K. 1992. Malaria: A Neglected Disease? *Parasitology* 104: S53–S69.

Mathur, K.K., G. Harpalani, N.L. Kalra, G.G.K. Murthy, and M.V.V.L. Narasimham. 1992. Epidemic of Malaria in Barmer District (Thar Desert) of Rajasthan during 1990. *Indian Journal of Malariology* 29: 1–10.

Miller, L.H. 1994. Impact of Malaria on Genetic Polymorphism and Genetic Diseases in Africans and African Americans. *Proceedings of the National Academy of Sciences USA* 91: 2415–19.

NAMP (National Anti Malaria Program). 1999. *Annual Report*. Delhi, India: Directorate of NAMP.

Nanda, N., H. Joshi, S.K. Subbarao, R.S. Yadav, R.P. Shukla, V.K. Dua, and V.P. Sharma. 1996. *Anopheles fluviatilis* Complex: Host Feeding Patterns of Species S, T, and U. *Journal of the American Mosquito Control Association* 12: 147–49.

NMEP (National Malaria Eradication Programme). 1986. *Malaria and Its Control in India,* Volume I. Delhi, India: NMEP, Government of India.

Nosten, F., T. Ter Kuile, T. Chongsuphajaisiddhi, C. Luxemburger, H.K. Webster, M. Edstein, L. Phaipun, K.L. Thew, and N.J. White. 1991. Mefloquine Resistant Falciparum Malaria on the Thai-Burmese Border. *Lancet* 337(8750): 1140–3.

Pattanayak, S., V.P. Sharma, N.L. Kalra, V.S. Orlov, and R.S. Sharma. 1994. Malaria Paradigms in India and Control Strategies. *Indian Journal of Malariology* 31: 141–99.

Raghavendra, K., K. Vasantha, S.K. Subbarao, M.K.K. Pillai, and V.P. Sharma. 1991. Resistance in *Anopheles culicifacies* Sibling Species B and C to Malathion in Andhra Pradesh and Gujarat States, India. *Journal of the American Mosquito Control Association* 7(2): 255–59.

Raghavendra, K., S.K. Subbarao, K. Vasantha, M.K.K. Pillai, and V.P. Sharma. 1992. Differential Selection of Malathion Resistance in *Anopheles culicifacies* A and B (Diptera: Culicidae) in Haryana State, India. *Journal of Medical Entomology* 29: 183–87.

Rajagopal, R. 1977. Malathion Resistance in *Anopheles culicifacies* in Gujarat. *Indian Journal of Medical Research* 66: 27–28.

Rawlings, P., P.R.J. Herath, and S. Kelly. 1985. *Anopheles culicifacies* (Diptera: Culicidae): DDT Resistance in Sri Lanka prior to and after Cessation of DDT Spraying. *Journal of Medical Entomology* 22: 361–65.

Rosenberg, R., and N.P. Maheswary. 1982. Forest Malaria in Bangladesh. II. Transmission by *Anopheles dirus. American Journal of Tropical Medicine and Hygiene* 31: 183–91.

Rosenberg, R., R.G. Andre, and L. Somchit. 1990. Highly Efficient Dry Season Transmission of Malaria in Thailand. *Transactions of the Royal Society of Tropical Medicine and Hygiene* 84: 22–28.

Sen, S.K., V.M. John, K.S. Krishnan, and R. Rajagopal. 1973. Studies on Malaria Transmission in Tirap District, Arunachal Pradesh (N.E.F.A). *Journal of Communicable Diseases* 5: 98–110.

Sharma, V.P. 1987. Community-Based Malaria Control in India. *Parasitology Today* 3(7): 222–26.

———. 1996a. Re-emergence of Malaria in India. *Indian Journal of Medical Research* 103: 26–45.

———. 1996b. Malaria: Cost to India and Future Trends. *South East Asian Journal of Tropical Medicine and Public Health* 27: 4–14.

———. 1998. Fighting Malaria in India. *Current Science* 75: 1127–40.

Sharma, V.P., and A.V. Kondrachine, eds. 1991. *Forest Malaria in South East Asia*. Delhi, India: Malaria Research Centre.

Sharma, V.P., and K.N. Mehrotra. 1986. Malaria Resurgence in India: A Critical Study. *Social Science and Medicine* 22: 835–45.

Sharma, V.P., C. Prasittisuk, and A.V. Kondrashin. 1991. Magnitude of Forest Related Malaria in the South-East Asia Region. In *Forest Malaria in South East Asia: Proceedings of an Informal Consultative Meeting*. WHO/MRC Publication. New Delhi, India: Malaria Research Centre.

Sharma, V.P., R.K. Chandrahas, M.A. Ansari, K. Srivastava, R.K. Razdan, C.P. Batra, K. Raghavedra, B.N. Nagpal, S.C. Bhalla, and G.K. Sharma. 1986. Impact of DDT and HCH Spraying on Malaria Transmission in Villages with DDT and HCH Resistant *Anopheles culicifacies. Indian Journal of Malariology* 23: 27–38.

Sharma, V.P., B.N. Nagpal, A. Srivastava, and N.L. Kalra. 1999. Malaria on Worker Efficiency in Tea Estates in Assam, India. In *Global Advances in Tea Science,* edited by N.K. Jain. New Delhi, India: Aravali Books International, 323–32.

Shukla, R.P., A.C. Pandey, and A. Mathur. 1995. Bionomics of Vector Anophelines in District Nainital, Uttar Pradesh. *Indian Journal of Malariology* 32: 119–28.

Singh, N., and V.P. Sharma. 1989. Persistent Malaria Transmission in Kundam Block, District Jabalpur (M.P.). *Indian Journal of Malariology* 26: 1–7.

Singh, N., O.P. Singh, and V.P. Sharma. 1996. Dynamics of Malaria Transmission in Forested and Deforested Regions of Mandla District, Central India (Madhya Pradesh). *Journal of the American Mosquito Control Association* 12: 225–34.

Singhanetra-Renard, A. 1986. Population Movement, Socio-economic Behavior and the Transmission of Malaria in Northern Thailand. *Southeast Asian Journal of Tropical Medicine and Public Health* 17: 396–405.

Subbarao, S.K. 1998. Anophelene Species Complexes in South-East Asia. Technical Publication No. 16. New Delhi: World Health Organization Regional Office for South-East Asia.

Subbarao, S.K., K. Vasantha, and V.P. Sharma. 1988. Responses of *Anopheles culicifacies* Sibling Species A and B to DDT and HCH in India: Implications in Malaria Control. *Medical and Veterinary Entomology* 2: 219–23.

Subbarao, S.K., N. Nanda, K. Vasantha, V.K. Dua, M.S. Malhotra, R.S. Yadav, and V.P. Sharma. 1993. Cytogenic Evidence for 3 Sibling Species in *Anopholes fluviatilis* (Diptera, Culicidae). *Annals of the Entomological Society of America* 87: 116–21.

Suvannadabba, S. 1991. Deforestation for Agriculture and Its Impact on Malaria in Southern Thailand. In *Forest Malaria in South East Asia,* edited by V.P. Sharma and A.V. Kondrachine. Delhi, India: Malaria Research Centre, 221–26.

Swaroop, S. 1946. Forecasting of Epidemic Malaria in the Punjab, India. *American Journal of Tropical Medicine* 29: 1–17.

Thein, H., and M.-M. Soe. 1989. Population Mobility and Malaria Contraction on Either Side of Bogo Yoma in Bogo Division, Myanmar. *Health Science Journal* 1: 118–21.

Trape, J.F. 2000. Antimalarial Drug Resistance in Africa: Epidemiological Background of a Disaster. In *Multi-Drug Resistance in Emerging and Re-emerging Diseases,* edited by R.C. Mahajan and A. Therwath. New Delhi, India: Narosa Publishing House, Chapter 19, 203–9.

Trigg, P.I., and A.V. Kondrachine. 1998. The Current Global Malaria Situation. In *Malaria: Parasite Biology, Pathogenesis, and Protection,* edited by I.W. Sherman. Washington, D.C.: ASM Press, 11–22.

van der Hoek, W., F. Konradsen, D. Perera, P.H. Amerasinghe, and F.P. Amerasinghe. 1997. Correlation between Rainfall and Malaria in the Dry Zone of Sri Lanka. *Annals of Tropical Medicine and Parasitology* 91: 945–49.

van der Hoek, W., F. Konradsen, D.S. Dijkstra, P.H. Amersinghe, and F.P. Amersinghe. 1998. Risk Factors for Malaria: A Microepidemiological Study in a Village in Sri Lanka. *Transactions of the Royal Society of Tropical Medicine and Hygiene* 92: 265–69.

White, N.J. 1999a. Antimalarial Drug Resistance and Combination Therapy. *Philosophical Transactions of the Royal Society of London B* 354: 739–49.

———. 1999b. Delaying Antimalarial Drug Resistance with Combination Therapy. *Parasitologica* 41: 301–8.

WHO (World Health Organization). 1990. *Practical Chemotherapy of Malaria.* Technical Report Series 805. Geneva, Switzerland: WHO.

Wijesundera, M.D. 1988. Malaria Outbreaks in New Foci in Sri Lanka. *Parasitology Today* 4: 147–150.

World Bank. 1993. *Investing in Health: World Development Indicators.* World Bank Development Report. Oxford, U.K.: Oxford University Press.

Yacob, K.B.M., and S. Swaroop. 1945. Investigation of Long Term Periodicity in the Incidence of Epidemic Malaria in the Punjab. *Journal of the Malaria Institute of India* 6: 39–51.

Yadav, R.S., T.R.R. Sampath, V.P. Sharma, T. Adak, and S.K. Ghosh. 1998. Evaluation of Lambdacyhalothrin-Impregnated Bednets in a Malaria Endemic Area of India. Part 3. Effects on Malaria Incidence and Clinical Measures. *Journal of the American Mosquito Control Association* 14: 444–50.

Boundaries, Health Impact Assessment, and Integrated Vector Management

Robert Bos

V.P. Sharma's chapter on the malaria situation in countries of the World Health Organization (WHO) South East Asia (SEA) Region evokes comments in three subject areas: boundaries, the opportunities offered by health impact assessment (HIA), and integrated vector management (IVM).

Boundaries

The politically determined boundaries of the WHO SEA Region make little sense in terms of malaria ecology, particularly the distribution of different vector species and species complexes. Although the problem may seem insignificant at first sight, it complicates work on contextual determinants with other United Nations agencies, because their regional division of the world does not coincide with that of WHO.

The fact that administrative and ecosystem boundaries usually do not coincide creates more important problems at the country level. In the collection of health (malaria) data, it confuses the analysis of possible ecological determinants of transmission, and in the delivery of health services, it may give rise to important differences in the health status of communities that inhabit the same ecosystem but are separated by administrative boundaries.

At a smaller scale—the urban environment—a similar phenomenon can be observed. This is relevant in the WHO SEA Region, where (as Sharma points out) urban malaria, transmitted by *Anopheles stephensi,* is an important public health problem. Part of this problem is found in peri-urban areas, the fringe area around big cities, with their particular mosaic of urban and rural environmental characteristics and intense human mobility. Peri-urban areas normally are outside of the jurisdiction of the municipal authorities; therefore, the delivery of adequate diagnostic, treatment, and vector control services are hampered or impossible.

The issue of climate change also raises the question of boundaries. Most models of climate change focus on long-term trends in average temperatures and rainfall. The impact of these changes is mainly a shift in the boundaries of potential malaria risk areas to higher altitudes and latitudes. For most parts of the SEA Region, these changes are not relevant (highlands excluded). However, trends in weather patterns—particularly the intensification of extreme weather conditions linked to El Niño–Southern Oscillation (ENSO)—are important. In unstable malaria areas of southeast Asia, they contribute to the patchiness of malaria in time and space. Other contextual determinants are linked to vector ecology (e.g., in Pakistan, waterlogged soil increases *Anopheles culicifacies* populations; in Bangladesh, waterlogged soil has no impact on *Anopheles minimus*). On the other hand, lowering the groundwater level in Bangladesh, as proposed under the Flood Action Plan, is expected to increase the risk of another vector-borne disease, leishmaniasis. Factors other than those linked to the physical environment also play a role, such as institutional or political; these other factors explain the fact that 61% of malaria mortality in the region occurs in Myanmar. They also explain the elevated malaria incidence among tribal groups in India.

Effective malaria control in the SEA Region is facilitated by a very strong knowledge base, going back to the beginning of the twentieth century. A reliable database on vector biology and ecology allows the attribution, in a qualitative and sometimes quantitative way, of malaria incidence to specific contextual determinants.

Briefly diverting from Southeast Asia to sub-Saharan Africa, conventional wisdom has it that the same approach of studying contextual determinants and manipulating them to reduce malaria transmission is generally not a feasible option in an African setting. This may be true at present for large parts of sub-Saharan Africa, but it is a mistake to discard options for transmission risk reduction in that part of the world categorically. Africa south of the Sahara is not an ecologically homogeneous region, and as our knowledge base increases, opportunities for malaria control through the manipulation of contextual determinants will present themselves (e.g., research on zooprophylaxis, the management of livestock, has been initiated for transmission risk reduction in areas with zoophilic *Anopheles arabiensis*). Furthermore, as the impact of the Roll Back Malaria initiative changes the local epidemiology of malaria (to different extents in different settings), opportunities for transmission risk reduction are likely to unfold. So, a rapid increase in our knowledge base of vector ecology and biology in Africa to the level found in the WHO SEA Region is a priority issue if we want to take maximum advantage of these opportunities.

Health Impact Assessment

Sharma referred to the Narmada Dam and its potential impact on malaria. Earlier this year, WHO (2000) completed a contribution to the World Commission on Dams, which was established in 1998 by the World Bank and the World Conservation Union to carry out an independent assessment of the development effectiveness of dams. The World Commission on Dams published its report (WCD 2000) in November, 2000, with a strong and prominent endorsement of health impact assessment (HIA) among the key best-practice elements in decisionmaking for the planning of dam projects. The WHO contribution focused on three concepts:

- Equity—Dams provide an important contribution to development, including to human health. Benefits (as well as risks), however, are not distributed equitably, and this issue should be addressed at the early planning stage. Vulnerable groups should be identified, and measures to minimize their health risks should be included.
- Economics—Environmental management for the reduction of health risks partly suffers from the concept of discounting of future costs, which works against capital investments in infrastructure development or improvement, even though past experience proves the sustainability of this approach, as well as its resilience in situations of political turmoil when regular health services may break down.
- Environment—Awareness is growing that health needs to be considered as a crosscutting issue in the context of environmental assessment. In the past, it was simply one of the items on the environmental impact assessment (EIA) checklist. The concept of an associated but separate HIA is increasingly gaining support.

HIA methodology categorizes risk factors, which may be useful to ensure a complete coverage of filters in models based on contextual determinants. They include community risk factors (e.g., genetic makeup, nutritional status, migration, immunity, occupation, and gender), environmental risk factors (physical as well as social environment), and institutional risk factors (capacity, capability, and jurisdiction). These risk factors can be considered in the prospective HIA of development projects, or they can be studied as part of a strategic risk assessment.

In this connection, the recent policy redirections by the World Bank are significant. In June 1999, the World Bank organized a brainstorming session to explore its comparative advantage in the Roll Back Malaria initiative. The conclusion was that the incorporation of malaria transmission safeguards the infrastructure projects for which loans are provided to client countries. This is compatible with the bank's mission as well as with the objectives of the Roll Back Malaria initiative. This position was reinforced by a May 15, 2000, press release from the World Bank, announcing the preparation of a new environment strategy aimed at integrating environmental concerns into its mainstream poverty alleviation and economic development efforts.

Important for the case of HIA, the press release states, among other things, that

- the emphasis is on incorporating sustainability into all the bank's activities to ensure that economic growth does not come at the expense of the people's health and future opportunities because of degraded natural resources and ecosystems;
- the draft strategy will call for a fresh look at the bank's policies on environmental safeguards, guidelines, regional environmental strategies, environmental sector work, and sector strategies such as the forest and water sectors;
- the main objectives improve human health by reducing people's exposure to environmental factors such as indoor and urban air pollution, water- and vector-borne diseases, and toxic substances.

From the perspective of WHO, the promotion of HIA policies and procedures has become a matter of urgency. Capacity building at the country level has been ongoing for several years (WHO/DBL 2001), the development banks are coming on board, and it is perhaps time to explore whether the private sector—particularly multinational companies—also can adopt HIAs in their development work. WHO's role in harmonizing methods, procedures, and policy will be crucial to its long-term success.

Integrated Vector Management

Experience in Southeast Asia shows how, under excessive chemical pressures on ecosystems (both through drugs aimed at the parasite and insecticides aimed at the vector), induction and spread of resistance can take place very rapidly. This undermines the sustainability of these chemicals as a resource to deal with really serious situations.

At the same time, there is a long history of successful environmental management for vector control in the WHO SEA Region. Community participation is a feasible approach in many of the cultures of the region. Therefore, there is fertile ground for the further development of integrated vector management (IVM). It requires the development and testing of decisionmaking criteria as well as procedures and methods of decentralized monitoring that will allow the deployment of a dynamic package of evidence-based control measures, including insecticides, where necessary.

Integrated pest management (IPM) in agriculture provides a workable starting point for the implementation of IVM strategies. IPM has evolved from a strategy based on economic thresholds to an ecosystem assessment aimed at ensuring ecosystem integrity while selectively suppressing pest species. The ecosystem model that IPM currently provides is arguably even more relevant for IVM than the IPM economic threshold model of 10 years ago.

Vector control concepts have evolved from integrated vector control (1983) to selective vector control (1994) and, most recently, to targeted vector control. Currently, a working definition of integrated vector management is under debate: IVM is a process of evidence-based decision-making procedures aimed to plan, deliver, monitor, and evaluate targeted, cost-effective, and sustainable combinations of regulatory and operational vector control measures, with a measurable impact on transmission risks, adhering to the principles of subsidiarity, intersectoriality, and partnership. In addition to a shift from centrally directed vector control programs to decentralized planning and implementation—which will allow effective consideration of locally important contextual determinants of malaria—a transition to IVM will also imply a change from a traditional emphasis on technical tools to an emphasis on development of managerial good practice.

Disclaimer

Opinions expressed in this chapter are the author's only and do not necessarily reflect the policies and views of the World Health Organization.

References

WCD (World Commission on Dams). 2000. *Dams and Development: A New Framework for Decision Making*. London: Earthscan Publications.

WHO (World Health Organization). 2000. *Human Health and Dams*. Submission to the World Commission on Dams (WCD). Document No, WHO/SDE/ESH/00.01. Geneva, Switzerland: WHO.

WHO/DBL (World Health Organization/Danish Bilharriasis Laboratory). 2001. Intersectoral Decision-Making Skills in Support of Health Impact Assessment of Development Projects. Document No. WHO/SDE/WSH/00.9. Geneva, Switzerland, and Charlottenlund, Denmark: WHO and DBL.

Chapter 9

Determinants of Malaria in the Middle East and North Africa

Andrei E. Beljaev

The *Middle East* is usually defined as "the lands around the southern and eastern shores of the Mediterranean Sea, extending from Morocco to the Arabian Peninsula and Iran and sometimes beyond" (*Encyclopaedia Britannica* 2000). This area roughly corresponds to the World Health Organization's (WHO's) Eastern Mediterranean Region, to which 23 countries belong (Afghanistan, Bahrain, Cyprus, Djibouti, Egypt, Islamic Republic of Iran, Iraq, Jordan, Kuwait, Lebanon, Libyan Arab Jamahiriya, Morocco, Oman, Palestine, Pakistan, Qatar, Saudi Arabia, Somalia, Sudan, Syrian Arab Republic, Tunisia, United Arab Emirates [UAE], and Yemen). The region spreads west to east from Morocco to Pakistan, and north to south from Iran to Somalia, thus including three sub-Saharan African countries (Djibouti, Somalia, and Sudan) that gravitate to the Middle East politically and culturally. Some countries that are outside the WHO Eastern Mediterranean Region but belong to the same geocultural entity are also considered in this chapter, when appropriate.

Malaria Situation in the Middle East

Historic Aspect

Since antiquity, malaria has played a major role in the communities around the Mediterranean Sea. Ancient and medieval physicians starting with Hippocrates described diseases that may be identified as different types of malaria. Mummies from predynastic Egypt (3200 B.C.) contain histidine-rich protein 2 (HRP-2), an antigen to the malaria parasite *Plasmodium falciparum*, strongly suggesting the presence of malaria at that time (Miller et al. 1994). However, it seems that *P. falciparum* spread massively in the Mediterranean only relatively recently (Ayala, Escalante, and Rich 1999; Coluzzi 1999).

More than once, the ravages of malaria have led to the disruption of the socioeconomic fabric of societies and the decline and disappearance of civilizations (Bruce-Chwatt 1965; McNeill 1979; Sherman 1998). Societies tried to protect themselves from malaria, and some of the activities (e.g., land reclamation and proper maintenance of irrigation systems) were instrumental in keeping malaria in check, despite ignorance of the cause.

On the other hand, malaria was an effective barrier to the colonization of Africa by European powers during the sixteenth through the nineteenth centuries. In contrast with the tropical and equatorial areas of the Americas and Asia, and despite the proximity of Africa to Europe, colonization of the interior of the "dark continent" became possible only after quinine (recommended in 1847 by A. Bryson for the British Navy) became available for chemoprophylaxis in the 1850s (Gelfand 1965).

The area of malaria distribution reached its maximum extent by the end of the nineteenth century and beginning of the twentieth century (Lysenko and Semashko 1968), when the whole of the Mediterranean and most of Europe were affected. During the first half of the twentieth century, malaria started to disappear from industrialized countries as a result of ecological change, increased availability of medical care, and improved quality of life. At the same time, malaria was still highly prevalent all over the Mediterranean, including the European portion. Limited attempts to control malaria by land reclamation started very early and were later complemented by larviciding and the use of drugs (Bruce-Chwatt and de Zulueta 1980). In the Middle East, malaria control received a boost during World War II, motivated mostly by the war effort (Leeson et al. 1950; Farid 1980). After the war, this process accelerated after two potent tools that had been used mostly for protection of troops became widely available for civil use: the drug chloroquine and the insecticide DDT revolutionized malaria control.

Very soon thereafter, the situation radically changed in most of the Middle East as countries implemented a malaria eradication strategy of indoor DDT spraying endorsed by the Eighth World Health Assembly in 1955 (WHO 1955). However, the eradication effort did not touch the stronghold of malaria in sub-Saharan Africa. In 1970, the WHO Expert Committee acknowledged that in large areas of tropical Africa, time-limited malaria eradication programs were often impracticable (WHO 1971).

In sub-Saharan Africa, the situation for malaria control started to change only in the early 1990s. The turning point occurred with the Interregional Conference on Malaria in Brazzaville, Congo, in October 1991, which endorsed a malaria control strategy in Africa (WHO/AFRO 1991). It was followed by the World Declaration on the Control of Malaria, adopted by the Ministerial Conference on Malaria in October 1992. The declaration committed the global community to controlling malaria, with special emphasis on the most affected countries, almost all of which were in sub-Saharan Africa (WHO 1992).

Almost all the countries of sub-Saharan Africa, including the three that belong to the WHO Eastern Mediterranean Region (Djibouti, Somalia, and Sudan), have expressed political commitment and have taken practical steps to control malaria. Awareness of the magnitude of the malaria problem in Africa is now universal. The highest level of commitment to malaria control was expressed at the Abuja Summit on Malaria on April 25, 2000.

Current Situation

The current status of malaria in the Middle East (Figure 9-1) reflects a half-century of organized efforts to control malaria. Depending on the degree of progress, three groups of countries are distinguished within the WHO Eastern Mediterranean Region.

Group 1. Malaria transmission was interrupted in nine Group 1 countries, starting in Cyprus in 1953 and ending in Tunisia in 1979; the other countries are Bahrain, Jordan, Kuwait, Lebanon, Libya, Palestine, and Qatar. Despite occasional episodes of transmis-

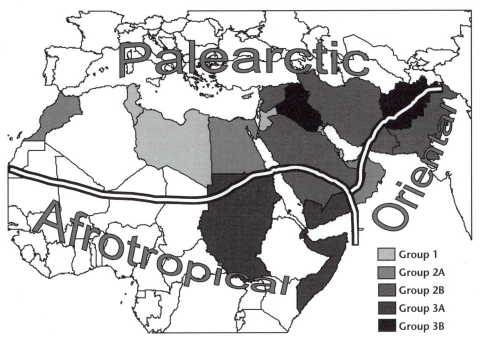

Figure 9-1. Status of Malaria Programs in the WHO Eastern Mediterranean Region, mid-2000

sion in some of these countries after malaria importation, this achievement has been sustained, and the countries are considered "transmission free." Group 1 countries make up about 7% of the population of the WHO Eastern Mediterranean Region.

Group 2. The majority of the population in the WHO Eastern Mediterranean Region (72%) lives in Group 2 countries, which consist of two subgroups in which malaria is effectively controlled. Of this percentage, 21% of the population lives in Group 2a countries (Egypt, Morocco, Oman, and UAE), where malaria eradication is under way and feasible in the near future. The remaining 51% live in Group 2b countries (Iran, Pakistan, Saudi Arabia, and Syria), where good progress was achieved during the initial stages of malaria eradication, and reduction of malaria transmission is feasible.

Morocco and Egypt came very near to interrupting transmission by the late 1970s. However, during the 1980s, common wisdom was to brand malaria eradication "a failure," and even the word "eradication" became unpopular. Without a clearly expressed goal of complete transmission interruption and strong political commitment, it was impossible to steer the programs through the consolidation phase when suppression of residual transmission requires many more resources per case than during the initial attack. Consequently, the malaria eradication process in these countries stagnated.

In May 1997, representatives of the five North African countries (Algeria, Egypt, Libya, Morocco, and Tunisia) agreed at a meeting of the WHO African Regional Office (AFRO) and the WHO Eastern Mediterranean Regional Office (EMRO) in Tunis, Tunisia, that a complete interruption of malaria transmission in the North African subcontinent was feasible by 2002 (WHO/EMRO 1997). At the time the meeting was held, malaria transmission continued only in a few well-defined residual foci in three Moroccan provinces, one focus in Algeria, and one district of the Fayoum governorate in Egypt. In

1996, the number of *Plasmodium vivax* cases of local transmission for each of the three countries was 57, 24, and 2, respectively, whereas *P. falciparum* was found only in Egypt (21 cases). Setting a clear target contributed to rapid progress thereafter. By 1999, malaria transmission apparently stopped in Egypt and continued only in Khouribga province (17 autochthonous cases) in Morocco. However, the situation in Libya is far from clear (because of insufficient surveillance), so the existence of residual transmission in Libya cannot be ruled out.

Even before the 1997 meeting in Tunis, Oman had set a malaria eradication goal in 1991 on its own initiative (Beljaev 1999). The approach was a success; the number of locally contracted cases diminished from 37,220 in 1990 to only 30 in 1999. In the UAE, where receptivity is low and malaria transmission depends on the situation in Oman, no autochthonous cases were detected in 1998–1999.

In the Group 2b countries, malaria control programs usually began to stagnate at the consolidation phase, when political interest in malaria control waned and the programs themselves were getting less and less flexible, more and more bureaucratized. This situation was compounded by newly emerging technical problems, such as increasing insecticide and drug resistance, and declining public interest in vector control. As a result, malaria in these countries regained its endemicity by spreading from a few residual foci. However, the endemicity usually stayed at a level well below that of the pre-eradication epoch. In other words, success of the malaria eradication campaign was sustainable to some extent, except in the case of a complete failure of political systems, as in Afghanistan.

Group 3. The Group 3 countries represent only 21% of the WHO Eastern Mediterranean Region but generate 14 million to 15 million cases of malaria—more than 95% of the total annual caseload in the region. They are subdivided into two subgroups: Group 3a, in the Afrotropical region (Djibouti, Somalia, and Sudan [south of the Sahara] and Yemen [ecologically close to sub-Saharan Africa]), and Group 3b (Afghanistan and Iraq), which experiences complex emergencies with *P. vivax* mostly (Afghanistan) or exclusively (Iraq).

In Group 3a countries, malaria is transmitted by very potent vectors. The impossibility of interrupting malaria transmission in these areas was shown as long ago as the 1960s (Bruce-Chwatt 1979). Additionally, the status of all these countries (or at least considerable parts of their territories) has been chronic complex emergency for many years. The four Group 3a countries participated in the Roll Back Malaria (RBM) initiative, a program of intensified support to control malaria, started in 1998 with special WHO and external funds. After the advent of RBM, these countries continued to receive support to strengthen malaria control programs, mostly in terms of rehabilitation and capacity building. The situation has markedly improved during the past few years with respect to training, drug supply, surveillance, and epidemic preparedness.

Malaria control in the Group 3b countries was quite successful during the eradication era. Unfortunately, the achievements of the eradication campaign in Afghanistan have been completely obliterated by civil war. In Iraq, a malaria epidemic broke out in the wake of the Gulf War; 100,000 cases were confirmed annually in 1994 and 1995. Despite its enormity, this epidemic was not as murderous as one would expect from the experience of a half-century ago, because *P. falciparum* had been effectively and sustainably eliminated from Iraq during the malaria eradication effort. Large-scale antimalaria measures with indoor residual spraying as a main tool brought the incidence down to 4,134 cases in 1999, despite many obstacles caused by difficult economic conditions and international sanctions.

Parasitic System of Malaria

Understanding why malaria control and eradication succeeded in some parts of the region and failed in others informs projections for future malaria distribution. The complexity and heterogeneity of malaria cause much confusion. In this chapter, I analyze the complexity of malaria from an ecological point of view.

Parasite Species

Although the word "malaria" is traditionally used in its singular form, its plural form, "malarias," would be more justified (as done by Coatney et al. in one of the fundamental treatises on malaria, *The Primate Malarias* [1971]). Human malarias stem from at least four different infections. Genetic studies indicate that these malaria species are only remotely related (Ayala, Escalante, and Rich 1999). They demonstrate striking differences in pathology, epidemiology, and public health significance.

Of four *Plasmodium* species, two (*Plasmodium falciparum* and *Plasmodium vivax*) are currently predominant in the Middle East. *Plasmodium ovale,* although not a rare parasite in West Africa and central Africa, was always restricted in its distribution (Lysenko and Beljaev 1969) and in the area under consideration, was reliably found only in central and southern Sudan. *Plasmodium malariae* became very rare and soon disappeared after the onset of mass antimalaria campaigns in the 1960s, except in some sub-Saharan areas, probably because of its high sensitivity to common antimalaria drugs quinine and chloroquine; absence of dormancy in the liver; and slow development, in both the human host and mosquitoes (Beljaev et al. 1986).

The differences between *P. falciparum* and *P. vivax* as relevant to malaria control may be summarized as follows:

- *P. vivax* is adapted to colder climates than *P. falciparum* because it has a lower threshold of development in the mosquito and may lie dormant in the form of hypnozoites.
- *P. vivax* can infect geographically remote vectors, whereas *P. falciparum* infects only vectors from the same geographic area (discussed in more detail later).
- *P. vivax* is better controlled by antimalaria drugs than *P. falciparum* is because it is highly sensitive to drugs; gametocytes disappear soon after blood schizontocides are administered, and the life span of gametocytes is short.
- *P. vivax* is less easily controlled by antivector measures than *P. falciparum* is because it lies dormant and the infection lasts longer.
- *P. vivax* is less of a threat to public health than *P. falciparum* is, because the disease it inflicts is less severe, almost never causes death, and does not leave lasting sequelae.

Vectors

Diversity of the Vectors. Within the genus *Anopheles,* which includes all species of mosquitoes that transmit malaria to humans, at least six subgenera are recognized. Of the six, only two are known to exist in the Old World, *Anopheles sensu stricto* (*s.s.*) Meigen and *Cellia* Theobald. The former subgenus is predominant in tropical and equatorial zones and is better adapted to transmit malaria than the latter.

Anopheles larvae typically grow in natural water bodies with clean, slow-moving, warm water and sufficient aquatic vegetation. However, the ecological requirements of particular species may deviate from typical conditions. Some species do not need aquatic vegetation and can breed in very small pools, such as hoof prints (*Anopheles gambiae sensu lato* [*s.l.*]), human-made containers such as overhead water tanks and water coolers (*Anopheles stephensi*), and relatively cold water (*Anopheles claviger*).

Very often, in tropical and equatorial zones, more than one vector species are prevalent in the same area. Although they inhabit the same geographic area, sympatric species occupy different ecological niches. A well-known pair that inhabits the Indian subcontinent is *Anopheles fluviatilis*, which breeds in the running water that is typical of the rainy season, and *Anopheles culicifacies*, which breeds in the small pools that are found during droughts. Together, these two species can ensure continuous transmission in relay and maintain much higher endemicity than if they occurred separately.

Much is still unknown about the distribution of the species, because many recognized "species" are, in fact, groups of related sibling species. Although they are very close or even identical morphologically, they may be very distinct ecologically and possess different susceptibility to *Plasmodia* and, hence, have different abilities to transmit malaria. For example, the *An. gambiae s.l.* complex, which includes seven established and several incipient species (Goetzee, Craig, and le Sueur 2000), includes the extremely efficient vectors *An. gambiae s.s.* and *Anopheles arabiensis* as well as a very poor one, *Anopheles quadriannulatus.*

Qualities of *Anopheles* as Malaria Vectors. Several characteristics determine whether a species is a competent vector. In order of importance, they are as follows.

- *Susceptibility* to parasites varies from a total incompatibility to a very high infection rate. Different susceptibility of the same vector to geographic variants of the same parasite has been reported. *P. falciparum* is much better adapted to local mosquito species than to those from afar. A well-known observation is the failure or a very low success rate in infecting European vectors with *P. falciparum* from sub-Saharan Africa. Sometimes parasites start their development in mosquitoes but cannot complete it. In parallel experiments with *P. falciparum* and *P. vivax* conducted in the USSR, *Anopheles atroparvus*, *Anopheles messeae*, and *Anopheles sacharovi* failed, with few exceptions, to develop sporozoites after feeding on carriers of *P. falciparum* gametocytes from sub-Saharan Africa and the Indian subcontinent. The same species were easily infected by *P. vivax* from sub-Saharan Africa, the Indian subcontinent, Southeast Asia, and South America (Dashkova 1977; Dashkova and Rasnicyn 1982). In Romania, *An. atroparvus* was easily infected by *P. vivax* from Southeast Asia but not by *P. falciparum* from sub-Saharan Africa (Teodorescu 1983). In the case of *P. falciparum*, only *Anopheles freeborni* from North America demonstrated high susceptibility for geographically remote strains (from Tanzania and South China) (Collins et al. 1981). In contrast, *P. vivax* seems more opportunistic and may be successfully picked up by vectors from geographically remote areas (Collins et al. 1980; Collins et al. 1985; Shute, Garnham, and Maryon 1980). However, a difference in susceptibility not amounting to a complete refractoriness has been observed in *P. vivax* as well, even within the same country. *Anopheles albimanus* from coastal Mexico is more susceptible to a phenotype of *P. vivax* from the coast, whereas *Anopheles pseudopunctipennis* is more susceptible to a phenotype prevalent at an altitude of 170 meters (Rodriguez et al. 2000).
- *Longevity* is important because the duration of sporogony is long—often longer than the life span of a mosquito. As a result, only a small fraction of mosquitoes that ingest infective blood survive long enough to develop infective sporozoites. Longevity depends on external conditions as well as on inherited properties of a

given species; for example, mosquitoes of the *An. gambiae* complex are known for their longevity.

- *Anthropophily* includes two aspects: predilection for human blood, and association of mosquitoes with human-made habitats. Predilection for human blood may be less important than is usually thought, because most *Anopheles* that are susceptible to *Plasmodia* are rather opportunistic and will feed on any available mammal host, including humans, if bigger mammals are unavailable. Only a few, such as *An. gambiae s.s.*, definitely prefer human blood.

- *Abundance*, which depends mostly on the prevalence of water bodies that are suitable breeding grounds for the species in question, is an important factor in defining the importance of a potential vector species. However, even mosquitoes that prefer atypical and rare breeding places may act as vectors and produce localized epidemics, provided that they are susceptible to *Plasmodia*. One example is *Anopheles plumbeus*, which breeds in accumulations of water in the hollows of old trees.

Human Host

Malaria has been a selective force in human evolution (Miller 1999). Clear evidence indicates that many of the red cell polymorphic hereditary traits (such as hemoglobin S, thalassemia, and G6PD deficiency) spread and accumulated in tropical human populations because of the selective pressure exerted by malaria. Many more such links are suspected. As an integral part of tropical ecosystems, malaria also had a profound effect on the behavior, socioeconomic activities, and distribution of human populations.

Systemic Organization

The parasitic system of malaria may be described in cybernetic terms as a self-regulating subsystem of an ecosystem. Disease, human factors (e.g., human-made malaria, malaria control activities, demographic effects, population distribution and activities, and poverty), and the natural environment (malariogenic conditions) interact through several feedback systems. Geography, humans, and malaria constitute a complex system. Consider three key factors:

- The distribution of the population is determined by geographic factors.
- Human activities transform the geographic environment.
- Malaria produces strong and durable demographic effects.

Such systems that have been evolving for millennia are usually well-equilibrated and resistant to change.

In tropical mountainous areas, for example, malaria encourages the population to occupy naturally malaria-free highlands and highland fringe at altitudes of about 2,000 meters (e.g., in Ethiopia [Roundy 1976] and New Guinea [Radford, Van Leeuwen, and Christian 1976]), where the population densities are higher than in more fertile but malarious valleys. On the other hand, human practices such as agricultural exploitation may increase (e.g., rice cultivation) or decrease (e.g., land reclamation) malaria transmission.

Antimalaria action is an important component of societal response to malaria, which might range from avoidance of malarious areas to attempts to modify the environment. With the development of a scientific and organized approach to malaria control, antimalaria action became an even more important part of this self-regulating system. After successes in malaria control, the feedback signal from malaria to society weakens (i.e., a decrease in malaria morbidity brings down public interest in malaria, thus weakening the vigor of antimalaria action). This response creates conditions for the return of malaria, which stimulates antimalaria action again. Such cycles may repeat several times. For example, Morocco was near complete interruption of transmission twice, in 1979 and 1983, and now approaches it again. The system often comes to a state of equilibrium, with malaria and antimalaria actions coexisting.

Spatial Organization

To be effective, malaria control requires a careful selection of measures that can be adapted to the prevailing epidemiological conditions.

Ecosystems and Physiographic Hierarchy. Following the ideas of Vernadsky expressed in the 1920s, modern ecologists considered *biosphere* an integration of living and non-living (i.e., biotic and abiotic) elements in which the exchange of matter and energy takes place (Lamotte and Duvigneaud 1999). This supersystem may be considered as an hierarchy of interacting *ecosystems* that may be described at different scales; both a drop of water and an ocean are ecosystems (Tansley 1935).

With some degree of simplification, ecosystems may be subdivided into a biotic part (*biocenoses*) and abiotic elements. Both parts are associated with a particular spatial unit (*biotope*). Although within the pairs of biocenoses and biotopes there is no rigid, strict one-to-one correspondence (because biocenoses are functional entities and biotopes are spatial units), biocenoses may be related to individual biotopes to some extent. This point is important, because biotopes may be relatively easily recognized in the field as part of the physiography, thus helping to identify particular biocenoses and ecosystems that are associated with them.

To the hierarchy of physiographic taxa (biotopes), a parallel hierarchy of ecosystems corresponds. Ecosystems of the same hierarchic level are, as a rule, interacting. In other words, the same individual organism may belong to several interacting biocenoses. Thus, ecosystems form a complex mosaic, often with a smooth transition from one to another. At each level, the spatial structure of ecosystems is heterogeneous, and this is one of the moving forces of the ecological process (Pickett and Cadenasso 1995).

Malaria, as a living system, may be described as a part of ecosystems of different levels. The structure of malaria is closely related to the structure of the biosphere, the physiographic structure of Earth's surface.

Hierarchy of physiographic taxa has been well developed by geographers, although there are some differences in approaches by different schools. For example, the Indian subcontinent is divided into six physiographic *divisions* (units of several hundred thousand square kilometers each) which contain a hierarchy of *subdivisions*, physiographic *provinces*, and *sections*, the latter taxon occupying an area of several hundred square kilometers (National Atlas and Thematic Mapping Organisation 1977). At even lower levels, this hierarchy has been well elaborated and used in applied research by the Russian school (Mikhailov 1985). The central element is usually a *landscape*, an area of several square kilometers, which includes a hierarchy of smaller units down to a *facia*, which may occupy a few square meters. At each of these levels, an ecosystem anchored to this physiographic taxon may be identified and considered.

Concept of a Biogeographic Region. One of the top hierarchical levels of this organization of ecosystems is a *biogeographic region*. Its concept was developed in the second half of the nineteenth century and took its shape in the work of A.R. Wallace in 1876 (*Encyclopaedia Britannica* 2000). According to this concept, the biosphere may be described as a hierarchy of divisions, starting from very big ones called *kingdoms* or *realms* of continent size, down to *regions* (considered in some classifications the top level) and *subregions*.

Depending on the interests of researchers who may focus on specific groups of living beings, biogeographical classifications for plants and animals (and particular groups of animals, such as mammals, birds, or insects) differ in detail. However, roughly, they are very similar. For example, the flora and fauna of the Afrotropical zoogeographical region are distinctive; many species are indigenous to the area. They include the largest living land animal, *Loxodonta africana* (African elephant) and tiny insects such as *Anopheles gambiae s.l.*, the malaria vector. The Afrotropical region has its own endemic human parasites, such as *Loa loa, Dipetalonema perstans,* and *Schistosoma intercalatum.* Afrotropical malaria also has its own specific characteristics (Coluzzi 1994).

The many geographic classifications of malaria are based on different principles. It probably would be more productive to use an already existing biogeographic classification as a basis, rather than to create a new one specifically for malaria. As indicated by Ramachandra Rao (1984), the present distribution of the members of the subfamily *Anophelinae* corresponds remarkably well with Wallace's classification of the regions. He distinguished seven regions. Most of the northern hemisphere is occupied by the Palearctic region, in Eurasia (Old World, "paleo-"), and the Nearctic region, in North America (New World, "neo-"). Together, these regions are often considered as one Holarctic region. To the south, in tropical areas, are the Neotropical (southern part of North America, Central America, and South America), Afrotropical (sub-Saharan Africa), Oriental (Indian subcontinent and Indochina), and Australasian (Australia and Oceania) regions. Finally, the Antarctic region is, for obvious reasons, out of our sphere of interest. The WHO Eastern Mediterranean Region encompasses parts of the Afrotropical, Oriental, and Palearctic biogeographic regions (see Figure 9-1).

Two subgenera of *Anopheles* are known to exist in the Old World: *Anopheles s.s.* and *Cellia*. The representatives of *Cellia* are, by and large, much more potent vectors of human malaria that are predominant in the Oriental region and particularly the Afrotropical region. In the Palearctic region, *Anopheles s.s.* are predominant.

Many facts illustrate a remarkable similarity of the vector fauna within these enormous ecogeographic regions. The *Anopheles maculipennis* complex, to which the major Palearctic malaria vectors belong, spreads from Morocco (represented by *Anopheles labranchiae*) to eastern Siberia (represented by *Anopheles beklemishevi* and *An. messeae*) and is also present in the Nearctic region. Outside these two regions, these vectors are absent. Similarly, the Afrotropical region is dominated by exceptionally effective vectors belonging to the *An. gambiae* complex that are unknown outside this region.

Wallace's classification adapted to malaria does not contradict the later classification by Macdonald (1957), with its 12 types. The former, however, seems more in line with the accepted biogeographic hierarchy; in Macdonald's classification, some of the divisions of a smaller rank are elevated to the rank of regions.

Depending on a particular researcher's animal or plant focus of interest, the borders of the zoogeographic regions may be traced in a slightly different ways. They are discussed below, with special consideration of the malaria ecosystem.

Borders of the Zoogeographic Regions in the Middle East. In Africa and Arabia, the border of Afrotropical malaria is determined by the northern border of *An. arabiensis*. This species is better adapted to arid conditions than are other species of the *An. gambiae* complex and is the only vector of significance in the Sahel of Africa and in the desert fringe of the southwest of the Arabian Peninsula. The Afrotropical region is separated from its neighbors by the great deserts of Africa and the Arabian Peninsula.

The western border of the Oriental region is less clear cut: "Some expectable overlap at the margins of the adjacent regions … is particularly seen in respect of the Oriental region which is not separated from its neighbours to the east and west by such insurmountable barriers as oceans or large deserts" (Ramachandra Rao 1984). Its western limit follows the Hindukush, then goes to approximately Bandar Abbas, Iran, and cuts off Oman with adjoining parts of the UAE and the island of Socotra. Although two important vector species of the Indian subcontinent transgress this line and may be found in many areas around the Persian Gulf (*An. stephensi* and *An. fluviatilis*), the full set of the major vectors of the western part of the Oriental region is found only to the east of this divide (notably, *An. culicifacies*). These three major vectors—*An. stephensi, An. fluviatilis,* and *An. culicifacies*—are, in fact, groups of sibling species whose composition in this western end of their range is far from clear. Studies supported by WHO/EMRO to determine whether sibling species of the Oriental fauna to the east and to the west of the regional divide are the same are under way.

The rest of the WHO Eastern Mediterranean Region is part of the Palearctic biogeographic region, Mediterranean subregion.

Eco-epidemiological Types of Malaria and Success of Its Control. Main characteristics of three eco-epidemiological types of malaria that correspond to these regions are given in Table 9-1.

Malaria is very well adapted to Afrotropical conditions. The main features of Afrotropical malaria are the predominance, high endemicity, and refractoriness to control measures of *P. falciparum*. These characteristics are mostly due to the presence of vectors belonging to the *An. gambiae* complex, primarily *An. gambiae s.s.* and *An. arabiensis*. These vectors are extremely effective because of their very high susceptibility to human *Plasmodia*, very long life span, close association with human beings (predilection for human blood and human-made habitats), and ability to build up high population densities.

Often these vectors work in concert with another powerful vector, *Anopheles funestus* (also a group of sibling species) (Besansky 2000). Even some of the species that are considered "secondary" in Africa, such as *Anopheles moucheti* and *Anopheles nili,* surpass some of the "primary" vectors from the other regions (Fontenille and Lochouaran 2000). The difference in vector quality explains why malaria is much more resilient in sub-Saharan Africa compared with areas with a similar climate, such as the Indian subcontinent and South America.

Malaria may be considered one of the essential components of the Afrotropical environment, which also includes poor agricultural productivity, poor health, poverty, political unrest, instability, and inefficient health programs. The elimination of malaria from the Afrotropical areas seems unrealistic in the foreseeable future, except in northern and southern fringe areas and in oceanic islands. Attempts to decrease malaria transmission may be risky if not sustained. It is feared that a decrease in force of falciparum malaria infection from very high to high and moderate levels may increase the incidence of cerebral malaria in children (Gupta et al. 1999) and shift the incidence of severe malaria from young children to adolescents and even young adults, which is perceived by the communities as an outright deterioration of the malaria situation.

Malaria is less difficult to control in the Oriental region than in the Afrotropical region. With good application of antimalaria measures, the transmission can probably

Table 9-1. Main Characteristics of Three Eco-epidemiological Types of Malaria in the Eastern Mediterranean Region

Region	Vector	Share of Plasmodium falciparum	Interruption of transmission
Afrotropical	Excellent	Predominant	Impossible
Oriental	Less effective	About half	Possible
Palearctic	Relatively weak	Almost absent	Relatively easy

be interrupted anywhere in the Indian subcontinent. However, maintaining this accomplishment has always been a problem, as setbacks in Pakistan, India, and Sri Lanka have demonstrated.

Malaria eradication was generally a success in the Palearctic region, from which *P. falciparum* disappeared almost completely (except in parts of Afghanistan and Tajikistan and, until recently, Egypt). The distribution area of *P. vivax* also shrank considerably. It is represented now by a big domain centered in northern Iraq with adjoining parts of Turkey, Syria, and Iran; another area in Azerbaijan, with adjoining parts of Iran and Armenia; and an area adjoining the Oriental region in Afghanistan and Tajikistan. Between, small foci are scattered in Iran and Turkmenistan. Small foci of *P. vivax* exist in Morocco and Algeria (one each), and some transmission may continue in Libya.

It appears from this overview that the outcome of the eradication and control effort depended not only on the capacities of the programs but also, very significantly, on the ecological conditions. The influence of the zoogeographic affiliation is particularly evident in the countries that straddle zoogeographic boundaries. In Iran, 83% of the malaria cases reported in 1998, including almost all cases of *P. falciparum*, were in the Oriental zoogeographic region (i.e., in the province of Sistan and Balochistan, the eastern part of Hormozgan, and the tropical part of Kerman, which accounts for 5% of the population of the country). In Saudi Arabia, malaria transmission has been interrupted everywhere except in the Afrotropical part in the southwest, where falciparum malaria is still a serious problem (Al-Seghayer 1996).

Crossing the Borders. Concern has been expressed regarding the possible reintroduction of malaria into malaria-free territories. There are two aspects of this problem: importation of malaria by gametocyte carriers, and the importation and establishment of more efficient vectors.

Importation of *P. falciparum* within the same ecosystems is highly probable. An outstanding historic example in the Palearctic region is the introduction of *P. falciparum* from southern Russia to Sol'-Vychegodsk (southern part of the Arkhangel region, 61°N, which is far to the north of the normal range of this parasite) (Lysenko and Kondrachine 1999). This importation occurred in the 1930s, in the course of a forced resettlement that coincided with an extremely hot summer, and produced a considerable malaria epidemic.

One example of a long-distance, continuous importation is the period of Soviet participation in the Afghan civil war (1979–1989). Malaria was brought back to regions all over the USSR on a large scale by demobilized soldiers (Sergiev et al. 1993), and secondary transmission of *P. vivax* was commonplace in the European (western) part of the USSR. All these outbreaks were effectively suppressed. In contrast, not a single case of reintroduction of *P. falciparum* was recorded.

Many obstacles concern the introduction of more efficient vectors. Importation by airplane has been documented many times, but the establishment of a breeding population in a new place is always problematic. Long-distance importation of adult *Anopheles* by land or sea transport is not easy, because the mosquitoes need to lay eggs every few days, and most do not breed in small containers. Accidental transportation of aquatic stages is also unlikely, because *Anopheles* larvae drown easily if water is disturbed. (This fact is known to every person who has tried to establish a colony from larvae collected in the field, then transported along a bumpy road.)

The low ability of *Anopheles* to propagate on ships is illustrated by comparison with *Aedes* species. *Anopheles* were unable to cross the Buxton line that separates New Guinea, Solomon Islands, and Vanuatu from the rest of Oceania, whereas *Aedes* easily could. An account by Melville (1847) dated to 1842 indicates that mosquitoes (not *Anopheles*) had invaded at least some of the islands only recently and hints at the possible routes of such invasion. He vividly describes his arrival at Imeeo (Moorea), an island close to Tahiti:

> We essayed a nap, but, alas, the plague, little anticipated, prevented. Unknown in Tahiti, the musquitoes [sic] here fairly eddied round us.... Some years previous, a whaling captain ... got into difficulty with [Imeeo] inhabitants.... He resolved upon taking signal revenge. One night, he towed a rotten old water-cask ashore, and left it neglected.... Hence the musquitoes [sic].

One may safely vouch that these mosquitoes, deliberately imported as an act of bioterrorism, were not anophelines.

In North Africa, much concern was expressed about the possibility of reintroducing *P. falciparum* across the Sahara (Bruce-Chwatt 1986). *P. falciparum* is regularly imported to North African countries from the south; however, not a single case of reestablished *P. falciparum* transmission has been documented, probably because of a low susceptibility of Palearctic mosquitoes to the Afrotropical *P. falciparum*. There is speculation, however, that the major North African vector, *Anopheles (Cellia) sergenti,* may be more susceptible to the Afrotropical *P. falciparum* by virtue of its belonging to the subgenus *Cellia*.

Importation of Afrotropical *Anopheles* by land, across the Sahara Desert, seems even less probable than by sea routes. But a corridor links sub-Saharan and North Africa: the Nile valley. It is probably through this route that another Afrotropical parasite, *Schistosoma mansoni,* spread to Lower Egypt in prehistoric times. The Afrotropical malaria vector also broke through at least once, resulting in a catastrophe. In early 1942, *An. gambiae* (*An. arabiensis,* according to modern taxonomy) started to spread in Upper Egypt. Immediately, transmission of malaria that had always been present in the area increased manifold. When an officer came to investigate the situation at Abu Simbel in May 1942, "he found the villages deserted and no human beings to be seen. All the inhabitants were ill and confined to their homes."

By its seriousness, this epidemic could be compared to the invasion of the Italo-German troops in northwestern Egypt that occurred at the same time (Shousha 1948). During 1942, *An. gambiae* was slowly spreading to the north, finally reaching a point 25 kilometers north of Asyut, some 700 kilometers from the entry point at the Sudanese border, in November 1942. The epidemic that followed resulted in many deaths in Upper Egypt in 1942 and 1943. Shousha (1948) estimated the number of malarial infections for these two years at 139,000 and related deaths at 10,100, whereas later estimates were 150,000 infections and 12,000 (Halawani and Shawarby 1957) to 180,000 (Farid 1980) deaths.

An. gambiae s.l. had survived two Upper Egyptian winters, despite occasionally cold weather. Shousha asserts that only vigorous antivector measures stopped it from invading the Nile Delta, where the winters are only marginally colder than in Upper Egypt.

However, no climatological data have been provided to support this view. It seems that the vector was not perfectly adapted to the alien environment, and its elimination was relatively easy—a feat unthinkable of in sub-Saharan Africa. In 1944, the number of deaths decreased to 1,789, even with much better surveillance. As soon as *An. gambiae s.l.* was eradicated in February 1945, the number of malaria deaths fell to 25 in 1945 and 6 in 1946 (Shousha 1948).

Realizing that Egypt is by no way exempt from such catastrophic events in the future, the government of Egypt closely collaborates with Sudan in monitoring and controlling malaria on both sides of the border in the so-called Gambia Project.

Lower Levels of Spatial Organization. At its highest level, the hierarchy of eco-epidemiological types of malaria closely follows the accepted classification of ecosystems. This is also true for lower levels of biogeographic hierarchy.

Although we have no Middle East example at hand, a study in Orissa, India (Beljaev et al. 1987), demonstrated that parasitological profiles obtained through primary health center laboratories were in remarkable agreement with the physiographic taxa. Patterns of malaria distribution were similar within each of the four physiographic provinces present in the state of Orissa and dissimilar between them. *P. falciparum* was moderately to very highly endemic in the provinces of Garhjat Hills and northern Eastern Ghats (hilly areas at an altitude typically from 300 to 900 meters) and quite rare in the provinces of Mahanadi Basin (internal plain) and Utkal plain (coast of the Bay of Bengal). *P. vivax* was mostly moderately but sometimes highly endemic in the first two provinces, and its endemicity was low, with one exception, on the plains. *P. malariae* was present only in the two hilly provinces.

Besides malaria, many other striking differences were apparent between (but not within) the provinces, for example, ethnic composition (mostly tribal populations in the two provinces with high level of malaria), type of human settlements, and land use. The transition between the provinces was sufficiently sharp to be noticed even by a traveler journeying through the area. Not only malaria but also lymphatic filariasis observed the physiographic boundaries. Its high prevalence in the coastal Utkal plain (where the level of malaria was low) was noticeable from the road, because people with elephantiasis could be seen along every mile of the route. Surgeons graphically advertised their skills in curing elephantiasis of the scrotum on billboards, apparent from roadside cafés at every corner of the plain, offering further evidence. The realm of filariasis stopped abruptly at the crossing of the landscape border from the Utkal plain to Eastern Ghats (the realm of malaria).

Needless to say, these differences had nothing to do with administrative borders. Using administrative districts as units for epidemiological analysis tended to blur and conceal otherwise sharp differences obvious at the physiographic approach. Physiographic provinces are large entities; however, the above approach works well also at lower levels of hierarchy (i.e., section, landscape, and the corresponding ecosystems).

Focus of Malaria as an Ecosystem. A still lower level of hierarchy is occupied by a focus of malaria. This concept is needed for understanding ecological relationships more deeply, developing a typology, and devising stratification. It also is paramount for malaria control programs that aim to limit or interrupt transmission, because the focus is a minimum entity: a unit that is the object of antimalaria action. Monitoring the situation by focus, with accurate identification of its functional status (e.g., active or nonactive, new or residual), is a cornerstone for success in interrupting transmission, a task that has been undertaken by several countries in the Middle East. The same concept is applicable to territories in the maintenance phase of malaria eradication, where "potential foci" (foci with imported cases but without proof of a local transmission) frequently appear.

Quite often, a *focus* is defined as a *territory*, that is, "a defined and circumscribed locality" (WHO 1963). However, this approach appears to not consider many important facets of a focus. An ecological definition as an ecosystem seems to be more meaningful. According to an early definition of this sort by Beklemishev (1947), the *focus* is an integration of the populations of the parasite and hosts that support its existence. Populations are understood as sets of interacting individuals of the same species that occupy the same territory. In other words, the notion of "territory" is implicitly included in the definition of a *focus,* and, consequently, the focus includes all the components of an ecosystem. Although corresponding to a definite territory, a focus is more than a mere territory.

This definition is applicable to any infectious disease but is particularly useful when applied to complex parasitic systems such as malaria or leishmaniasis, which may include dozens of interacting species of parasites and hosts. A focus of malaria is tied down to a biotope, which centers around a locality but also includes mosquito breeding, feeding, and resting places that gravitate to the settlement as well as places frequented by people during their activities, especially at night.

In Figure 9-2, populations are represented by shapes that contact and even overlap each other. Even in this very simplified form (e.g., assuming that there is one vector species [whereas there usually are several] and only one parasite species), the diagram illustrates several important concepts:

- The population of a vector consists of two hemipopulations, aquatic (larval) and airborne (adult), and only the airborne vector is in contact with humans and other animal hosts.
- Although animal hosts do not harbor human malaria parasites, they may play important roles as components of a focus that supports the vector population.
- Most of the malaria parasite population is harbored in humans.

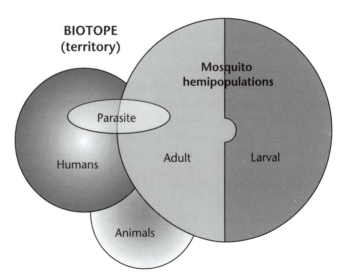

Figure 9-2. Focus of Malaria as an Ecosystem

The boundaries of a focus are fuzzy because of the movement of human hosts. For example, a human can be found, with a varying (but predictable) degree of probability, in a house, in a field, or in a particular part of the forest. For practicing epidemiologists, fuzzy boundaries are nuisances that complicate their surveys and make the identification of foci a messy task. However, trying to simplify the model by assuming that a human inhabits only a residence may lead to serious misjudgement. Malaria is regularly transmitted outside the house, and even outside the home village.

To draw exact boundaries of a focus is impossible because it would contradict Heisenberg's principle of uncertainty. It follows from this principle that it is impossible to observe the world without disturbing it. Applied to a complex system such as a focus, this principle implies that the more precisely the status of the system is studied, the more the system is disturbed and the less realistic the results.

In some situations, subunits called *microfoci* may be recognized within the focus. This practice may be of a practical interest when a full cycle of mosquito breeding and feeding is possible within a single household. This situation can be observed in semi-arid areas, where virtually every household in the village stores water in pits of a considerable size. When such pits can support mosquito breeding (the case of *An. sacharovi* in Azerbaijan), female mosquitoes rarely leave the household. If malaria were imported into such a microfocus, it would spread mostly within it, leading to a clustering of cases and a patchy distribution of malaria within a focus.

Like most ecosystems, foci are seldom isolated. They interact through an exchange of hosts, that is, humans or mosquitoes. Such interacting foci may be independent (remaining at the same level of activity even when isolated from the neighboring foci) or dependent (waning or disappearing if the supply of parasites from outside stopped). A "pseudofocus" represents an extreme degree of dependency, that is, an ecosystem in which there are no conditions for transmission and where malaria exists only because it is imported from the outside. Within a landscape, groups of foci constitute a complex mosaic of ecosystems that may be considered an ecosystem of a higher level.

Quite often, for the sake of simplicity, a malaria focus is equated with a locality within administrative boundaries. There may be a fallacy in this assumption, because such "villages" may in fact be groups of households more or less separated from each other and where the transmission takes place more or less independently. This approach may be particularly misleading in mountainous areas where the same "village" may consist of parts that lie at different altitudes, some below and some above the altitudinal limit of malaria.

Application of the Ecogeographic Approach in Antimalaria Programs. To make use of an ecogeographic approach, the known ecosystemic entities must be given a malariologic interpretation. After that, it is possible to classify them relative to malaria, in other words, to simplify and generalize the view of complex mosaics of landscapes or foci. The next logical step would be to devise and apply particular sets of antimalaria measures to each type of landscape or focus. Several successful programs were based on this approach, most systematically in Tajikistan in the 1950s and 1960s, and in North Vietnam in the 1960s (Lysenko and Semashko 1968).

This is a top-down approach to characterizing malaria (i.e., from the existing structure of geographic units). A bottom-up approach is also possible (i.e., collection of information for every geographic point, describing vector and parasite species, meteorology, human characteristics, and so on). However, it seems that the latter approach demands many more resources.

Attempts have been made to apply qualimetric methods used in industry to measure the "quality" of the territories from the point of view of their suitability to malaria. On this basis, an integrated indicator of malariogeneity was developed, and the territory of the USSR mapped accordingly (Alekseeva and Martynova 1977; Kamenskij, Martynova, and Alekseeva 1978; Soprunov 1988).

Eco-epidemiological Determinants of Malaria

As in the case of any parasitic disease with a complex life cycle, the distribution of malaria depends first on the natural environment, that is, on physiographic and biogeographic factors. At the same time, as with any anthropophosis, malaria is strongly influenced by various human-related factors.

When trying to outline various groups of factors and their practical importance, as given below, we understand that this kind of anatomic dissection kills the living system. The complicated tangle of factors includes malaria as its very active component, which itself alters those factors.

Belonging to an Eco-epidemiological Type

As the above examples from the Middle East demonstrate, belonging to a particular eco-epidemiological type is the primary descriptor of malaria on a small scale (e.g., zoogeographic region or subregion). However, this approach works at lower levels of ecosystems as well, down to foci, which may be usefully typologized according to several criteria.

This descriptor already contains an integrative characteristic that includes indications on vector species, climate, behavioral and cultural characteristics of the human population, and, to some extent, human genetic background. The advantage of this approach is that there is no need to build up the typology anew, specifically for malaria. This work has been already done for other purposes by generations of physico- and biogeographers. The task of a malariologist would be only to add malariological dimension to the already existing framework.

Meteorological Factors

Temperature. The major factor influencing the development of mosquitoes and the malaria parasites within them is temperature. An important question is which of the two organisms is more sensitive to the temperature, that is, through which of them—the parasite or the vector—temperature would act as a limiting factor.

Mosquitoes are less sensitive to low temperatures than parasites are. In northern Eurasia, *An. messeae* can breed at a water temperature above 10 °C and may attack at 7 °C (Lysenko and Kondrachine 1999), whereas the lower threshold temperature for *P. vivax* sporozoite development is 16 °C, although the parasites can survive for a few days at lower temperatures (Moshkovsky and Rashina 1951). The northernmost findings of *Anopheles* were at the latitudes of 68–69°N (in Finland, Sweden, and Russia), whereas the northern limit of malaria was only 64–66°N in Russia. Malaria was prevalent in the regions where average daily temperatures were above 15 °C for more than 30 days a year (Lysenko and Semashko 1968; Lysenko and Kondrachine 1999).

Because *Anopheles* is better adapted to the cold weather, a swath of "anophelism without malaria" occupied parts of northern Europe and northern Asia in the pre-eradication era. When temperature is slightly above the threshold, parasite development in mosquitoes is so slow that only few survive to the infective stage. For example, at average daily temperatures of 18 °C, the development of *P. vivax* sporozoites takes about 30 days, which is well beyond the median life span of mosquitoes. In this case, malaria transmission cannot be excluded, but it takes place at a very low level.

Low temperatures are practically the only reason why malaria transmission is impossible for most of the year in temperate and subtropical zones. Malaria transmission stops for a few months a year because of low temperatures even in parts of the tropical zone, for example, in Egypt and the plains of Pakistan and northern India.

For equatorial and tropical ecosystems, temperatures are not very important, because they are above the development threshold all year. However, some temperatures are too high for mosquitoes and *Plasmodia*. Average daily temperatures above 33 °C are usually considered deleterious for parasites and mosquitoes alike. Even so, mosquitoes are able to find suitable microclimates and survive in small numbers even when temperatures measured at the meteorological station seem all too prohibitive. Such conditions exist in summer in arid and semi-arid tropical areas, for example, in the plains of the African Horn and south of the Arabian Peninsula.

In tropical and equatorial zones, low temperatures are a limiting factor only at high altitudes. Little is known about the development of tropical strains of parasites at low temperatures, and their requirements may not be necessarily the same as the well-studied requirements of the parasites from Europe. However, the fact that *An. gambiae s.l.* could survive temperatures below 10 °C in Upper Egypt, well below the temperature threshold of the Palearctic *P. falciparum* (Shousha 1948), seems to indicate that low temperatures affect primarily the spread of the parasites, not vectors, in the Afrotropical region as well. If the same mechanism acts there as in the north, the existence of a belt of anophelism without malaria may be expected at particular altitudes.

This issue is key to elucidating the mechanism of outbreaks of "highland malaria" at altitudes where transmission is possible only during short periods when temperatures are exceptionally high. At lower altitudes, such outbreaks may be yearly events. These epidemics are believed to be due to a yearly repopulation of the highlands by the vector. This idea seems farfetched. The same seems to be true regarding the assertion repeated recently in several media reports about global warming: that *Anopheles* species are invading the highlands, hence, malaria epidemics.

A more plausible explanation is that a limited population of vectors is present there all the time, but malaria is absent because the temperature is insufficient for parasite development. Elevated temperatures allow parasite development in the already present mosquitoes (whose population also benefits from the rise of temperature). If this mechanism is in place, no additional time is required to establish a breeding population of vectors, which may explain the explosive nature of such epidemics. This hypothesis warrants applied research aimed at studying

- the mechanisms of overwintering of *An. gambiae*,
- the bionomics of *An. gambiae* near its altitude limit, and
- the development of tropical strains of *Plasmodia* at low temperatures.

Hydrological Factors. Water-related factors influence malaria in two ways: by ensuring the availability of breeding places and by maintaining a level of humidity sufficient for the survival of vectors that require humidity of not less than 50%.

Low rainfall is not critical for malaria in all situations. Malaria used to be present in desert oases, where, by definition, the amount of rainfall is less than 200 millimeters per year. The endemicity was high and fairly stable. In North African countries, the oases of the Sahara were the last refuges of malaria when the rest of the countries' territories (in Algeria, Egypt, Libya, and Tunisia) had already been made malaria-free.

The effect of rainfall depends on the breeding habits of mosquitoes. It may boost the proliferation of species breeding in running water and suppress those that prefer stagnant water and small pools. Most spectacular is the effect of heavy rainfall in semi-arid and arid areas. For example, consider Djibouti city, which was malaria-free before the mid-1980s. Later agricultural development along the Oued Angouli River within the city limits created a lot of potential breeding places. These sites were "activated" immediately after the heavy rains, which occur irregularly—usually once a year. The rains were followed by epidemics that started three to four weeks after the rain (unpublished observation).

The level of water in rivers is important mostly for arid areas of the Middle East. River elevation due to rainfall hundreds of kilometers away has been known to produce epidemics in Khartoum (Sudan) and in the Somali valleys of Juba and Shebelle.

Human-Related Factors

Development. Since time immemorial, malariogenic conditions have been affected by human development activities. The same activities may lead to a propagation of malaria or to its limitation, as a few examples from the Middle East demonstrate (Table 9-2).

Implementation of industrial projects is often conducive to malaria transmission, a phenomenon well studied in India (Sharma 1991). Some types of industries are particularly associated with malaria, for example, brick production in the Fayoum oasis in Egypt (Bassiouni et al. 1999). Excavation for clay around the kilns creates borrow pits that are readily flooded because of the high level of subsoil water and the use of large quantities of water in the technological process. These pits are productive breeding places for *Anopheles sergenti*. The factories tend to concentrate in particular areas of the oasis, probably because of the quality of the clay, which depends on local geology. This is an example of how malaria is indirectly conditioned by physiography via a particular human activity.

Warfare and Armed Conflicts. It is a well-established fact that malaria has played a major role in the history of wars. During the Second World War, the British Army accorded top priority to malaria prevention in the Mediterranean and Middle East, particularly in Iran, Iraq, and Palestine (Leeson et al. 1950). Heavy fighting in southern Italy during the period between the landing of Anglo-American troops in September 1943 and the complete retreat of the Germans from the area in June 1944 resulted in a series of serious epidemics among the civil population that also affected the troops in 1944 and 1945. The factors contributing to the epidemics were the disintegration of public health systems and an increase in vector breeding, which resulted from the destruction of dams, discontinuation of maintenance of irrigation and drainage systems, abandonment of cultivation, and numerous bomb craters (Merzagora, Corbellini, and Coluzzi 1996).

Recently, the Middle East has been plagued by armed conflicts, which were the leading cause of malaria flare-ups during and after the civil war in Afghanistan; the Gulf War; and internal conflicts in southern Sudan, Somalia, Djibouti, and Yemen. Conflicts lead to the destruction of the health infrastructure, and conducting control activities becomes impossible as a result of combat; landmines; shortages of essential funds, supplies, and equipment; and the displacement of huge masses of population. Even in the

Table 9-2. Activities That May Lead to the Limitation or Propagation of Malaria

Activity	Limits malaria	Favors malaria
Increased agricultural land use	If it reduces the number of swamps and unnecessary water collections	If highly water-demanding crops such as rice are introduced or if crops are cultivated within city limits (e.g., Khartoum, Djibouti)
Irrigation	If it is properly arranged and maintained	If there is seepage, or when artificial lakes' beds are not prepared before the filling, leaving expanses of shallow water
Road construction	If it improves accessibility to health services	If it creates additional breeding in borrow pits and through water logging in the absence of proper culverts
Urbanization	If it improves housing, making houses less accessible for mosquitoes, reduces breeding surfaces, and makes the remaining water bodies unsuitable for breeding by lining the bank or because of pollution	If it creates slums, with crowding and unprotected housing; by chaotic spread of residential colonies when housing is constructed faster than drainage and water supply (e.g., Khartoum); by increased breeding places during the construction phase
Drilling for water or providing piped water supply	If it reduces the need for storage of water in open tanks within the households	If it is poorly maintained (e.g., spillage, broken pipes)

absence of active fighting, surveillance usually breaks up because of de facto independence of parts of the national territories from the central governments.

Wars also can seriously undermine malaria control in countries that send troops abroad, as demonstrated by the increase in malaria importation to the USSR during and after Soviet military intervention in Afghanistan (Sergiev et al. 1993).

Migrations. Migrations are a normal fact of life of communities, and they cause some malaria-related problems even in affluent societies (e.g., intensive importation of malaria by job seekers from abroad is a problem in the countries around the Persian Gulf). Migrations in the course of economic development and especially warfare create even more problems. Common in these two situations are the displacement of large groups, often over long distances, and habitation in crowded and unsanitary conditions, with a meager means of existence. Among the many diseases that plague migrants, malaria plays a leading role. Malaria is aggravated in the process of population movement from high-endemic to low-endemic areas and vice versa—even between the high-endemic areas, which leads to a mixing of parasite populations originating from different areas and the exchange of parasites with an antigenic structure not experienced previously.

At present, the malaria problem associated with migration is of greatest importance among the refugees from Afghanistan to Pakistan and Iran, from southern Sudan to the Khartoum area, and from Somalia to Yemen. This immigration seriously aggravates the malaria situation in the host countries.

Organized resettlement also has its malariological consequences. Concentrating populations in big villages in an attempt to curtail guerilla activities (as in Iraq in the 1980s) might limit malaria transmission, but the dissolution of those villages was one of the factors leading to the resurgence of malaria in northeastern Iraq after the Gulf War. People scattered toward their old villages, often destroyed by that time, and restarted irrigation for rice cultivation under very primitive conditions (unpublished information from J.A. Najera, WHO, 1994). On the other hand, forced resettlement from nonmalarious to malarious areas usually is catastrophic (e.g., in Ethiopia) (Prothero 1994; Kloos 1990).

One example of malaria reintroduction by the workforce occurred in Lebanon. In 1996, four cases of vivax malaria were contracted locally in urbanized areas: two in greater Beirut and two in Jounieh. The source could be traced to Syrian construction workers who lived in the same semiconstructed houses where they worked and had no access to health services (Kassatsky 1997). Outbreaks were small because of the scarcity of breeding places in the urban setting for the vector, *An. claviger,* and the vector's preference for feeding near the breeding places.

Recent Epidemiological Change

Malaria is a self-regulating system that adapts to changing epidemiological factors; consequently, epidemiological patterns of malaria keep changing. Below are some of the changes that occurred during the lifetime of people who started their careers during the heyday of malaria eradication in the 1960s.

Directions of the Changes. The changes went in both directions, some diminishing malaria transmission, others enhancing it. Decreased malaria transmission was often beneficial, but not always. For example, a transition from a highly endemic situation to decreased, but still continuing transmission was usually accompanied by a delay in the development of immunity and decreased immune protection from overt attacks of malaria. At the same time, populations at risk continued to receive infective bites, maybe several times per year instead of several hundred times. Malaria that previously affected mostly young children (in whom it was an ill-defined part of a mixture of multiple diseases) gradually became more noticeable to the public. The population became more aware of higher attack rates in adults, the appearance of severe and fatal malaria in adolescents, and increased difficulty in treatment (due to increased drug resistance).

Changes in the Parasitic System Induced by Malaria Control. Malaria control programs achieved various degrees of malaria suppression. Not uncommonly in the Palearctic region, *P. falciparum* transmission could be interrupted while *P. vivax* transmission continued (e.g., in Azerbaijan, Iraq, Morocco, Syria, and Turkey and in most of the territory of Iran). As a result, the *P. falciparum*-free areas with continuing transmission of *P. vivax,* which were confined to the fringe of the area of malaria distribution in cold climates in the past, became commonplace in more warm climates as well. This selective elimination of *P. falciparum* was sustainable everywhere in the Middle East except in Tajikistan, where *P. falciparum* reappeared after a massive importation by Afghan refugees. There are no examples of *P. falciparum* reintroduction from afar.

Spread of *P. falciparum* resistance to chloroquine continued, and nowadays some degree of resistance is present almost wherever this species is still endemic in the Old World. The only exception known to us was the last Egyptian focus of malaria in Fayoum. Although no formal susceptibility tests have been done in the area, the treatment of cases with chloroquine never presented any problems.

The proportion of *P. falciparum* increased in highly endemic areas, at the expense of other species. One of these species, *P. malariae,* became quite rare in the Middle East, probably because of an increased use of antimalaria drugs to which *P. falciparum* is usually less responsive. This occurrence does not contradict the disappearance of *P. falciparum* in the Palearctic areas, because it occurred mostly under the impact of anti-vector measures that affect primarily *P. falciparum,* which is more sensitive to the climatic conditions.

Many human-made epidemics have occurred after haphazard, unsustained indoor residual spraying campaigns in Africa. One of them was a malaria control program in Gezira, an important agricultural area of Sudan, where intensive vector control was carried out for 10 years but was abruptly stopped in 1989. As a result, malaria prevalence among children, as measured by the slide positivity rate (the number of malaria-positive test slides per number of people examined, multiplied by 100), increased from 0.5% in 1988 to 33% in 1994 (Najera, Kouznetsov, and Delacollette 1998).

Changes Brought by Socioeconomic Processes. The most important changes are the presence of malaria control programs in every country and the world community's commitment to controlling malaria. One of the most significant outcomes is the widespread availability of antimalaria drugs and their use by laymen, which limits, to some extent, the deleterious effects of malaria. Community action against malaria also has increased.

On the other hand, human-made malaria linked to various economic activities, economic crisis, civil strife, and wars is playing a more prominent role than before. Increased population movement—for economic and political reasons—is increasing malaria importation by migrants within or between countries.

It is true that the deterioration of economic and living conditions favors malaria, but not always. Degradation of the environment that is often observed in parallel to urbanization (what is aptly called *poubellisation* in French-speaking Africa) leads to the disappearance of water accumulations suitable for *Anopheles* breeding because of heavy pollution, thus decreasing malaria transmission, sometimes almost to zero (Trape and Zoulani 1987). Such is the case of big urban agglomerations in tropical Africa, in which areas of low or no transmission have emerged while the countryside remains highly malarious (Gérard 1988).

Climatic Change. After long disputes, global warming finally has been accepted by the majority as a reality (Jackson 1995). Feared possible repercussions include a spread of malaria to the temperate areas and the highlands of tropical and equatorial zones. However, conclusions are not unanimous. Some predict the return of malaria to the industrialized world. One of the extreme predictions is that in the future, *P. ovale* and *P. malariae* will spread to northern Europe and occupy the whole of Scandinavia (Martin and Lefebvre 1995); the authors of this prediction appear to have ignored the facts that these two species require higher temperatures than *P. vivax* to survive and that ecological factors other than temperature limit the spread of malaria. Others doubt that the global warming would lead to any drastic change (Taubes 1997). Reiter (2000) asserts that because *P. falciparum* was widespread in Europe during the Little Ice Age (sixteenth through eighteenth centuries), high temperature is not the main factor in the spread of malaria, and hence, the doomsday scenarios are farfetched.

The concern that global warming would lead to a spread of malaria at higher altitudes in the tropics (Patz et al. 1996) is supported by several observations. Malaria has appeared at altitudes where it has not been previously known in Kenya (Some 1994;

Ouma, Rapuoda, and Beret 1995) and Rwanda (Loevinsohn 1994). During the early 1990s, such "highland epidemics" were documented in Burundi, Ethiopia, Madagascar, Swaziland, and Zimbabwe (Benzerroug, Beljaev, and Barakamfitiye 1994). Evidence indicates that during the Yemeni epidemics of 1996 and 1997, malaria was particularly murderous at an altitude of about 2,000 meters, which is considered an upper limit for malaria. However, this epidemic was very poorly documented. Surprisingly, in most of the publications about epidemics at high altitude, no meteorological records are given, and quite often, even the altitude is not indicated.

In the countries of the African Horn and in the south of the Arabian Peninsula, increased rainfall—often in the wake of a prolonged drought—also has contributed to severe epidemics in Djibouti, Ethiopia, northern Somalia, parts of Sudan, and Yemen. These episodes are not unprecedented and are long remembered by people as "malaria years." However, because of insufficient documentation, it is difficult to say whether those episodes have become more frequent than before.

Practical Use of Predictors of Malaria Incidence

The need for monitoring predictors of malaria risk arises for different reasons. The most obvious one is to forecast changes in the level of transmission and the outcome of interventions. The second is to indirectly assess malariogeneity, which may give more realistic estimates of the burden of malaria than surveillance data. A rule that states that "the more prevalent the malaria, the less adequate the surveillance" is true not only because of the weakness of surveillance systems in highly malarious countries but also because the disease tends to be less conspicuous in highly endemic situations.

Criteria for Selection of Indicators

Quite often, recommendations are given to monitor all conceivable factors that may have any relation to malaria. Following such advice would exceed the capacities of any surveillance system.

Because most of the above factors are interlinked and evolve in parallel, increasing their numbers would not lead to a commensurate improvement of the forecast. The monitoring of some factors requires a prohibitive amount of effort. Other factors are very variable in space and time; hence, the data obtained from observational posts would not always represent the conditions in the point we are interested in. For example, monitoring of humidity is often recommended. However, this factor strongly depends on rainfall and temperature; in other words, these two meteorological factors already contain most of the information required. Moreover, humidity varies depending on biotopes, and the data obtained from a meteorological station may not be representative. Thus, it is important is to select the most informative factors to avoid redundancy and improve representativeness.

Many of the factors causally related to malaria are not measurable directly. Quite often it would be more practical to replace them with proxies (i.e., other factors that are easier to observe and measure). This is the concept of indicators that is widely used in the earth sciences. In ecology, the term *indicator* refers to "a group of plants or animals whose presence acts as a sign of particular environmental conditions" (*Oxford English Dictionary* 1989). This definition may be expanded to include any factor that is conspicuous, easily obtainable, and closely associated with the condition in question (e.g., a particularly conspicuous kind of vegetation or a pattern of land use). This association is not necessarily causally determined; sometimes the condition and the indicator are independent of each other but both are caused by a third, hidden factor; hence, they would develop in parallel.

It is important that these indicators be easily available (e.g,. from a map, census report, or meteorological record) and be more or less independent from the other selected indicators (to reduce redundancy). Remote sensing that became popular recently for the monitoring of ecological conditions is, in fact, based on the monitoring of such proxy indicators. One indicator that is causally related to malaria in the Oriental region is sympatric occurrence of *An. culicifacies* and *An. fluviatilis*. It is an indicator of high malariogenic potential. One indicator that is not in direct cause–effect relationship with malaria is the proportion of particular ethnocultural groups in the general population.

In the early 1980s, I had the opportunity to study the latter indicator in India. The proportion of tribal population among the general population excellently correlated with the burden of falciparum malaria (unpublished observation, 1980–1985). The interaction of this indicator and malaria is complex and bidirectional. Populations belonging to the so-called scheduled tribes in India are mostly descendants of the pre-Aryans who preserved many ancient traits of social organization, economy, and culture. They occupy hills with a high level of malaria transmission, and those hills are avoided by other population groups mostly because they are malarious. However, the tribes are better adapted to survive malaria because of several protective hereditary traits and may survive in very malarious environments. Their economy is based on slash-and-burn agriculture and exploitation of the forest, both practices associated with an increased risk of malaria. Their beliefs make them reluctant to accept modern medicine and disease control. Their custom of decorating the walls of their houses with elaborate patterns of multicolor clays make them reject spraying with insecticides, which would damage their art. In addition, a language barrier makes health education difficult.

These factors are so intertwined that it is difficult to analyze them separately. However, one may argue whether this analysis is needed. It may be sufficient to note that the percentage of tribal population is a good indicator of malaria and use it as such. Interestingly, a committee identified areas that were to be included in the *P. falciparum* Containment Program in India (1979–1989) that almost exactly corresponded to the areas with a high proportion of tribal population, even though the committee did not use this factor as a criterion for selection.

Another important indicator of malaria is altitude. Its relationship with malaria is indirect, mostly through the temperatures that make successful development of sporozoites difficult or impossible due to the extreme cold at the altitude or, sometimes, extreme heat near the sea level. Altitude is simpler to use than the meteorological record, because data on altitude are available for any geographic point and may be easily read from topographic maps, whereas temperature data are interpolations of measurements obtained from a relatively rare network of meteorological stations. Moreover, the altitude determines not only the temperatures but also other factors that may be related to malaria, such as rainfall patterns and types of breeding places. Therefore, as an indicator, altitude contains more information than temperature alone.

Practical Use of Meteorological Indicators in Malariology

Careful monitoring of meteorological events, which was the trademark of successful malaria control programs from the 1920s to the 1960s, was abandoned during the eradication campaign in most (but not all) countries. Unfortunately, monitoring was not revived when the eradication policies were abandoned in the 1970s.

Enumeration of these factors may be found in any treatise on malariology, but it is very rare that practical methods for their use are suggested. As a result, in practice, the wealth of meteorological information that exists in any country is exploited very poorly by the public health sector. Monitoring of meteorological factors is important at medium and large scales (province and district) and in real time.

A score of temperature indicators are used by meteorologists. Among them, the average daily temperature should be retained. In contrast, the practice of using annually averaged temperatures to project the prevalence of malaria is misguided. What matters is existence of a temperature range suitable for the development of the plasmodium and the mosquito lasting for the appropriate length of time (two to three weeks). In Siberia, despite a low annual average temperature, summer temperatures are high enough for malaria to spread. In Scotland, where the average annual temperature is much higher, the summer temperatures are too low for malaria to find a foothold.

Rainfall is essential for the availability of breeding places, except in river valleys. Not only the overall amount of precipitation is essential, but also its speed; a large amount of rain that falls over a few hours flushes out breeding places, whereas the same amount spread over a few days is beneficial for breeding. For this reason, rainfall should be monitored daily.

Meteorology in Programs Aimed at Interrupting Transmission and Preventing Reintro-duction of Malaria. Most malaria interruption and malaria prevention programs operate under conditions in which malaria transmission is seasonal because of low temperatures. In such situations, a method that assesses characteristics of the malaria season may be used (Moshkovsky 1946). Among those, the most important characteristics are the beginning and end dates of the period during which parasite development in mosquitoes is possible, the date of the first effective infection of humans, and the date of the last effective infection of mosquitoes. The method is also useful for epidemiological analysis of cases in territories with no or limited malaria transmission (i.e., in consolidation and maintenance phases of malaria eradication), answering questions such as the following:

- If a case is imported on a given date, when can the first introduced case, if any, be expected to emerge?
- When there are two cases, can the second originate from the first one?
- Was the given case of *P. vivax* contracted during the current transmission season, or is it a result of the last years' transmission (a late manifestation)?

The method also permits the calculation of the duration of the complete cycle of parasite development from the moment of the infection of the vector until the moment of gametocyte maturation in the next host. This cycle includes the following elements:

- time needed for sporozoite maturation (a variable depending on the temperature and the parasite species),
- average incubation period (10 days for *P. falciparum* and 15 days for *P. vivax*), and
- average period from the onset of symptoms to gametocyte maturation (12 days for *P. falciparum* and 0 days for *P. vivax*).

The possible number of such sequential cycles during one transmission season is an indicator of the quality of the climate regarding malaria transmission. In the climatic

Table 9-3. Temperatures Required for the Completion of Sporogony in Three *Plasmodium* Species

Species	Lower threshold of development (°C)	Base temperature (°C)	Required sum of temperatures above the base temperature (degree days)
P. vivax	16	14.5	105
P. falciparum	18	16	111
P. malariae	18	16	144

conditions of the former USSR, *P. vivax* might complete one to seven cycles of transmission annually (Shipicina 1964), and these cycles were used to stratify the country.

Moshkovsky's method is based on the concept of agricultural science that holds that the growth of a plant is dependent on the total amount of heat to which it is subjected during its lifetime, accumulated as *degree days* (*Encyclopaedia Britannica* 2000). By analyzing the speed of development of *Plasmodia* in controlled experiments, Moshkovsky found that the same concept is applicable to developmental stages of parasites in mosquitoes and calculated the parameters for *P. falciparum, P. vivax,* and *P. malariae* (Moshkovsky 1946; Moshkovsky and Rashina 1951). For each parasite species, the fundamental parameters are threshold temperature (temperature below which the parasite does not develop), base temperature, and the sum of temperatures above the base temperature required to complete sporogony (Table 9-3).

At threshold temperatures, parasite development takes an indefinitely long time. Practically, the development of *P. vivax* requires at least 16 °C, and that of *P. falciparum* and *P. malariae* requires at least 17–18 °C. At temperatures above 30 °C, the conditions for parasite development worsen, and at 37 °C, parasites die rapidly.

The formula for the duration of development (in days) is

Required sum of temperatures/(Average daily temperature – Base temperature)

For example, at 19 °C, the development of *P. falciparum* would be determined as

111 degree days/(19 °C – 16 °C) = 37 days

Here 3 °C (19 °C – 16 °C) is the *effective temperature* that is accumulated by the parasite during a day. At variable temperatures, the effective temperatures are calculated for each day and added together. Only days with temperatures above the threshold are counted (i.e., above 16 °C for *P. vivax* and above 18 °C for *P. falciparum* and *P. malariae*). A sum of temperatures equal to the required sum signals the end of sporozoite maturation.

Some standard instructions to the field epidemiologists in the USSR are still in force in Russia. For example, they record mean average daily temperatures (obtained from the yearly data for the whole period of meteorological observation) and the average date of the mass emergence of the first generation of adult mosquitoes from the breeding places. They also maintain the same data for the current year. They compare the two sets to determine whether the current year is more favorable or less favorable for malaria transmission than on the average. If cases occur, they must determine when the secondary cases are likely to emerge, if at all.

Long experience in the (former) USSR shows that the method may be a useful tool for epidemiological analysis, although the results should not be taken too literally. Several uncertainties make the conclusions less than foolproof:

- The initial basic measurements were made on a limited number of strains. There is no absolute certainty that tropical strains would behave in the same way as the temperate ones. Hence, it is not clear whether this method may be used in mountainous areas of the tropics.
- Temperatures used are from the nearest meteorological station, not from the mosquitoes' resting places, and the average daily temperatures inside and outside buildings may vary by several degrees.
- Data on the impact of the temporary reduction of the temperature below the development threshold have not been quantified. It is known only that after a short temperature decrease, sporozoites recover and continue their development. Sporozoites of *P. vivax* are more tolerant to the drops in temperature than those of *P. falciparum,* more mature sporozoites are more tolerant, and lower temperatures kill more sporozoites.

Epidemic Control. Epidemics are particularly dangerous in tropical arid and semi-arid areas (where epidemics are triggered by rainfall) and at high altitudes (where epidemics are triggered by an elevation of temperature, sometimes with increased rainfall).

Meteorological records spanning several decades are available for most countries, at least for those that have orderly airports. The work that is yet to be done is to inventory past epidemics. This task is not very difficult in principle, because epidemics usually leave an imprint on the collective memory. Even if public health records do not exist, malaria epidemics are usually reported in the media. The proposed course of action would be to compare the meteorological record and the record of epidemics to determine what was particular in meteorology during the period preceding the epidemics, to watch for the same meteorological combination to recur, to produce a forecast, and to act. The time for action is ample, because it takes at least three weeks for an epidemic to start after a good rainfall.

In arid and semi-arid areas occupying the valleys of big rivers, such as the Nile, the malaria situation may depend more on the water level (i.e., flooding) than on the rainfall. These data are also widely available. For mountainous countries, exact knowledge of the cut-off limit of malaria, historically and currently, is essential. The altitude should be used as a primary indicator for delineating the epidemic-prone areas. A malaria-free stratum would be bordered by a stratum of irregular epidemics, followed by a stratum of frequent epidemics, followed by an endemic stratum.

Use of Phenology

Phenology is "the study of the times of recurring natural phenomena, especially in relation to climatic conditions" (*Oxford English Dictionary* 1989) Examples are the fruiting of plants; the foliation and defoliation of trees; the arrival, nesting, and departure of birds; and, closer to our subject, events in the life of mosquitoes. The most important life events of mosquitoes in temperate areas are the date of the first emergence of female mosquitoes after hibernation, the date of the mass emergence of the first generation of mosquitoes, and the date of the mass retreat of hibernating females into hiding places. These variables should be monitored prospectively, to characterize the current year, as well as retrospectively, to characterize the average or normal date for these events.

These data should be used in conjunction with the meteorological data. For example, in central and northern Russia, vector mosquitoes of the first generation are already available when temperatures are not yet favorable for sporozoites. In this case, an average daily temperature of 16 °C would be the starting point for computations using

Moshkovsky's formula. In central Asia, the opposite is true: in early spring, the temperature is high enough, but adult mosquitoes are still not there. In this case, the starting point would be the time of mass emergence of adult mosquitoes, and not the arrival of warm weather.

It would be attractive to find a phenological indicator that would coincide with important events in the lives of mosquitoes or parasites, yet be more conspicuous and more readily observable—such as the blossoming of a particular plant. Such a discovery would greatly simplify observations.

Conclusion

This review of the determinants of malaria in the WHO Eastern Mediterranean Region and some adjoining areas illustrates the usefulness of an ecological approach to studying the epidemiology of malaria and to planning malaria control. This approach integrates malariology into a broader context of ecology and geography.

Acknowledgement

The author expresses gratitude to Varvara Mironova for discussing matters related to biogeography.

Disclaimer

Opinions expressed in this chapter are the author's only and do not necessarily reflect the policies and views of the World Health Organization.

References

Alekseeva, Z.M., and I.Z. Martynova. 1977. Methodology of the assessment of indicators of natural and social factors influencing the distribution of malaria [in Russian]. *Meditzinskaja Parazitoloija i Parazitarnye Bolezni* 46: 289–94.

Al-Seghayer, S.M. 1996. Malaria control in the Kingdom of Saudi Arabia. *Saudi Epidemiological Bulletin* 3(1): 4.

Ayala, F.J., A.A. Escalante, and S.M. Rich. 1999. Evolution of *Plasmodium* and the recent origin of the world populations of *Plasmodium falciparum*. *Parassitologia* 41: 55–68.

Bassiouni, H.K., A.E. Beljaev, O.M. Awad, and M.H. Ahmed. 1999. Parasitological profile of the surveyed population for malaria in an endemic area in Fayoum governorate, Egypt. *Journal of the Egyptian Public Health Association* 74(1-2): 28–46.

Beklemishev, V.N. 1947. The problem of typization of malaria foci and some types of malariogenic landscapes [in Russian]. *Meditzinskaja Parazitoloija i Parazitarnye Bolezni* 16(9): 231–42.

Beljaev, A.E. 1999. Oman goes for eradication. *World Health* 51(3): 29.

Beljaev, A.E., J.A. Brohult, G.K. Sharma, and K.C. Samantaray. 1987. Studies on the detection of malaria at primary health centres. Part 3. Parasitological profile of population surveyed for malaria through passive case detection. *Indian Journal of Malariology* 24: 97–106.

Beljaev, A.E., V.M. Rybalka, A.Y. Lysenko, R.G. Abrashkin-Zhuchkov, M.I. Alexeyeva, L.P. Arsen'eva, O.V. Babaeva, Y.P. Gorbunova, N.G. Dashkova, and B.A. Koshelev. 1986. *Plasmodium vivax*: Further observations on polymorphism in relation to the duration of exoerythrocytic development [in Russian]. In *Malaria Parasites of Mammals,* edited by T.V. Beyer et al. Academy of Sciences of the USSR *Protozoology* series, No. 11. Leningrad, USSR: Nauka, 140–57.

Benzerroug, E.H., A. Beljaev, and D. Barakamfitiye. 1994. Paludisme en Afrique: Considérations épidémiologiques et économiques. In *La Lutte Contre le Paludisme en Afrique Francophone: Prendre l'Initiative,* edited by J.F. Naimoli and P. Nguyen-Dinh. USAID-CDC, 6–10.

Besansky, N.J. 2000. Complexities in the analysis of cryptic taxa within the genus *Anopheles*. *Parassitologia* 41: 97–100.

Bruce-Chwatt, L.J. 1965. Paleogenesis and paleo-epidemiology of primate malaria. *Bulletin of the World Health Organization* 32: 363–87.

———. 1979. Man against malaria: Conquest or defeat? *Transactions of the Royal Society of Tropical Medicine and Hygiene* 73(6): 605–17.

———. 1986. North Africa: New caravans of the old Sahara. *Lancet i* Apr. 19: 903–4.

Bruce-Chwatt, L.J., and J. de Zulueta. 1980. *The Rise and Fall of Malaria in Europe*. Oxford, U.K.: Oxford University Press.

Coatney, G.R., W.E. Collins, M. Warren, and P.G. Contacos. 1971. *The Primate Malarias*. Bethesda, MD: National Institutes of Health, U.S. Department of Health, Education, and Welfare.

Collins, W.E., P.G. Contacos, W. Chin, M.H. Jeter, and P.E. Briesh. 1980. Transmission of *Plasmodium vivax* from Vietnam by four different anophelines. *American Journal of Tropical Medicine and Hygiene* 29(3): 473–5.

Collins, W.E., P. Nguyen-Dinh, J.C. Skinner, and B.B. Sutton. 1981. Infectivity of a strain of *Plasmodium falciparum* from Hainan, People's Republic of China, to different anophelines. *American Journal of Tropical Medicine and Hygiene* 30(3): 538–40.

Collins, W.E., J. Skinner, W.A. Krotosky, F.B. Cogswell, R.W. Gwadz, J.R. Broderson, S.F.M. Nancy, P. Mehaffey, and B.B. Sutton. 1985. Studies of the North Korean strain of *Plasmodium vivax* in *Aotus* monkeys and different anophelines. *Journal of Parasitology* 71(1): 2.

Coluzzi, M. 1994. Malaria and the Afrotropical Ecosystems: Impact of Man-Made Environmental Changes. *Parassitologia* 36: 223–7.

———. 1999. The clay feet of the malaria giant and its African roots: Hypotheses and inferences about origin, spread and control of *Plasmodium falciparum*. *Parassitologia* 41: 277–83.

Dashkova, N.G. 1977. New data on the susceptibility of the mosquitoes of the genus *Anopheles* to imported strains of human malaria parasites [in Russian]. *Meditzinskaja Parazitoloija i Parazitarnye Bolezni* 46(6): 652–7.

Dashkova, N.G., and S.P. Rasnicyn. 1982. Review of the data on the susceptibility of mosquitoes of the fauna of USSR to imported strains of malaria parasites. *Bulletin of the World Health Organization* 60(6): 22–6.

Encyclopaedia Britannica. 2000. http://www.britannica.com (accessed August 2001).

Farid, M.A. 1980. The malaria programme: From euphoria to anarchy. *World Health Forum* 1(1-2): 8–33.

Fontenille, D., and L. Lochouaran. 2000. The complexity of the malaria vectorial system in Africa. *Parassitologia* 41: 267–71.

Gelfand, M. 1965. Rivers of death in Africa. *Central African Journal of Medicine* 11(Suppl.): 1–46.

Gérard R. 1988. Spécificités urbaines du paludisme en Afrique tropicale. *Ecologie Humaine* 6(2): 3–20.

Goetzee, M., M. Craig, and D. le Sueur. 2000. Distribution of African malaria mosquitoes belonging to the *Anopheles gambiae* complex. *Parasitology Today* 16(2): 74–77.

Gupta, S., R.W. Snow, C. Donnelly, and C. Newbold. 1999. Acquired immunity and postnatal clinical protection in childhood cerebral malaria. *Proceedings of the Royal Society of London, Series B* 266: 33–38.

Halawani, A., and A.A. Shawarby. 1957. Malaria in Egypt. *Journal of the Egyptian Medical Association* 40(11): 753–92.

Jackson, E.K. 1995. Climate change and global infectious disease threat. *Medical Journal of Australia* 163: 570–4.

Kamenskij, E.I., Z.I. Martynova, and Z. Alekseeva. 1978. Use of operation-qualimetric methodology for the assessment of malariogenicity of territories [in Russian]. *Meditzinskaja Parazitoloija i Parazitarnye Bolezni* 47(5): 61–9.

Kassatsky, A.I. 1997. *Malaria Outbreak in Lebanon*. Unpublished EM/MAL/247/E/R/04.97/20. Geneva, Switzerland: World Health Organization. Eastern Mediterranean Regional Office.

Kloos, H. 1990. Health aspects of resettlement in Ethiopia. *Social Science and Medicine* 30(6): 643–56.

Lamotte, M., and P. Duvigneaud. 1999. Biosphère. In *Dictionnaire de l'écologie*. Paris, France: Encyclopaedia Universalis/Albin Michel.

Leeson, H.S., W.H.R. Lumsden, J. Yofe, and T.T. Macan. 1950. *Anopheles and Malaria in the Near East.* London, U.K.: H.K. Lewis and Co. Ltd., 223.

Loevinsohn, M.E. 1994. Climatic warming and increased malaria incidence in Rwanda. *Lancet* 343(8899): 714–20.

Lysenko, A.J., and A.E. Beljaev. 1969. An analysis of the geographical distribution of *Plasmodium ovale. Bulletin of the World Health Organization* 40(3): 3.

Lysenko, A.J., and A.V. Kondrachine. 1999. *Malariology* [in Russian]. WHO/MAL/99/1089. Geneva, Switzerland: World Health Organization.

Lysenko, A.J., and I.N. Semashko. 1968. Geography of malaria. A medico-geographic profile of an ancient disease [in Russian]. In *Itogi Nauki: Medicinskaja Geografija 1968.* Moscow, USSR: VINITI, 25–146.

Macdonald, G. 1957. *The Epidemiology and Control of Malaria.* London, U.K.: Oxford University Press.

Martin, P.H., and M.G. Lefebvre. 1995. Malaria and climate: sensitivity of malaria potential transmission to climate. *Ambio* 24(4): 200–7.

McNeill, W.H. 1979. *Plagues and Peoples.* Harmondsworth, Middlesex, U.K.: Penguin Books.

Melville, H. 1847. *Omoo: A Narrative of Adventures in the South Seas.* London, U.K.: John Murray.

Merzagora, L., G. Corbellini, and M. Coluzzi. 1996. *L'Altra Battaglia di Cassino.* Cassino, Italy: Università degli studi di Cassino.

Mikhailov, N.I. 1985. *Physico-geographic Regionalization* [in Russian]. Moscow, USSR: Moscow University.

Miller, L.H. 1999. Evolution of the human genome under selective pressure from malaria: Applications for control. *Parassitologia* 41: 77–82.

Miller, R.L., S. Ikram, G.J. Armelagos, R. Walker, W.B. Harer, C.J. Shiff, D. Baggett, M. Carrigan, and S.M. Maret. 1994. Diagnosis of *Plasmodium falciparum* infections in mummies using the rapid manual ParaSight-F test. *Transactions of the Royal Society of Tropical Medicine and Hygiene* 88(1): 31–2.

Moshkovsky, S.D. 1946. On the dependency of the speed of development of *Plasmodia* of malaria on the temperature. Part 1 [in Russian]. *Meditzinskaja Parazitoloija i Parazitarnye Bolezni* 15(6): 19–28.

Moshkovsky, S.D., and M.G. Rashina (eds.). 1951. *Epidemiology and Medical Parasitology for Entomologists* [in Russian]. Moscow, USSR: Medgiz.

Najera, J.A., R.L. Kouznetsov, and C. Delacollette. 1998. *Malaria Epidemics.* WHO/MAL/98/1084. Geneva, Switzerland: World Health Organization.

National Atlas and Thematic Mapping Organisation. 1977. Physiographic regions. In *National Atlas of India,* 2nd edition. New Delhi, India: Government of India, Plate 41.

Ouma, J.H., B. Rapuoda, and J.C. Beret. 1995. Patterns of malaria epidemics in the highland areas of Kenya. *American Journal of Tropical Medicine and Hygiene* 53(Suppl. 2), abstract no. 551.

Oxford English Dictionary. 1989. OED2, version 1.11 [CD-ROM].

Patz, J.A., P.R. Epstein, T.A. Burke, et al. 1996. Global climate change and emerging infections. *Journal of the American Medical Association* 275: 3.

Pickett, S.T.A., and M.L. Cadenasso. 1995. Landscape Ecology: Spatial Heterogeneity in Ecological Systems. *Science* 269: 331–4.

Prothero, R.M. 1994. Forced movement of population and health hazards in Tropical Africa. *International Journal of Epidemiology* 23(4): 657–64.

Radford, A.J., H. Van Leeuwen, and S.H. Christian. 1976. Social aspects in the changing epidemiology of malaria in the Highlands of New Guinea. *Annals of Tropical Medicine and Parasitology* 70(1): 11–23.

Ramachandra Rao, T. 1984. *The Anophelines of India.* Delhi, India: Malaria Research Centre, Indian Council of Medical Research.

Reiter, P. 2000. From Shakespeare to Defoe: Malaria in England in the Little Ice Age. *Emerging Infectious Diseases* 6: 1.

Rodriguez, M.H., L. Gonzalez-Ceron, J.E. Hernandez, J.A. Nettel, C. Villarreal, K.C. Kain, and R.A. Wirtz. 2000. Different prevalences of *Plasmodium vivax* phenotypes VK210 and VK247 associated with the distribution of *Anopheles albimanus* and *Anopheles pseudopunctipennis*. *American Journal of Tropical Medicine and Hygiene* 62(1): 122–7.

Roundy, R.W. 1976. Altitudinal mobility and disease hazards for Ethiopian populations. *Economic Geography (USA)* 52(2): 103–15.

Sergiev, V.P., A.M. Baranova, V.S. Orlov, et al. 1993. Importation of malaria into the USSR from Afghanistan, 1981–89. *Bulletin of the World Health Organization* 3/4: 385–8.

Sharma, V.P. 1991. Environmental management of malaria in India. In *Malaria: Waiting for the Vaccine,* edited by G.A.T. Targett. New York: John Wiley & Sons, 49–66.

Sherman, I.W. 1998. A brief history of malaria and discovery of the parasite's life cycle. In *Malaria,* edited by I.W. Sherman. Washington, DC: ASM Press, 3–10.

Shipicina, N.K. 1964. The season of malaria transmission and malarious zones of the Soviety Union [in Russian]. In *Problemy medicinskoj parazitologii i profilaktiki infekcij,* edited by SH. D. Moshkovsky. USSR Ministry of Health, Martzinovsky Institute of Medical Parasitology and Tropical Medicine, 258–276..

Shousha, A.T. 1948. Species eradication. The eradication of *Anopheles gambiae* from Upper Egypt, 1942–1945. *Bulletin of the World Health Organization* 1(2): 309–34.

Shute, P.G., P.C.C. Garnham, and M. Maryon. 1980. The Madagascar strain of *Plasmodium vivax.* *Archives de l'Institut Pasteur de Madagascar* 47(1): 173–83.

Some, E.S. 1994. Effects and control of highland malaria epidemic in Uasin Gishu District, Kenya. *East African Medical Journal* 71(1): 2–8.

Soprunov, F.F. (ed.). 1988. *Malaria Control.* Moscow, Russia: U.N. Environment Programme, Centre for International Projects GKNT.

Tansley, A.G. 1935. The Use and Abuse of Vegetational Concept and Terms. *Ecology* 16(3): 284.

Taubes, G. 1997. Apocalypse not. *Science* 278: 1004–6.

Teodorescu, C. 1983. Essais d'infection expérimentale d'une souche de *Anopheles atroparvus* indigène aux espèces de *Plasmodium* d'importation. *Archives Roumaines de la Pathologie Expérimentale et Microbiologie* 42(4): 365–70.

Trape, J.F., and A. Zoulani. 1987. Malaria and urbanization in Central Africa: The example of Brazzaville. 3. Relationships between the urbanization and intensity of malaria transmission. *Transactions of the Royal Society of Tropical Medicine and Hygiene* 81(6, Suppl. 2), 19–25.

WHO (World Health Organization). 1955. *Eighth World Health Assembly, Mexico, 10–27 May 1955.* Official Records of WHO No. 63. Geneva, Switzerland: WHO.

———. 1963. *Terminology of Malaria and of Malaria Eradication.* Geneva, Switzerland: WHO.

———. 1971. *Expert Committee on Malaria, 15th Report.* WHO Technical Report Series No. 467. Geneva, Switzerland: WHO.

———. 1992. *World Declaration on the Control of Malaria.* Geneva, Switzerland: WHO.

WHO/AFRO (World Health Organization, African Regional Office). 1991. *Strategies for Malaria Control in the African Region and Steps for Their Implementation.* Brazzaville, Congo: WHO/AFRO.

WHO/EMRO (World Health Organization, Eastern Mediterranean Regional Office). 1997. Malaria Coordination Meeting in North Africa, Tunis, Tunisia, 26–28 May 1997. Unpublished document WHO-EM/MAL/249/E/L. Alexandria, Egypt: WHO/EMRO.

Chapter 10

Determinants of Malaria in Sub-Saharan Africa

Jonathan St. H. Cox, Jean Mouchet, and David J. Bradley

T he determinants of malaria vary on many scales throughout the world in their effects as well as their occurrence. In many regions, one could argue that there is little justification for considering malaria at a continental scale; often the differences within a continent are too great and diverse. But for Africa, a good case can be made: the vector species are limited in number but widely spread across the continent, and malaria itself has a relatively coherent epidemiology throughout much of sub-Saharan Africa. In particular, because Africa is the home of the most efficient anopheline transmitters of malaria and because transmission reaches much higher levels than elsewhere in the world (with only local exceptions), the characteristics of African malaria are more extreme than observed elsewhere. In addition, the responses to changes in determinants may be different, or more subtle, than may be suspected elsewhere.

The determinants of African malaria and the consequences of changing intensities of those determinants can be understood only in light of the dynamics of African malaria. There often is a quantitative mismatch between the shift in a determinant and the effect produced on malaria, however the latter is measured.

In this chapter, we first analyze how malaria is defined and measured. This explanation is necessary because historically, measurement has focused entirely on transmission. However, recently, other variables have been considered, many of which are more relevant to the populations most affected, in the long or short run. We then address the dynamics of malaria in Africa as the basis for subsequent discussion. Several other general principles of the analysis also are presented.

Malaria and Its Measurement

Malaria must be defined and measured if the effects of possible determinants on it are to be examined. Because the attention of the early researchers and first modelers was on the control of transmission, the first measure of malaria was the basic case reproduction rate (BCRR), as introduced by Ross and developed by Macdonald for malaria. More accurately called the *basic case reproduction number,* BCRR is very similar to the secondary attack rate that follows one case of malaria in a nonimmune population. It is an excellent measure of malaria at the margins of its occurrence in space or time (e.g., in situations where the environment is only marginally suitable for malaria transmission, or where malaria has just begun to spread in its invasion of a nonimmune population or is in the last stages of an eradication program). The target for researchers concerned with systematic climate change has been situations where the environment is only marginally suitable, and the key climate change–malaria models have used the Ross–Macdonald formulation as a starting point. Transmission models have been formulated in terms of BCRR, which is usually represented in equations as R_0.

Researchers more concerned with the risk to nonimmune people introduced into a steady-state endemic situation have instead used the mean number of potentially infective bites per person per night (or per year) as a convenient measure. It is more easily understood but not so appropriate for changing conditions, because it is merely a static description of a dynamic steady state. However, this measure is more easily understood than R_0, which has no obvious correlate in the endemic situation.

Both these measures are of infection. But in the African endemic situation, where the majority of children from infancy to adolescence have parasitemia on most days of the year, there may be more concern for the incidence of disease. To define an attack of clinical malaria in the holoendemic situation is profoundly difficult. The parasites are usually present anyway; the fever of malaria under these circumstance is not pathognomonic; and evidence indicates that African children suffer four febrile attacks each per year on average, even in the absence of malaria.

So, how is a clinical attack of malaria to be defined? It may be diagnosed on a combination of fever and a high malaria parasite count in the blood, where "high" is a locally defined age-specific parasite density. Epidemiologically, an "attributable fraction" approach can be used, but this approach requires adequate study populations and substantial effort. Moreover, simple attacks of clinical malaria rarely lead to death. The causes of malaria mortality are profound anemia in the very young and cerebral malaria in all ages from the very young upward. Although the latter point is of immense importance, population-based measurements of the incidence of cerebral malaria are hard to make.

When endpoints are used, the problem is different. Deaths may be recorded or surveyed in various ways, and death is an unequivocal state. In the absence of autopsies in the field, it is hard to reliably ascribe deaths to malaria; however, some limited success has been attained by verbal autopsy. Moreover, measures applied vigorously and successfully to control highly endemic malaria usually reduce the overall death rate by more than the number of deaths ascribed to malaria, so malaria appears to contribute to deaths ascribed to other primary causes. A dynamic model of malaria with disease as the dependent variable has not yet been developed, but it could conceptually be considered relevant for highly endemic situations, even though data are inadequate to construct such a model.

Malaria can be measured in many ways, all with relevance to some situations and all with some drawbacks in operational use. At the edges of transmission, infection and disease become nearly synonymous, because parasitemia is usually accompanied by illness in nonimmune people. In contrast, much of Africa is subject to stable holoendemic malaria, and the effects of environmentally driven changes in transmission cannot be seen as increased prevalence of parasitemia. But there is concern as to whether malaria as a disease may worsen—an outcome that will depend on the shape of the relationship between transmission and disease.

For many decades, this relationship has been viewed as moving to an asymptote at moderately high transmission levels, so that changes in transmission at the top (holoendemic) level have been viewed as neutral in their effects on disease. Recently, although several very detailed studies of communities at different levels of endemic transmission in West Africa have supported this orthodox view, queries have been raised from two quarters.

First, the use of insecticide-treated mosquito nets has substantially reduced clinical malaria attacks, even under very high endemicity. Second, data comparing areas with high transmission rates and very high transmission rates have shown a decrease in severe anemia mortality and an increase in cerebral malaria as transmission falls somewhat (Snow et al. 1997). Whether this shift indicates a paradoxical effect of rising mortality with falling transmission at these levels is a more controversial hypothesis, and extensive data related to defined populations are needed to be able to indicate the effects of transmission changes on disease at highly endemic levels. The issue is not irrelevant to consideration of the effects of changing environmental determinants.

Principles of the Analysis

Relationship to Processes

In considering malaria determinants in Africa, we sought to relate them to the known processes that influence the transmission cycle and the sequence of events that lead to disease and death. This stepwise approach is a relatively cautious one and may miss the sweeping broad assertions of relationship that can come from simple regression of one variable on another. However, the ability to use relationships and to extrapolate wisely to predict the consequences of interventions or of environmental or social changes depends on having insight into the processes concerned. The biological or social plausibility of the relationships of determinants to malaria should not be ignored.

Inclusion of Control Measures

The determinants of malaria and its consequences include the measures that are intended to affect transmission or to treat illness. Conventional practice has been to categorize them apart from other determinants. We reject this separation for some purposes and include them in our analysis for several reasons.

First, there is no clear barrier between activities deliberately undertaken to control malaria and activities that are undertaken for different purposes but affect the level of malaria as an infection or a disease. People may buy bed nets for malaria control or to ward off nuisance insects, or even for purposes of privacy or social conformity. The presence of the net and the way it is used will determine the effect on malaria, not the motivation that led to its use. Similarly, the presence of a ceiling in a hut may affect the anopheline biting rate, but ceilings are only very rarely built with this end in mind.

Second, as we emphasize the need to consider health impacts in all aspects of socioeconomic development, the boundaries between deliberate malaria control actions and aspects of environmental planning that have favorable health impacts along with other positive effects become increasingly blurred. The boundary between healthy living and disease control is inevitably unclear.

Third, the population consequences of multiple individual health acts cannot be ignored, especially in relation to genetic change of the pathogen, most notably, the emergence of heritable drug resistance. Chloroquine is given for fever ("clinical malaria") and has been so used throughout Africa for many decades. Much of the fever is not due to malaria, but over time, the malaria parasites have developed resistance against chloroquine. Misdirected control measures can have major effects on the epidemiology and population genetics of malaria parasites and their anopheline vectors. They are part of the determinants of malaria.

Historical Dependence of Some Determinants

Although some malaria determinants can simply be applied as modifiers on the major climatic determinants, others are highly dependent on previous historical processes. An extreme example is the absence of anophelines from some islands of Polynesia and Micronesia, not because they are necessarily geographically unsuitable but because the genus does not seem to have reached them. A far-off, possibly unique event did not happen. One could posit some general rule (e.g., that islands more than a certain distance from others have a lowered risk, or probability of no malaria), but such a method is an unsound way of dealing with rare historical incidents.

A more common situation for which this approach may be appropriate concerns historically determined risks. Drug resistance to chloroquine appears to arise only with great rarity. It can be argued plausibly that chloroquine resistance originally only arose twice—once in the Thai–Vietnam border area, and once in Colombia—and that all subsequent initial chloroquine resistance has been spread genetically from these two sites. In this case, the chance of drug resistance occurring at a given place depends on a set of local patterns of malaria transmission and drug use as well as on the distance from a location where the genes for that kind of resistance are prevalent.

This argument also can be applied to the presence of malaria parasites. If an area of central Asia, far from current transmission, changes environmentally to become highly suitable for malaria transmission, it may take a long while for parasites to be introduced by migrants or to gradually spread from the nearest, but distant, focus of current infection. In contrast, if environmental circumstances become more favorable for malaria transmission at the high altitudes of a tropical mountain whose low slopes abound in uncontrolled holoendemic malaria, parasites will tend to spread rapidly. Thus, models of the impact of climate change on the spread of malaria must account for contagious processes.

Dynamics of Malaria in Africa

The key determinant of the dynamics of malaria transmission in Africa is the great efficiency of African vectors relative to those of other continents. This vector system is responsible for very high inoculation rates and is remarkably stable in a wide range of environmental conditions. African vectors also appear to be relatively flexible in exploiting landscape changes brought about by anthropogenic activity (Coluzzi 1984).

Coluzzi (1984) estimates that together, *Anopheles funestus, Anopheles gambiae,* and *Anopheles arabiensis* account for 95% of all infective bites in the Afrotropical region. On a broad scale, we would expect the distribution of transmission to mirror that of these species. Other malaria vectors, including *Anopheles nili, Anopheles moucheti,* and the saltwater breeders *Anopheles melas* and *Anopheles merus,* are relatively inefficient but may have important effects at the local level. In forested areas of Cameroon, for example, *An. moucheti* has been as efficient as *Anopheles gambiae sensu stricto (s.s.),* although its distribution is limited to the slow-running rivers of central Africa.

According to Mouchet et al. (1998), stable malaria has an inertia that tends to absorb environmental changes caused by human activities. However, that buffering capacity has its limits, even in Africa, and the degree of local environmental changes needed to effect the transition from stable to unstable malaria is uncertain. Some heavily built-up areas near the center of Africa's large cities and mining areas with strictly enforced environmental health regulations have very little transmission. However, experience has shown that in most endemic areas, significant reductions in malaria transmission are difficult to achieve, whether by trying to eliminate breeding sites at the research level in Tanga, Tanzania, or by reducing mosquitoes in West Africa, where less than one mosquito per house maintains endemicity. The findings from bed net studies and Snow et al. (1997) suggest that even under conditions of persistent, stable, highly endemic malaria, environmental changes can change the frequency of febrile attacks or of the prevalent type of severe malaria while having little effect on parasitemia. This area needs much more research attention in terms of determinants, interventions, and clinical research.

The chief determinants of unstable malaria are the factors that vary the level of transmission, whereas the main determinant of stable holoendemic malaria in sub-Saharan Africa is human acquired immunity. It provides a dynamic regulation of malaria levels, producing the "inertia" described by Mouchet et al. (1998).

The extremely efficient African vector mosquitoes, together with a favorably warm climate, lead to very high values of BCRR and of the steady-state entomological inoculation rate (EIR), which is the mean number of mosquito bites infectious for malaria received by the average inhabitant per unit of time (e.g., per year or per night). If transmission is considered in terms of BCRR, a value of 1 means that transmission is just at replacement level: for every individual infected with malaria who recovers or dies, another incident case appears. This situation is very unstable. If transmission decreases, the malaria ceases to renew itself in the human population and tends to die out. However, if the BCRR increases, so will malaria—except as limited by slowly acquired human immunity.

A BCRR value of 10 means that each case will give rise to 10 more, and the resulting exponential increase will lead to a large epidemic until either all the population is infected or the transmission falls as a result of changed environmental circumstances. When the BCRR remains high, the forces of immunity in the affected population will gradually regulate the spread of infection and the level of transmission. This process is seen most clearly in Africa because the BCRR there is so high; it may exceed 1,000 in parts of the savannas of western and eastern Africa. Under these circumstances, the steady-state EIR (i.e., the risk to a nonimmune visitor) may exceed 300 infective bites per year. The features of this very high degree of endemicity must be understood if we are to understand the likely effects of environmental change (including climate change) on the situation.

What leads to this remarkably high transmission level? Three main variables of anopheline ecology determine the BCRR level:

- the density of female mosquitoes,
- the frequency with which each mosquito feeds on human blood, and
- the longevity of the adult mosquito.

Of these variables, density is the least influential, because there is a simple linear relationship between it and transmission. Changes in the human blood–feeding behavior have a greater effect: because one bite is required to infect the mosquito and another bite is required to infect another person, transmission is proportional to the square of the probability of feeding on human blood. Mosquito longevity is even more crucial because of the exponential survival curve of the adult female mosquitoes; the chance of surviving through one day is raised to the power of the number of days that elapse between the day the mosquito becomes a carrier of malaria parasites and the first day it becomes infectious to humans.

Therefore, transmission is proportional to the 10th power (or thereabouts) of the chance of surviving through one day, and mosquito longevity is a crucial factor in determining the efficacy of a malaria vector. The three major African vectors are all long-lived. In addition, *An. gambiae* and *An. funestus* are intensely anthropophilic—they have a marked preference for feeding on humans rather than other vertebrates, hence the intense transmission.

Very high BCRRs are responsible for the key features of malaria in much of sub-Saharan Africa. Humans tend to become infected at a very early age, so the vast majority of the population is parasitemic in the first year or even the first month of life. Repeated and overlapping infections are usual, so most children have falciparum malaria parasites in their blood on most days from infancy to age 10. Parasite counts in the blood peak in infancy or early childhood and are reduced gradually by progressively acquired immunity to the red cell forms of the infection.

The price of this immunity may be very high; in the absence of chemotherapy, it may lead to a mortality as high as 5% of all births. It also is very difficult to control because up to a 99.9% reduction in transmission may be needed to keep the BCRR below 1 and thus eradicate malaria. In the Nigerian savanna, eradication has proved beyond the capability of spraying homes with residual insecticides combined with the administration of chemotherapy. Changes in the environment related to climate or land and water resource development have a smaller effect and therefore rarely can disturb the stable malaria transmission of the African forest and savanna. Only toward the margins of environmental suitability (e.g., areas of relatively low temperatures associated with high altitudes or latitude, or in desert areas, where mosquito breeding is highly restricted) does the BCRR fall to a level at which malaria becomes unstable and is more readily susceptible to environmental variation.

Climatic Determinants

Temperature

Environmental temperature affects the development and survival of malaria vectors and, perhaps more significantly, the duration of *Plasmodium* development within the invertebrate host. In simple terms, the duration of sporogony increases hyperbolically with decreasing environmental temperatures to a point at which parasite development ceases altogether. This critical temperature varies by parasite species. For *Plasmodium falciparum*, the most abundant parasite in sub-Saharan Africa, laboratory studies have estimated it to be in the range of 16–19 °C (Macdonald 1957; Detinova 1962). In practice, transmission is commonly assumed to be limited to months in which the average temperature is above this threshold (Molineaux 1988). In Africa, these temperature limits commonly are reached only at high altitudes (discussed below) and at high latitudes.

If a relatively conservative temperature threshold of 18 °C is assumed, then most of tropical Africa experiences temperatures suitable for malaria transmission at least 10 months per year (Plate 10-1*). However, extensive areas in which temperatures are sub-optimal for six months or more are found in the high-latitude fringes of southern Africa (Botswana, Namibia, South Africa, Zambia, and Zimbabwe) and in highland fringe areas

---

*Color plates for this chapter appear following page 190.

of Madagascar. In these areas, the effects of low average temperatures may be compounded by those of frost. In Zimbabwe, for example, Leeson (1931) found that *Anopheles gambiae sensu lato* (*s.l.*) disappeared when minimum air temperatures fell below 5 °C. The limits of vector distributions in South Africa also appear to be determined by those of frost (e.g., de Meillon 1934). In regions near the equator, the effects of low temperatures are likely to be restricted to discrete highlands areas in Burundi, Democratic Republic of the Congo, Ethiopia, Kenya, Rwanda, Tanzania, and Uganda (Plate 10-1). The geographical transition from areas where suitable temperatures persist year-round to areas where temperatures are limiting for significant periods is often sharp.

It is often difficult to compare large-scale and small-scale effects, because environmental changes may be described in different terms. The macroscale effects of climate are usually given in terms of temperature, precipitation, and humidity. Smaller-scale environmental changes include water and land resource changes, such as irrigation and deforestation. Comparability is improved if these changes are also described in terms of their effects on microclimate.

Lindblade et al. (2000) described microclimatic effects in a recent analysis of land use changes in the highlands of southwest Uganda. At 1,500–2,400 meters, the landscape comprises parallel ridges separated by steep-sided valleys, at the foot of which were extensive papyrus swamps half a century ago. To increase food production, some 85% of these swamps have been drained and used to grow crops. There is widespread concern that malaria has increased in the area, most notably in a recent epidemic apparently linked to the El Niño climatic oscillation.

The hypothesis that malaria outbreaks were due to swamp cultivation goes back to the 1940s (e.g., Steyn 1946; Vincke and Jadin 1946). Lindblade et al. (2000) compared measurements of microclimatic and anopheline bionomics from villages beside the valley bottoms, both near the papyrus swamps and near the drained cultivated areas. Eight villages were studied in each category, and indoor-resting mosquitoes were caught for eight months, beginning in the rainy season. Mean indoor resting densities, predominantly of *An. gambiae s.l.*, were almost twice as high beside the drained swamps (0.36 mosquitoes/house) as near the papyrus (0.19 mosquitoes/house). However, this difference did not reach statistical significance; one village was responsible for a substantial part of the difference. There also were nonsignificant differences in sporozoite rates and in the EIRs (sevenfold) between the villages. A regression analysis indicated that temperature differences between the villages were a main contributor to the different transmission parameters.

Rainfall

Although several studies have demonstrated an association between *An. gambiae* abundance and rainfall (e.g., Charlwood et al. 1995), a direct, predictable relationship does not exist. *An. gambiae* can breed prolifically in temporary, turbid water bodies such as hoof prints or rain puddles, whereas *An. funestus* prefers permanent water bodies. However, both temporary and permanent water bodies depend on adequate rainfall; therefore, there is good reason for using rainfall to indicate the probable presence of vectors, vector survival, and the potential for malaria transmission (Craig, Snow, and Le Sueur 1999).

The geographic pattern of annual rainfall in sub-Saharan Africa is illustrated in Plate 10-2. The highest amounts are found in coastal areas of Cameroon, Liberia, Madagascar, Nigeria, and Sierra Leone, but annual totals in excess of 1,000 millimeters are characteristic of much of the interior of the continent. The driest areas are southwest Africa

(Botswana, Namibia, and South Africa), parts of the African Horn (Somalia and sections of Ethiopia and Kenya), and the northern Sahel. In these regions, the longevity of adult vectors is likely to be negatively affected by low humidity; relative humidity in excess of 60% is generally deemed necessary for effective malaria transmission (Molineaux 1988).

The effects of quite dramatic climatic events on the level of malaria transmission may depend on their timing. Catastrophic flooding in Mozambique consequent to abnormally high rainfall levels in March 2000 clearly illustrates this point. By late April, malaria transmission had not risen unusually, contrary to what had been predicted in the lay media. The heavy rains had washed out anopheline breeding places, and much of the country remained under water; this is not the breeding habitat for the *An. gambiae* complex, nor is it ideal for *An. funestus*. The breeding habitats were likely to be created as the floods receded, but because the flooding was so extensive, breeding would not be very high until after the temperature had fallen to winter levels unsuitable for malaria transmission. Had the timing of the floods been different, the malaria hazard could have been far greater.

Thus, at the limiting temperatures for malaria transmission, the timing of rainfall hazards may be crucial, and the consequences may vary greatly by season. Increased rainfall in the arid zones will have a much greater effect on transmission. Near the equator, even though extra rainfall may augment mosquito breeding and potentially raise malaria transmission, malarial morbidity may be only modestly affected because of the already high levels of transmission and human immunity.

Climate-Based Models of Malaria Transmission

The potential effects of geographical variations in climate on continental patterns of malaria transmission risk have been well illustrated by models developed within the Mapping Malaria Risk in Africa project (MARA; Snow, Marsh, and Le Sueur 1996). MARA's climate-based malaria distribution model has been developed using a simple numerical approach for defining the geographical limits of transmission based on the biological constraints of temperature and rainfall (Craig, Snow, and Le Sueur 1999). This method uses fuzzy logic to represent whether, under average climate conditions, rainfall or temperature is expected to limit malaria transmission at a given site in any given month. The aggregated annual picture (Plate 10-3) is based on the premise that several contiguous months of "suitable" climate conditions are required to constitute a malaria transmission season. The legend in Plate 10-3 therefore corresponds to the maximum model value that can be sustained over a five-month period (or three months in areas above 8°N, where relatively high environmental temperatures at the onset of the rainy season cause vector populations to increase particularly quickly).

It is important to recognize that the MARA model is based on long-term climate averages (Hutchinson et al. 1995) and provides an essentially static picture of malaria transmission potential under expected climatic conditions. The model may, as a result, underestimate the significance of malaria in epidemic-prone areas (where transmission usually depends on unexpected meteorological conditions). Moreover, because it is a purely climate-based model, it does not account for the distribution of human populations or the likely presence of nonclimatic risk factors. Therefore, although the model corresponds well with existing stratification and expert opinion maps on the broad scale, significant anomalies do occur. For example, because the MARA model does not account for the rather patchy population distribution of sub-Saharan Africa (Plate 10-4), it may give a misleading impression of the risk of disease in sparsely populated areas.

Climate Change

Given the stability of transmission in many parts of Africa, climate change probably will not yield significant shifts in malaria epidemiology in most areas. The potential impact in fringe transmission areas is likely to be somewhat variable, however. In many areas (particularly desert fringe), the effects of climate change will be limited by very low population densities. In other areas (e.g., Madagascar, South Africa, and Zimbabwe), malaria surveillance and control in fringe localities may be sufficient to mitigate any increases in transmission brought about by climate change. The fringe areas of most concern are the highlands of Madagascar and of eastern and central Africa, which support relatively large human populations (Plate 10-4). Because of the sensitivity of transmission to temperature in these areas, relatively small changes in the climate of highland areas may lead to significant increases in the local altitudinal limits of malaria transmission, thereby putting large numbers of immunologically naive people at risk of infection.

Although the evidence is patchy, data for certain highland localities suggest that malaria has become progressively more serious, especially since the early 1990s (Loevinsohn 1994; Tulu 1996; Malakooti, Biomndo, and Shanks 1998; Mouchet et al. 1998; Cox et al. 1999). To what extent these data are a reflection of a more general, regional, or continental trend is unclear. The role of climate change is also uncertain; whereas epidemics have clearly been associated with abnormal weather events, as yet, little evidence indicates that they are a feature of longer-term shifts in climate conditions. In the rare instances where changes in malaria transmission intensity have been correlated with climate change, evaluating the contribution of confounding (nonclimatic) factors has been difficult. For example, recent increases in highland malaria transmission have been observed at a time when, for one reason or another, basic health services and malaria control activities have been in decline. This problem is likely to be compounded by emerging drug resistance and, in certain instances, by uncertain drug supplies. Under such conditions, a rise in observed morbidity and mortality may not necessarily reflect an increase in malaria transmission but nevertheless represents a significant problem for national malaria control programs.

Changes in climate and environment do not always increase malaria transmission. For example, meteorological data from the marshy areas of the Niayes (Senegal) indicate that rainfall in the period 1980–1990 was nearly 30% below the 1931–1960 average and that the rainy season became progressively shorter over the same period (Mouchet et al. 1996). Entomological surveys carried out in 1991–1992 indicated that *An. funestus,* previously a significant vector, had all but disappeared from the area, and *An. gambiae s.s.* also had declined—more than the less efficient *An. arabiensis* (Faye et al. 1995). These changes in vector populations were thought to be responsible for a marked decline in malaria transmission; parasite rates among local children fell from 40–80% in the late 1960s to less than 10% in 1991–1992. Similar trends were observed in the Niger River valley, Zinda, and Dilla areas of Niger, where a 29% decrease in annual rainfall (measured at Niamey) between the periods 1950–1959 and 1981–1990 was considered largely responsible for dramatic decreases in malaria prevalence rates (Mouchet et al. 1996).

Altitude

Although altitude has long been recognized as an important determinant of malaria endemicity (e.g., Hirsch 1883), the transmission factors that are directly or indirectly affected by altitude are actually of more epidemiological significance. The most obvious and important of these factors is environmental temperature, which is negatively correlated with altitude, but rainfall also tends to vary negatively with elevation at high altitudes (e.g., Lauscher 1976). Even though past researchers have been tempted to define altitudinal thresholds for malaria transmission on this basis, for Africa as a whole or for specific regions (e.g., Schwetz 1942; Wilson 1949; Lindsay and Martens 1998), this tendency should be resisted for two reasons.

First, the relationship between altitude and temperature is often oversimplified and in practice may vary substantially over time and space. At the continental scale, the effect of latitude is important, and its significance in the context of malaria has long been recognized (e.g., Gill 1923). In addition to its effect on mean annual temperature, latitude influences the relative importance of seasonal and diurnal variations in climate; the latter tends to predominate in tropical highlands. Highland temperature regimes also are affected by continentality. Specifically, diurnal and annual temperature ranges tend to decrease with increasing proximity to large water bodies, whereas the incidence of cloud and mist increases, significantly reducing temperature.

Second, the assumption that temperature is the sole or principal factor limiting malaria transmission in highland areas may not always be valid. The significance of other transmission factors is suggested by the existence of altitudinal limits of transmission that are far below what would be expected on the basis of temperature alone in many parts of Africa. Large areas of the highlands are too dry; in some areas, local topographical characteristics offer too few breeding sites; in yet other areas, the ecology is not conducive to supporting anopheline populations.

Land Cover and Land Use Change

Surface Water

The availability of suitable sources of surface water for vector breeding is a prerequisite for malaria transmission. In many parts of Africa, surface water is scarce—either because of the general aridity of the climate or because local topographical characteristics preclude the pooling of water (e.g., de Zulueta et al. 1961). In other cases, existing water sources may be rendered unsuitable as breeding sites for specific species depending on the availability of light and shade and the type of vegetation present.

In fringe transmission areas, the distribution of suitable breeding sites for efficient vectors is likely to have a profound influence on patterns of malaria transmission. A good historical example is provided by parasitological and entomological surveys carried out in highland areas of southwest Uganda. In southern Kigezi (now Kabale district), the surveys of Garnham, Wilson, and Wilson (1948) revealed hyperendemic conditions around Lake Bunyonyi (1,920 meters), where entomological surveys indicated that *An. funestus* was the principal malaria vector present. Away from the lake areas, where *An. gambiae s.l.* was determined to be the main vector, spleen rates dropped off rapidly. Subsequent studies carried out in Kigezi as part of the preeradication effort (de Zulueta et al. 1961, 1964) also showed pockets of endemic malaria around Lakes Bunyonyi, Mutanda (1,800 meters), and Kimbuga (1,600 meters). The absence of permanent malaria foci in highlands beyond these areas was attributed to an "almost complete lack of water collections" in areas above 1,200 meters (de Zulueta et al. 1961).

The anomalous picture created by the presence of hyperendemic sites at high altitudes in sub-Saharan Africa is illustrated in Figure 10-1. Parasite and spleen rates in the vicinity of Lake Bunyonyi are atypical of the general trend of decreasing levels of transmission intensity with increasing altitude. However, such pockets of high transmission

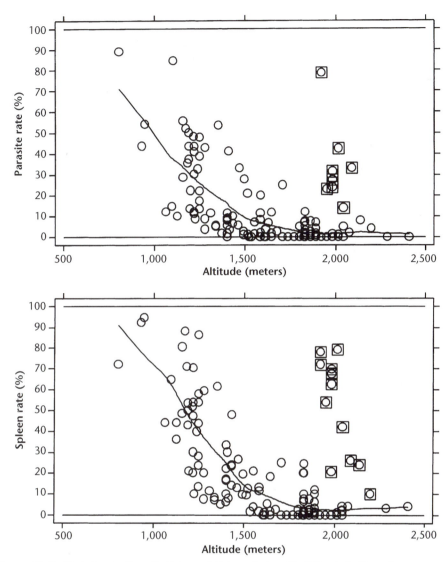

Figure 10-1. Variation in Parasite Rate and Spleen Rate with Altitude in Uganda

Circles in boxes indicate survey results (observations) from the vicinity of Lake Bunyonyi.

Sources: Historical data are taken from various published and unpublished sources (Cox et al. 1999).

are not unique to Uganda. In Kenya, for example, Roberts (1964) referred to focal swamps in which vectors were perennially present and from which they would spread, given suitable meteorological conditions. Spleen rates in the vicinity of these swamps were typically 50% higher than in the surrounding areas.

The natural distribution of breeding sites may be transformed by the creation of new water sources, such as dams (see later), or by modifications to existing water bodies that render them more suitable to anopheline breeding. In southwest Uganda, for example, the entomological results of Goma (1958) and others indicated that in its natural condition, much of the permanent swamp was unsuitable for vector breeding. From the early 1940s, large areas of swamp were cleared of their natural vegetation for agriculture, and these operations were accompanied by large increases in both the number of malaria vectors and malaria incidence (Steyn 1946). A similar phenomenon was observed in neighboring Rwanda and Burundi (e.g., Vincke and Jadin 1946), where swamp cultivation was considered to be primarily responsible for the spread of malaria to higher slopes (Meyus, Lips, and Caubergh 1962).

Impounded Waters

The seasonal scarcity of water in savanna areas and the Sahel, together with opportunities to harness larger rivers to provide hydropower and stores of water to allow dry season irrigation, have led to extensive dam construction in the semi-arid areas of Africa.

Initially, attention was directed to a series of large dams that created huge lakes, with significant and often adverse effects on populations from the inundated areas. Kariba (Zambia and Zimbabwe), Volta (Ghana), Kaiingi (Nigeria), and the Aswan High Dam (Egypt) are notable examples. These dams were the subjects of international concern and financing and, after early health disasters, the objects of research studies and attempts to mitigate the problems. Advice was not always well founded. In the case of the Volta Dam, initial advice was based on U.S. experience in the Tennessee valley, where the periodic abrupt lowering of water levels by siphons or opening sluices had stranded mosquito larvae and prevented their development. Subsequent better advice (sought when the original suggestions proved impossible to implement for so vast an impoundment) drew attention to the likely creation of breeding sites for *An. gambiae* by lowering the water level and exposing great expanses of muddy shore with puddles. However, the initial holoendemicity of malaria in the area before dam construction indicated that although the mosquito population might rise subsequent to dam construction, the level of malaria endemicity was unlikely to change much. This was in fact the result, and the disease changes mostly affected infections such as schistosomiasis rather than malaria. The African experience differs vastly from that of India, where dam construction has been followed by malaria epidemics.

One particular concern was raised concerning the Aswan High Dam and Lake Nasser, which extends for hundreds of miles south into the Sudan. Twice in the twentieth century, *An. gambiae* has penetrated north into Egypt from the Sudan. For example, in the late 1940s, penetration was followed by massive malaria epidemics controlled by Fred L. Soper, who was able to eradicate *An. gambiae* locally and restore the situation. It was believed that Lake Nasser would facilitate the northward passage of *An. gambiae,* with terrible consequences for Egypt. However, these feared consequences have not materialized.

Greater and more justified concerns have surrounded the construction of small dams on a huge scale in Africa. One state in Nigeria had more than 550 small dams constructed in a few years. International financing is not involved, and health risks are rarely considered. Dams that are in areas previously too arid for much malaria transmission or at altitudes at which malaria is unstable may produce adverse results.

Parasitological data have been collected as a part of an ongoing project to assess the impacts of small-scale irrigation dams in Tigray, Ethiopia, where hundreds of such dams are planned (Ghebreyesus et al. 1998). Although irrigation dams have increased malaria transmission in lowland Ethiopia (e.g., Meskal and Kloos 1989), less is known about their potential impacts in the highlands. Preliminary data from Tigray suggest that parasite rates in the vicinity of dams are significantly higher than those in outlying areas. Dam construction has had similar demonstrable effects on local levels of malaria transmission in Kenya (e.g., Khaemba, Mutani, and Bett 1994) as well as in Rwanda and Burundi (e.g., Meyus, Lips, and Caubergh 1962).

Irrigation and Rice

Water resource developments for agriculture in Africa include irrigation schemes on all scales, from the huge area of the Gezira in Sudan, which extends more than 100 kilometers, to small furrows constructed by peasant farmers. Although irrigation is often expected to be followed by malaria outbreaks on other continents, in Africa, many irrigation schemes are constructed in areas of holoendemic malaria, where the addition of mosquitoes may increase the biting nuisance but have little effect on malaria transmission. In highland or extremely arid areas where malaria is unstable or rare, irrigation may indeed facilitate transmission, but this result should not be assumed to be universal.

The Gezira Irrigation Scheme, developed to grow cotton, has increased malaria problems by unintentionally providing mosquito breeding sites in its canals (no drains were built to remove the excess water that would otherwise evaporate, leaving behind salts and eventually salinizing the land; the Blue Nile River water that feeds the scheme has such low salinity that drains were not expected to be needed to protect agricultural interests). Malaria transmission was effectively controlled when cotton was the only crop and discipline over cultivation and water management was very strict. However, with the rise of chloroquine resistance and less rigid management, the problem has increased. In the analogous West African situation at the Office du Niger in Mali, the surrounding area has seasonally transmitted holoendemic malaria. Within the irrigation scheme, malaria transmission is close to perennial, but the actual level of disease is no higher.

In The Gambia, the introduction of irrigated rice into the Middle River region (as distinct from the swamp rice grown throughout the country) has had a complex effect. Irrigation in the dry season causes a second annual peak of mosquito abundance, in addition to that after the rains. But the second peak is not accompanied by any increase in malaria transmission (Lindsay et al. 1991). Whether this difference is due to short mosquito survival in the hot weather, temperatures too high for the malaria parasites to survive in the mosquitoes, or even different mosquito cytotypes is not fully clear.

Therefore, the issue of rice cultivation is perhaps more complex in Africa than elsewhere, and the effects of irrigation on malaria are sometimes counterintuitive. The malaria outcome (in terms of transmission rates and prevalence of the disease) resulting from modification of a transmission factor varies depending on preexisting levels of transmission.

Although rice cultivation has greatly increased populations of *An. gambiae* in West Africa, patterns of malaria have remained relatively unaffected. In Burkina Faso, for example, sporozoite rates in rice-cultivated areas were one-tenth of those in surrounding savanna areas (where the mopti cytotype is dominant), so although vector densities were 10 times higher, inoculation rates effectively remained unchanged (Robert et al. 1985, Favia et al. 1997). In Burundi, at intermediate altitudes, rice cultivation has been linked to increases in the population and vectorial capacity of *An. arabiensis* (but not *An. funestus*) and to the existence of highly localized, hyperendemic pockets in otherwise unstable transmission areas (Coosemans et al. 1984).

The positive association between rice cultivation and increased risk of malaria transmission has perhaps been demonstrated most strongly in Madagascar, where rice fields have supported relatively high concentrations of *An. funestus* and *An. arabiensis*. The rapid development of rice cultivation in the highlands, together with the influx of workers from malaria-endemic parts of the country, was thought to be responsible for extensive epidemics of malaria in the late nineteenth century. High levels of malaria transmission prevailed until 1949, when control measures (DDT spraying, drug chemo-prophylaxis, and the administration of chemotherapy) were introduced (Laventure et al. 1996). By the early 1960s, malaria was widely believed to be eradicated; DDT operations ceased, and malaria treatment centers were later closed down. What followed was described by Mouchet et al. (1997) as a gradual "reconquest" of the highlands by malaria, which culminated in severe epidemics in 1986–1988.

Deforestation

In its natural state, forest vegetation is usually unsuitable for malaria vectors, particularly *An. gambiae* complex, although *An. moucheti* is a forest mosquito. However, anophelines may quickly colonize areas that have been disturbed sufficiently to allow direct sunlight on small temporary water collections that are suitable for larval development (Coluzzi 1994). In southern Cameroon, for example, forest clearance for cultivation, village settlements, and road systems has been associated with the invasion of malaria vectors such as *An. gambiae s.s.* and, to a lesser extent, *An. nili* and *An. moucheti* (Livadas et al. 1958).

In Africa, deforestation is usually associated with increases in *Plasmodium falciparum* transmission, but the scale of this increase depends on the degree of disturbance and the human populations involved. Effects of deforestation are likely to be most extreme when clearance is accompanied by urbanization, as described by Coluzzi et al. (1979). In south Nigeria, *An. arabiensis* was able to colonize urban areas including Benin City and Sapele to create what Coluzzi et al. called islands of "derived savanna."

The effects of deforestation on disease will depend on existing levels of malaria endemicity in surrounding areas and the degree of immunity among the new settlers. Where forests are being cleared by local residents in hyperendemic settings, patterns of disease are unlikely to be altered radically, despite local changes in transmission intensity.

Urbanization

The ecological processes associated with urbanization should, in theory, limit malaria transmission by reducing the opportunities for vector breeding and the degree of contact between humans and vectors. Improved access to health care and malaria control measures (e.g., bed nets) also should contribute to a reduced burden of malaria disease. Evidence from the field largely bears out this theory but also suggests that the existence of diverse epidemiological situations in most urban areas makes generalization difficult. In most cases, human settlement initially favors the multiplication of breeding sites and the perennial presence of high densities of *An. gambiae*. But as urban areas become more established and human and building densities rise, potential vector breeding sites become increasingly scarce. This situation may be compounded by the canalization of streams and other sources of surface water and by the effects of pollution.

The intensity of malaria transmission within an individual city therefore may be quite variable, depending on the degree of development within specific localities. It is illustrated by results of entomological and parasitological surveys carried out in Ouagadougou, Burkina Faso (Sabatinelli et al. 1986), and Brazzaville, Congo (Trape and Zoulani 1987a,b; Trape 1987). In both cases, levels of transmission were generally lower in town areas than in the surrounding countryside, but variation between different urban sites was considerable. Trape and Zoulani (1987a) demonstrated that although the average Brazzaville inhabitant receives 22.5 infective bites per year, in individual districts, this figure varied from more than 100 infective bites per year to less than 1 bite every three years.

Where larval habitats do exist in urban areas, high transmission rates are likely to be focused on restricted areas, given the limited dispersal of *An. gambiae* in densely populated areas. In Ouagadougou, for example, malaria prevalence rates were significantly different in groups of children living in houses only 300 meters apart (Sabatinelli et al. 1986).

In cases where the environmental modifications associated with urbanization lead to a change in the composition of local vector species, the effect on levels of malaria transmission may be more difficult to predict. In Cotonou, Benin, transmission rates in many peri-urban sites are reportedly higher than in outlying rural areas because the increased availability of freshwater collections has increased populations of *An. gambiae s.s.* relative to those of the less efficient *An. melas*, which is a saltwater breeder (Akogbeto et al. 1988). Urbanization in Accra, Ghana, was allegedly responsible for the complete disappearance of *An. funestus* while the relatively inefficient *An. arabiensis* remained widespread in many urban localities because it was better able to adapt to breeding in polluted water (Chinery 1984).

Human, Genetic, and Socioeconomic Determinants

Human Determinants

Human population heterogeneity is another major determinant of malarial consequences, though less so of malarial transmission. In a nonmigrant population under steady levels of malaria transmission, age will be a surrogate for malarial immunity, and the population can be viewed as a whole in its responses to changing environmental determinants of malaria transmission. But the genetic heterogeneity of the human population in genes that affect responses to malaria or a diverse migration history of some elements of the human population may render the effects of malaria and of changes in transmission level more complex.

Migration, always a feature of African malaria (Prothero 1977), is even more evident today. By mixing gene pools and creating populations heterogeneous in their past histories of malaria, migration must be considered part of the determining factors for human malaria.

Genetic Determinants

The picture of the basic science of malaria has become more coherent in the last few years. Malaria can be viewed biomedically as the population genetics of three interacting populations: human hosts, vectors, and malaria parasites. Each is more polymorphic in genetic expression than was previously realized. Although the main human genetic determinant of infection is the Duffy blood group system (which affects susceptibility of red cells to *Plasmodium vivax* infection), many other polymorphisms affect pathogenesis and the severity of disease, most notably, the hemoglobinopathies (of which sickle-cell anemia is best known). More recently, polymorphisms of the tumor necrosis factor gene and its regulation have been found to affect the risk of severe malaria.

The blood group antigens and hemoglobinopathies have been mapped in some detail for Africa, and they clearly act as a filter on the species of malaria parasite to be found in a given area and on the frequency of severe and complicated malaria. Because the West African indigenous population is largely Duffy-negative, vivax malaria is very scarce in that part of Africa; *P. vivax* is rather widely replaced by *Plasmodium ovale*. Climate and other environmental changes appear unlikely to significantly affect the frequency or geographical distribution of the Duffy antigens. However, one might expect some degree of increase of the sickling gene in areas of Africa (largely hill areas) invaded by *P. falciparum* as a result of environmental change, so there will be a reciprocal interaction of host genotype and parasite intensity. This process will be slow and imperfect. Therefore, in the short run, host polymorphism should be viewed as modifying the determinants of malaria.

Socioeconomic Determinants

Attempts to model climate change effects that also incorporate different socioeconomic development scenarios have been undertaken by the Hadley Climate Centre in the United Kingdom. However, the effect of these socioeconomic variables on malaria is by indirect routes that vary geographically in their effects, depending on the mosquito vector species involved. In particular, economic growth is unlikely to have a major beneficial effect on the distribution of malaria in Africa, although it is likely to reduce mortality by enabling people to afford medicines and seek medical assistance for their children. If incomes rise substantially, the state may be able to run malaria control programs, but programs would be expensive if they were to substantially affect transmission in tropical Africa. In the more temperate climate of Zimbabwe and South Africa, costs of effective transmission control are more modest; consequently, it is feasible to attempt transmission control on a long-term basis, and eradication remains a stated goal in Zimbabwe.

Unlike some tropical infections, the individual and household behavior of people who become more prosperous is not enough to eliminate malaria, even though such people may reduce their individual risk by using bed nets, screening their windows, obtaining prompt treatment, using mosquito repellents, and even taking chemoprophylactic drugs. Even organized control measures by residual insecticide spraying cannot stop transmission in the Sahel, but they can well do so in highland and other unstable malaria areas and in some urban situations.

The public and private construction works of prosperity may increase risk because building sites may breed mosquitoes in the rainy season, and "borrow pits" along newly constructed roads are a notorious source of anophelines. However, better-constructed houses diminish transmission; the insertion of ceilings tends to reduce vector resting sites, and screens and air conditioning have an even greater effect.

Historically, socioeconomic development has been associated with decreases in malaria morbidity and mortality, particularly when these developments were associated with environmental modifications that limited contact between vectors and humans (Coluzzi 1994). This was the experience in Europe and parts of North Africa, but one probably should be less hopeful for sub-Saharan Africa because of vector characteristics.

Conclusion

The chief determinants of unstable malaria in Africa are the factors that vary the level of transmission, whereas the main determinant of stable holoendemic malaria (the disease, not parasitemia) in sub-Saharan Africa is human acquired immunity.

Although the general distribution of endemic malaria in Africa is strongly related to climate, transmission over large parts of the continent is likely to be relatively unaffected by climate change, either because they are already holoendemic for malaria or because current climate conditions are so unsuitable that very extreme shifts in rainfall or temperature would be necessary to create conditions conducive for transmission. Areas where malaria transmission is "sensitive" to long- or short-term climatic variations therefore are likely to be limited to the current edges of the malaria distribution associated with high altitudes, high latitudes, or desert fringes. The precise effect of climate change in these areas will depend on the extent to which malaria surveillance and control can mitigate the effects of increased transmission. At the local level, the influence of nonclimatic risk factors (such as changes in land use or land cover) may dominate over that of climate.

The overall picture of malaria in sub-Saharan Africa that emerges is of a limited number of areas at the limits of altitude or latitude (both surrogates for temperature or rainfall) for malaria transmission where the resulting unstable malaria is highly susceptible to small changes of environmental and other variables. These areas (especially those at higher altitudes) are of greater importance than their relative surface area would suggest because of the population density located there.

The remaining malarious areas—the bulk of the African continent south of the Sahara—are highly endemic stable malaria where the consequences of environmental and social change on transmission will be less apparent because of immunological damping in the heavily infected population. Such changes that might occur are in fact controversial or rather uncertain. However, they should not be ignored.

A truism of epidemiology is that small changes in common diseases make more difference to the public health than large changes in rare diseases. Changes within the uncertainty levels for holoendemic areas might well exceed in mortality and morbidity effects those more apparent and dramatic epidemics that could occur at the edges of transmission. Although much can be predicted and the effects of many variables other than "simple" climate variations and changes can be assessed with some confidence, the areas of our uncertainty in highly endemic malaria need much more analytical attention before reasonable predictions become feasible.

References

Akogbeto, M., M. Di Deco, R. Romano, and M. Coluzzi. 1988. Analasi comparativa del ruolo vettore per la malaria di *Anopheles gambiae* e *Anopheles melas* nella zona lagunare costiera del Benin. *Parassitologia* 30(Suppl. 1): 7–8.

Charlwood, J.D., J. Kihonda, S. Sama, P.F. Billingsley, H. Hadji, J.P. Verhave, E. Lyimo, P.C. Luttikhuizen, and T. Smith. 1995. The rise and fall of *Anopheles arabiensis* (Diptera: *Culicidae*) in a Tanzanian village. *Bulletin of Entomological Research* 85(1): 37–44.

Chinery, W.A. 1984. Effects of ecological changes on the malaria vectors *Anopheles funestus* and the *Anopheles gambiae* complex of mosquitoes in Accra, Ghana. *Journal of Tropical Medicine and Hygiene* 87: 75–81.

Coluzzi, M. 1984. Heterogeneities of the malaria vectorial system in tropical Africa and their significance in malaria epidemiology and control. *Bulletin of the World Health Organization* 62(Suppl): 107–113.

———. 1994. Malaria and the afrotropical ecosystems: Impact of man-made environmental changes. *Parassitologia* 36(1/2): 223–227.

Coluzzi, M., A. Sabatini, N. Petrarca, and M.A. Di Deco. 1979. Chromosomal differentiation and adaptation to human environments in the *Anopheles gambiae* complex. *Transactions of the Royal Society of Tropical Medicine and Hygiene* 73(5): 483–497.

Coosemans, M., M. Wery, B. Storme, L. Hendrix, and B. Mfisi. 1984. Epidemiologie du paludisme dans la plaine de la Ruzizi, Burundi. *Annales de la Société Belge de Médecine Tropicale* 64(2): 135–158.

Corbett, J.D., and R.F. O'Brien. 1997. *The Spatial Characterization Tool*. Temple, TX: Blackland Research Center, Texas A&M University.

Cox, J., M. Craig, D. Le Sueur, and B. Sharp. 1999. *Mapping Malaria Risk in the Highlands of Africa*. Durban, South Africa: MARA Collaboration.

Craig, M.H., R.W. Snow, and D. Le Sueur. 1999. A climate-based distribution model of malaria transmission in sub-Saharan Africa. *Parasitology Today* 15: 105–111.

de Meillon, B. 1934. Observations on *Anopheles funestus* and *Anopheles gambiae* in the Transvaal. *Publications of the South African Institute of Medical Research* 6: 195.

de Zulueta, J., G.W. Kafuko, J.R. Cullen, and C.K. Pedersen. 1961. The results of the first year of malaria eradication project in northern Kigezi, Uganda. *East African Medical Journal* 38: 1–26.

de Zulueta, J., G.W. Kafuko, A.W.R. MacRae, J.R. Cullen, and C.K. Pedersen, and D.F.B. Wasswa. 1964. A malaria eradication experiment in the highlands of Kigezi, Uganda. *East African Medical Journal* 41: 109–120.

Deichmann, U. 1996. African Population Database. Washington, DC: World Resources Institute/ U.N. Environment Programme.

Detinova, T.S. 1962. *Age-Grouping Methods in Diptera of Medical Importance*. Geneva, Switzerland: World Health Organization.

Favia, G., A. della Torre, M. Bagayoko, A. Lanfrancotti, N. Sagnon, Y.T. Toure, and M. Coluzzi. 1997. Molecular identification of sympatric chromosomal forms of *Anopheles gambiae* and further evidence of their reproductive isolation. *Insect Molecular Biology* 6(4): 377–383.

Faye, O., O. Gaye, D. Fontenille, G. Hebrard, L. Konate, N. Sy, J.P. Herve, Y. Toure, S. Diallo, and J.F. Molez. 1995. La sécheresse et la baisse du paludisme dans les Niayes du Sénégal. *Cahiers Santé* 5(5): 299–305.

Garnham, P.C.C., D.B. Wilson, and M.E. Wilson. 1948. Malaria in Kigezi, Uganda. *Journal of Tropical Medicine and Hygiene* 50: 156–159.

Ghebreyesus, T.A., M. Haile, A. Getachew, T. Alemayehu, K.H. Witten, A. Medhin, M. Yohannes, Y. Asgedom, Y. Yeebiyo, S.W. Lindsay, and P. Byass. 1998. Pilot studies on the possible effects on malaria of small-scale irrigation dams in Tigray regional state, Ethiopia. *Journal of Public Health Medicine* 20(2): 238–240.

Gill, C.A. 1923. The relation of malaria to altitude. *Indian Journal of Medical Research* 11: 511–542.

Goma, L.K.H. 1958. The productivity of various mosquito breeding places in the swamps of Uganda. *Bulletin of Entomological Research* 49: 437–448.

Hirsch, A. 1883. *Handbook of Geographical and Historical Pathology. Volume 1: Acute Infective Diseases*. London, U.K.: Sydenham Society.

Hutchinson, M.F., H.A. Nix, J.P. McMahon, and K.D. Ord. 1995. *Africa: A Topographic and Climatic Database*. Canberra, Australia: Centre for Resource and Environmental Studies.

Khaemba, B.M., A. Mutani, and M.K. Bett. 1994. Studies of anopheline mosquitoes transmitting malaria in a newly developed highland urban area: A case study of Moi University and its environs. *East African Medical Journal* 71(3): 159–164.

Lauscher, F. 1976. Weltweite typan der hohenabhanm gigkeit des niederschlags. *Wetter und Leben* 28: 80–90.

Laventure, S., J. Mouchet, S. Blanchy, L. Marrama, P. Rabarison, L. Andrianaivolambo, E. Rajaonarivelo, I. Rakotoarivony, and J. Roux. 1996. Le riz source de vie et de mort sur les plateaux de Madagascar. *Cahiers Santé* 6(2): 79–86.

Leeson, H.S. 1931. *Anopheline Mosquitoes in Southern Rhodesia*. London, U.K.: London School of Hygiene and Tropical Medicine.

Lindblade, K.A., E. D. Walker, A.W. Onapa, J. Katungu, and M.L. Wilson. 2000. Land use change alters malaria transmission parameters by modifying temperature in a highland area of Uganda. *Tropical Medicine and International Health* 5(4): 263–274.

Lindsay, S.W., and W.J.M. Martens 1998. Malaria in the African highlands: Past, present and future. *Bulletin of the World Health Organization* 76(1): 33–45.

Lindsay, S.W., H.A. Wilkins, H.A. Zeiler, R. J. Daly, V. Patrarca, and P. Byass. 1991. Ability of *Anopheles gambiae* mosquitoes to transmit malaria during the dry and wet seasons in an area of irrigated rice cultivation in The Gambia. *Journal of Tropical Medicine and Hygiene* 94(5): 313–324.

Livadas, G., J. Mouchet, J. Gariou, and R. Chastang. 1958. Peut-on envisager l'éradication du paludisme dans la région forestière du sud Cameroun? *Rivista di Malariologia* 37: 229–256.

Loevinsohn, M.E. 1994. Climatic warming and increased malaria incidence in Rwanda. *Lancet* 343(8899): 714–718.

Macdonald, G. 1957. *The Epidemiology and Control of Malaria*. London, U.K.: Oxford University Press.

Malakooti, M.A., K. Biomndo, and D.A. Shanks. 1998. Reemergence of epidemic highland malaria in the highlands of western Kenya. *Emerging Infectious Diseases* 4(4): 671–676.

Meskal, F.H., and H. Kloos 1989. Vector-borne disease occurrence and spread as affected by labour migrations to irrigation schemes in Ethiopia. *Demography and Vector-Borne Diseases,* edited by M.W. Service. Boca Raton, FL: CRC Press, 225–236.

Meyus, H., M. Lips, and H. Caubergh. 1962. L'état actuel du problème du paludisme d'altitude au Ruanda-Urundi. *Annales de la Société Belge de Médecine Tropicale* 42: 771–782.

Molineaux, L. 1988. The epidemiology of human malaria as an explanation of its distribution, including some implications for its control. In *Malaria: Principles and Practice of Malariology*, volume 2. Edited by W.H. Wernsdorfer and I. McGregor. New York: Churchill Livingstone, 913–998.

Mouchet, J., O. Faye, J. Juivez, and S. Manguin. 1996. Drought and malaria retreat in the Sahel, West Africa. *Lancet* 348(9043): 1735–1736.

Mouchet, J., S. Laventure, S. Blanchy, R. Fioramonti, A. Rakotonjanabelo, P. Rabarison, J. Sircoulon, and J. Roux. 1997. La reconquête des Hautes Terres de Madagascar par le paludisme. *Bullétin de la Société de Pathologie Exotique* 90(3): 162–168.

Mouchet, J., S. Manguin, J. Sircoulon, S. Laventure, O. Faye, A.W. Onapa, P. Carnevale, J. Julvez, and D. Fontenille. 1998. Evolution of malaria in Africa for the past 40 years: Impact of climatic and human factors. *Journal of the American Mosquito Control Association* 14(2): 121–130.

Prothero, R.M. 1977. Disease and mobility: A neglected factor in epidemiology. *International Journal of Epidemiology* 6(3): 259–267.

Robert, V., P. Gazin, C. Boudin, J.F. molex, V. Ouedraogo, and P. Carnivale. 1985. La transmission du paludisme en zone de savane arborée et en zone rizicole des environs de Bobo Dioulasso (Burkina Faso). *Annales de la Société Belge de Médecine Tropicale* 65(Suppl. 2): 201–214.

Roberts, J.M.D. 1964. The control of epidemic malaria in the highlands of western Kenya. Part II. The campaign. *Journal of Tropical Medicine and Hygiene* 61: 191–199.

Sabatinelli, G., A. Bosman, L. Lamizana, and P. Rossi. 1986. Prevalence du paludisme a Ouagadougou et dans le milieu rural limitrophe en période de transmission maximale. *Parassitologia* 28(1): 17–31.

Schwetz, J. 1942. Recherches sur la limite altimetrique du paludisme dans le Congo orientale et sur la cause de cette limite. *Annales de la Société Belge de Médecine Tropicale* 22: 183–208.

Snow, R.W., K. Marsh, and D. Le Sueur. 1996. The need for maps of transmission intensity to guide malaria control in Africa. *Parasitology Today* 12: 455–457.

Snow, R.W., J.A. Omumbo, B. Lowe, C.S. Molyneux, J.O. Obeiro, A. Palmer, M.W. Weber, M. Pinder, B. Nahlen, C. Obonyo, C. Newbold, S. Gupta, and K. Marsh. 1997. Relation between severe malaria morbidity in children and level of *Plasmodium falciparum* transmission in Africa. *Lancet* 349(9066): 1650–1654.

Steyn, J.J. 1946. The effect on the anopheline fauna of cultivation of swamps in Kigezi District, Uganda. *East African Medical Journal* 23: 163–169.

Trape, J.F. 1987. Malaria and urbanization in central Africa: The example of Brazzaville. Part IV. Parasitological and serological surveys in urban and surrounding rural areas. *Transactions of the Royal Society of Tropical Medicine and Hygiene* 81(Suppl. 2): 26–33.

Trape, J.F., and A. Zoulani. 1987a. Malaria and urbanization in central Africa: The example of Brazzaville. Part II: Results of entomological surveys and epidemiological analysis. *Transactions of the Royal Society of Tropical Medicine and Hygiene* 81(Suppl. 2): 10–18.

———. 1987b. Malaria and urbanization in central Africa: The example of Brazzaville. Part III: Relationships between urbanization and the intensity of malaria transmission. *Transactions of the Royal Society of Tropical Medicine and Hygiene* 81(Suppl. 2): 19–25.

Tulu, A.N. 1996. *Determinants of Malaria Transmission in the Highlands of Ethiopia: The Impact of Global Warming on Morbidity and Mortality Ascribed to Malaria.* London, U.K.: London School of Hygiene and Tropical Medicine, 296.

Vincke, I.H., and J.B. Jadin. 1946. Contribution à l'étude de l'anophelisme en pays d'altitude. *Annales de la Société Belge Médicine Tropicale* 26: 483–500.

Wilson, D.B. 1949. Malaria incidence in central and south Africa. In *Malariology* (volume 2), edited by M.F. Boyd. Philadelphia, PA: Saunders, 800–809.

PART 3

A Changing Context

Chapter 11

Climate Variability, Climate Change, and Malaria

Reid E. Basher and Mark A. Cane

The original purpose of this chapter was to provide regional climate scenarios for the near future (2050). Climatic elements directly or indirectly affect several stages of the malaria cycle; hence, climate is an important factor in the geographical distribution of the disease and in its seasonal and episodic variations. However, present scientific knowledge does not allow reliable regional or local predictions of climate conditions decades ahead, which would be of great interest to malaria research and management.

Some useful generic scenarios can be provided, particularly for temperature, where there is much more confidence than for the water-related factors such as rainfall, soil moisture, lying water, and stream flow. Because the magnitude of current seasonal-to-interannual climate variations is comparable to the climate variations projected for the 2050s, the opportunity to understand, predict, and manage the large fluctuations of malaria incidence that can occur at these time scales is immediate. The ability to manage malaria during existing seasonal climate variations will be an essential adaptation tool in a world whose climate is projected to warm even more over the next half-century.

In this chapter, we survey the current knowledge of climate variability, including anthropogenic (human-made) climate change and the El Niño–Southern Oscillation (ENSO) system. Specific attention is given to the development of the climate models that predict the ENSO system one or two seasons ahead.

The evolution of the global climate system over future decades and centuries can be projected by using complex computer-based physical models of Earth's atmosphere, oceans, and terrestrial surfaces. For this purpose, the models are configured to gloss over the details of the short-term and local features of climate to concentrate on the long-term impacts of specific increases in greenhouse gas concentrations. The climate models can be configured to predict climate variations at the seasonal-to-interannual time scale. These variations are important to malaria risk. The field of oceanic temperature anomalies is the driving factor while the greenhouse gas concentrations remain fixed. The models involve a high level of uncertainty and may give only general scenarios or outlooks, rather than firm predictions.

The Intergovernmental Panel on Climate Change (IPCC) concluded that long-term regional climate cannot be projected with any confidence. Therefore, firm projections of the 2050s climate for malaria scenario building are not possible. However, we argue for a strong focus on the seasonal-to-interannual time scale, where considerable climate knowledge and, in some cases, usefully accurate predictions may be used to enhance malaria research and ongoing public health management over the next decade. Adaptation to the future impacts of climate change will largely involve using the knowledge and tools currently available to manage existing variability and extremes in climate. To this end, we review the nature of seasonal-to-interannual climate variability and predictability, especially that associated with the ENSO system.

Climate and Human Health

Within the issue of climate change, considerable attention has been focused on the link between climate and health (Houghton et al. 1996). Several key health concerns have been identified, including vector-borne diseases (McMichael et al. 1996). The IPCC summarized the likely impacts of climate change on human health as follows:

> Climate change could affect human health through increases in heat-stress mortality, tropical vector-borne diseases, urban air pollution problems, and decreases in cold-related illnesses. Compared with the total burden of ill health, these problems are not likely to be large. In the aggregate, however, the direct and indirect impacts of climate change on human health do constitute a hazard to human population health, especially in developing countries in the tropics and subtropics; these impacts have considerable potential to cause significant loss of life, affect communities, and increase health-care costs and lost work days. (Watson, Zinyowera, and Moss 1998)

The impacts depend on not only the direct climatic sensitivity of the particular health issue under consideration but also many other environmental and socioeconomic changes (e.g., land use change, civil strife, and migration) that can mediate or exacerbate the effects of climate change or alter the intrinsic vulnerability of populations to the effects of climate change that occur. For example, IPCC noted that the percentage of the developing world's population living in cities is expected to exceed 50% by 2020 and that serious urban environmental problems such as air pollution (e.g., particulates, surface ozone, and lead), poor sanitation, and problems in water quality and potability are often associated with these cities (Watson, Zinyowera, and Moss 1998). IPCC stated that new and resurgent vector-borne and infectious diseases such as dengue, malaria, hantavirus, and cholera appear to have increased widely and globally. It did not clarify what, if any, role that climate has played in these increases. However, most natural disasters are related to climate, associated with droughts or floods. An increase in disease in the more vulnerable population is typically among the significant human impacts of natural disasters.

In the case of malaria (and dengue), the climatic sensitivities of many parts of the disease cycle are reasonably well known and can be modeled to some extent. For example, model-based geographical projections indicate that global mean increases in temperature in the upper part of the IPCC-projected range (3–5 °C by 2100) would increase the geographical zone of potential malaria transmission and would expand the affected proportion of the global population from approximately 45% to approximately 60% (Watson, Zinyowera, and Moss 1998). The transmission rate in areas where malaria is currently endemic could increase by about 50 million to 80 million additional cases annually. If this rate were to increase, the IPCC prediction that "compared with the total

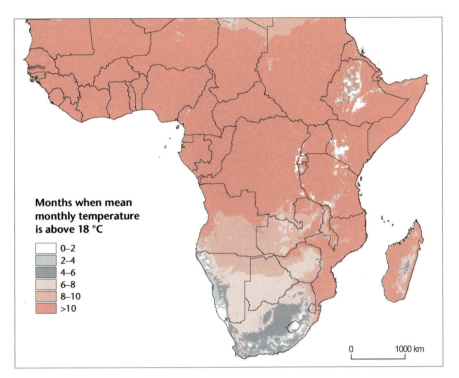

Plate 10-1. Average Number of Months in the Year When the Mean Monthly Temperatures Are Above 18 °C

Sources: Data are from Hutchinson et al. (1995) and Corbett and O'Brien (1997).

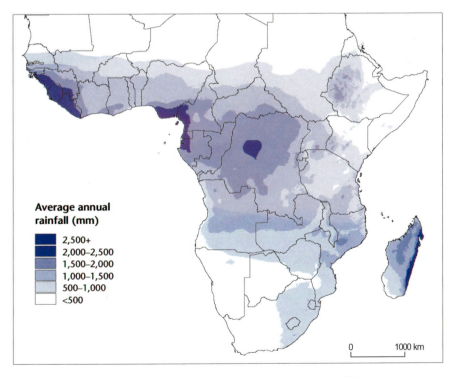

Plate 10-2. Distribution of Average Annual Rainfall for Sub-Saharan Africa

Sources: Data are from Hutchinson et al. (1995) and Corbett and O'Brien (1997).

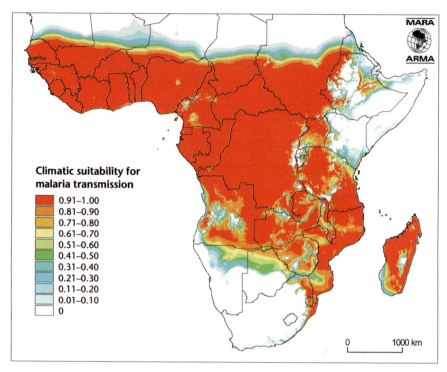

Plate 10-3. MARA Climate Suitability Model for Malaria

Note: Larger values indicate higher risk of malaria transmission.

Source: Craig, Snow, and Le Sueur 1999.

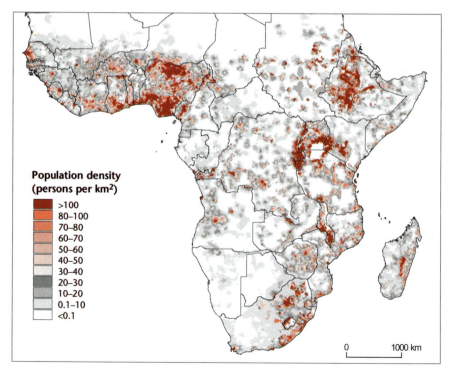

Plate 10-4. Human Population Distribution for Sub-Saharan Africa, 1990

Source: Deichmann 1996.

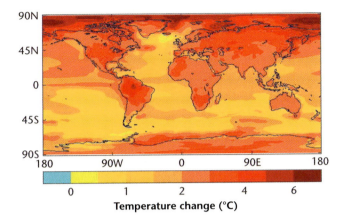

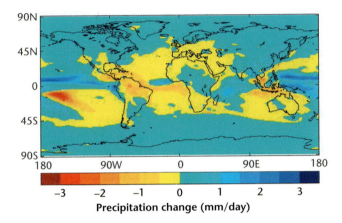

Plate 11-1. Temperature and Precipitation Changes, 2050s Minus Present Day

Note: Changes in annual mean surface temperature (*top*) and annual mean precipitation (*bottom*) are projected for the 2050s relative to 1961–1990 means, using a model from the Hadley Centre with the IPCC business-as-usual scenario of greenhouse gas emissions.

Source: Hadley Centre for Climate Prediction and Research, Meteorological Office.

burden of ill health, these problems are not likely to be large" clearly would not apply to the tropical and subtropical developing countries affected by such increases.

One critical factor in determining the health impacts is the nature of the sensitivity of the disease characteristics to the climatic elements. For malaria, highly nonlinear (exponential) responses to temperature (Patz et al. 1998) are evident, indicating that, all other things remaining equal, small changes in temperature will have a large effect on malaria incidence. Regardless of whether temperature predictions are available, the evidence of variability and trends in past climate records (Karl 1999) is clear: temperature variations and change will play a crucial role in not only the long-term risks (such as those reported above) but also the seasonal and episodic risks. Information about historical temperature probabilities, recent temperature patterns, and seasonal temperature forecasts therefore could become useful for current research and public health management (Bouma and van der Kayy 1996).

The incidence of disease vectors will be affected by changes in water body characteristics such as running or ponding water for larvae growth. Changes in the frequency of storms and rain events and in the amount and patterns of rainfall also will affect the incidence of vector-borne diseases. This issue is more complex than temperature is, because water body characteristics are nonlinearly related to the regularity of rainfall, the incidence of droughts and floods, and human behavior such as land use practices and saving rainwater in containers during dry periods. Again, this knowledge of climate applies to long-term risks as well as to seasonal and episodic risks. In the latter case, climate experts and population health managers can collaborate to research the processes involved with a view to monitoring, predicting, and managing the seasonal and other climate events.

Variation of the climate at seasonal and longer-term scales also might create "climatic windows of opportunity" that allow the introduction and establishment of vectors or disease agents in previously unaffected areas, directly or indirectly through stresses such as drought or flood, which raise the vulnerability of populations to an existing risk. Moreover, people and populations weakened by malaria are more vulnerable to other health stresses and to stresses that arise from their reduced ability to work, which, in turn, may be related to climate (e.g., drought or flood). The potentially significant aggregate economic impacts of a malaria-weakened population will further reduce the ability of nations to address the public health issues involved.

Natural Variability, Anthropogenic Change, and Climate Models

By a wide margin, most disasters are related to climate, associated with droughts or floods (we use the U.S. Agency for International Development definition of *disaster* [Dilley and Heymann 1995]). Among the significant human impacts that result from natural disaster, increased incidence of disease in the affected population is typical.

The great Indian famine of 1877–1878 is one case in point. More of the estimated 6 million to 8 million deaths appear to have been due to malaria and other diseases than to starvation (Whitcombe 1993). The spread of malaria was aided by the British policy of herding the population into camps to facilitate food distribution. In addition, the vector population was likely to have been larger than normal, because mosquitoes recover more rapidly from the drought than their predators do (Bouma and van der Kayy 1994). In addition, 1877 was the year of a very large El Niño event, and droughts in India are now known to be likely consequences of these interannual climate anomalies (Ropelewski and Halpert 1987).

The Indian famine example illustrates several points about the relationship between climate variations and malaria. Although variation and change in climate directly influence the malaria cycle by changing temperature and water-related factors (e.g., rainfall, soil moisture, lying water, and stream flow), indirect effects may be even more important. Forecasting the incidence of malaria as a function of solely climatic factors such as temperature and water availability is too simplistic. Forecasting schemes must account for a range of ecological factors that affect the life cycle of parasite and vector as well as account for social factors, such as the vulnerability of groups and the ability of society to take countermeasures. In complex ways, climate variability and climate change can substantially affect the resilience of a social system. The interactions of natural disasters and society are not easily predicted.

Quite often, local climate disasters are associated with and embedded in the shifts of the global patterns of climate variation. ENSO is the largest, best known example of such shifts. It gives rise to extensive droughts, floods, and other climate anomalies (Watson, Zinyowera, and Moss 1998; Dilley and Heymann 1995; Ropelewski and Halpert 1987; Fagan 1999; WMO 1999). It also influences the incidence of forest fires, hurricanes, severe winter storms, and other localized climate events. For example, during El Niño, the number of Atlantic hurricanes usually is below average, but the probability of a typhoon striking Shanghai is higher than average. As part of the La Niña (cold) phase of the ENSO cycle, the U.S. Southwest typically experiences a severe drought.

Various climate records show variability at every time scale: daily, seasonal, interannual, decadal, centennial, and millennial. These climate anomalies typically are generated by mechanisms internal to the climate system, not by external causes—human or otherwise. They are related to the loss of predictability in chaotic dynamic systems, as evidenced by climate models' high sensitivity to initial conditions. This characteristic of the climate system means that most (but not all) climate variations are inherently unpredictable. It is responsible for the irregularity of the ENSO cycle. Although interannual variability is smaller in amplitude than the regular seasonal cycle, its unpredictability is far more difficult for societies to cope with. This is especially true of its extreme forms (e.g., drought, flood, and severe storms).

Climatologists generally regard climate variability as occurring in a relatively few preferred spatial patterns with very large scales. None believe that these patterns are all there is to the climate system, but it may yet become apparent that these few patterns are all that can be predicted and all the rest is random noise. The North Atlantic Oscillation (NAO) is a good example of such a pattern (Hurrell 1995). Historically, the NAO has been defined by the difference between sea-level atmospheric pressure at the Azores and Iceland. Pressure at these two locations tends to fluctuate out of phase; when the Icelandic low is anomalously low (and the Azores high is anomalously high), the winds over the Atlantic tend to be stronger than normal and tend to bring warm, wet weather to Europe. Such conditions extend to the Middle East, giving, for example, greater rainfall in Turkey and thus enhanced flow in the Tigris–Euphrates system (Cullen and deMenocal 2000).

When the anomalies of the Azores and Icelandic pressures switch, the climatic conditions are roughly opposite to those listed above. The NAO is defined in the atmosphere, but it corresponds to definite patterns in sea surface temperature (SST) of the northern Atlantic Ocean. There also are connections to the tropical Atlantic sector, possibly affecting West African rainfall and Atlantic hurricane activity. The NAO pattern swings back and forth about every 2 years, but longer swings take place at nearly 10 years, and paleo-proxy indicators such as tree ring growth suggest still longer periods. The cause of the NAO has not yet been satisfactorily explained.

The ENSO system, however, can confidently be attributed to interaction between ocean and atmosphere in the tropical Pacific Ocean. Changes in the subsurface ocean lead to changes in SST, which lead to changes in the atmosphere, which induce further changes in the ocean. Increases in ocean temperatures of up to 4 °C occur over sizeable areas of the eastern Pacific Ocean. Large amplitude variations result because this chain of interaction is self-reinforcing; that is, there is positive feedback. In an El Niño year, the powerful, extensive zone of convection normally centered over Indonesia moves out into the central equatorial Pacific. The consequent change in atmospheric circulation results in worldwide changes in climate. The publicity surrounding the 1997–1998 El Niño made these global impacts famous—and sometimes notorious. ENSO impacts are unambiguously forced from the tropics.

Outside the tropics, the effects of ENSO tend to fall into well-defined patterns. In particular, the proximate cause of the variations over North America is a change in the Pacific–North America (PNA) pattern, a set of four atmospheric circulation cells centered near Hawaii; over the northern Pacific Ocean; over Alberta, Canada; and over the Gulf Coast. However, the PNA also fluctuates without an ENSO change to force it, and as with the NAO, it seems useful to think of the PNA as a preferred mode of atmospheric variability that can be forced in more than one way.

The view that climate variations take the form of a few fixed patterns has implications for global warming scenarios. Greenhouse gas forcing may preferentially excite certain phases of these modes and thus change the odds of our seeing particular forms of climate variability. It is well established that the global mean surface temperature has warmed over the past few decades. Much of that warming is in high latitudes in the northern hemisphere and may be viewed as a simultaneous locking-in of the PNA and NAO patterns. Of course, this occurrence does not tell us whether the pattern was forced by greenhouse gases or has just occurred naturally. In either case, given the prevalence and importance of the patterns, a major part of the climatic response to greenhouse forcing will inevitably manifest as a preference for particular phases of these dominant modes. It would change the frequency and duration of drought and floods associated with each mode, and one might expect much of the action to originate in the tropics.

Natural variability affects climate change issues in at least three ways. First, climatic "noise" masks the signal of secular change. Second, natural variability provides a historical record against which to calibrate and validate climate models. Third, the pattern of natural variability may be altered by climate change, with potentially important consequences. For example, changes in mean conditions may change the frequency or the intensity of ENSO-related drought. A study with one of the more believable climate models indicates that increased greenhouse gases will increase the frequency of ENSO extremes (Timmermann et al. 1999). The possibility of climate change altering natural variability raises the question of what climate models may realistically predict. Making a deterministic prediction for, say, 2051—or the decade of the 2050s, for that matter—is inherently impossible. The most that one should expect to forecast is a probability distribution of possible climate outcomes. In particular, one may hope to predict how climate change will bias the climate system. ENSO research provides examples of predictions of this kind, where a warm (El Niño) event biases the rainfall over much of South America but does not determine it uniquely.

Increased greenhouse gases may have a greater effect on climate variability than on mean climate; that is, the frequency of different regimes may be changed markedly, even while no unprecedented climate states occur and the mean climate barely changes (Palmer 1993). This possibility would create a different detection problem from the one that currently dominates the literature. In accord with this paradigm, we speculate that climate change may express itself in part as a change in the ENSO cycle. This idea is widespread, but there is no consensus on what form this change would take. The lack of consensus is, in part, a consequence of differences in models and a lack of confidence in what they predict. The comprehensive, coupled general circulation models of the ocean and atmosphere that are used in seasonal-to-interannual forecasting are, in fact, rather similar. They incorporate state-of-the-art knowledge of climatic processes, but how this knowledge is parameterized is subtly different. As with small differences in initial conditions, the chaotic model climate system can amplify a small difference in the representation of a particular process to become a large difference in the predicted climate. A genuine improvement in a particular process parameterization may degrade the overall model performance by freeing some other imperfect component to stray farther from the true path.

Seasonal-to-interannual climate prediction imposes a discipline on the process by forcing constant comparison of the model forecast with reality. This comparison is especially effective when the forecasts are made public. One of the difficulties with climate change modeling is the lack of any possible similar measure of the quality of the models. Model results for the past century can be compared with historical data, however, and some models are clearly better than others. The best models show a genuine ability to reproduce natural climate variations, capturing the global impacts of ENSO and the NAO. They even do a credible job of simulating the Indian monsoon. High-resolution regional models have shown great ability to capture local features by using the output of global models as boundary conditions.

Climate models do not do a perfect job of predicting natural variability, so their predictions cannot be fully trusted for a year ahead, let alone for a world subjected to global warming. This being so, do the models provide reliable information to use in studies of future impacts of climate change? The reasonable, informed answer is yes—with caveats. They add information, but one must remember the model flaws and the limited predictability of the climate system and recognize the information as a statement of altered future probabilities, not of a certain outcome. People routinely take actions based on imperfect information. Investors (and other savvy gamblers) look for an edge; these climate models are good enough now to give us an edge. It should be borne in mind that the objective is not to closely define the climate of the 2050s (an impossibility) but to better inform today's policy decisions with respect to the future effects of climate change.

For current models to provide reliable guidance, their biases must be clearly understood. For example, do their simulations of natural variability overpredict or underpredict extreme events? One could reasonably presume that their greenhouse predictions are biased in the same way. Complete sets of biases of each model are not known in detail; however, some of them can be documented by comparison with the climate record of the past century. A particularly serious overall bias of our current climate change models is evidenced from a consideration of the paleoclimate record: very large and very rapid changes in climate have occurred (see the next section), and neither model nor theory can account for them. Perhaps current climate models are overly damped and thus unrealistic in predicting only gradual change under the impact of human activity. They likely understate the probabilities of rapid and extreme change. Unfortunately, societies are far less able to adapt to rapid changes than to gradual ones. As a result, the inability of models to simulate rapid change may inspire a misplaced confidence in human ability to cope with the consequences of global warming.

Past and Future Global Climate Change*

Extensive scientific studies have shown that human activities, especially the burning of fossil fuels and changes in land use and land cover, have the potential to alter some key features of the climate (Houghton et al. 1996; McMichael et al. 1996; Watson, Zinyowera, and Moss 1998; IPCC 1998). The principal change is an increase in the concentrations of long-lived greenhouse gases, which tend to warm the atmosphere. Aerosols, formed mainly from the burning of sulfur-containing fuels, have a cooling effect in some regions that partly counteracts the warming effect. Because of the enormous heat capacity of the world's oceans, the climate system requires many hundreds of years to reach a new equilibrium after a change in greenhouse gas concentrations. The warming effect of increased greenhouse gases therefore will not become fully evident for many generations, whereas the effects of the higher human emissions of greenhouse gases projected for the next century will compound the warming for centuries ahead.

IPCC consensus predictions based on models of the global climate system and on plausible scenarios of future emissions of greenhouse gases and aerosols indicate that by 2100, the mean annual global surface temperature will increase by 1–3.5 °C, global mean sea level will rise by 15–95 centimeters, and the spatial and temporal patterns of precipitation and the intensity of the hydrological cycle will change (Houghton et al. 1996). The rates of change over years and decades are not predicted to be smooth and steady but appear quite variable because of the superposition of the natural climate variability. The model results predict larger temperature increases in continental regions than in oceanic regions and in higher latitudes than in the tropics (Plate 11-1, top†). Regional differences in the patterns and timing of change probably will be significant. These very large scale, fundamental changes in the climate system probably would affect major features of climate—such as ENSO, tropical cyclone characteristics, and the Asian monsoon—but scientific evidence is not conclusive as to what these effects will be.

Separate analyses of historical databases of measured climatic elements have shown various climate trends over the past century or two, some consistent with the model-based predictions. Average temperature over the past 100 years has increased in almost all parts of the world, by up to 3 °C (Karl 1999), and most of the highest record-setting global-average annual mean temperatures have occurred in the past 10 years. The magnitude of the global average increase (0.5 °C/100 years) is reasonably consistent with climate model projections. Some studies argue that this global trend lies outside of any natural variability. The historical temperature records do not increase linearly with time but exhibit rises and falls over decades (Karl 1999). The trends generally show spatial coherence over thousands of kilometer ranges, but large gaps in data coverage are apparent over much of the malaria-affected regions of tropical Africa and tropical South America (Karl 1999).

It is useful to rank the available information on detected and predicted trends (from most certain to least certain).

- Factors for which there is a relatively high degree of confidence:
  - Atmospheric carbon dioxide concentration is rising and will continue to rise under currently likely socioeconomic and greenhouse gas emissions scenarios.

---

*This section was written prior to the publication of the Third Assessment Report by the Intergovernmental Panel of Climate Change (IPCC). The qualitative statements given here are unlikely to change greatly, but some of the quantitative estimates may be subject to revision.

†Color plates for this chapter appear following page 190.

— Global mean air temperature and global mean sea level exhibit rising trends whose rates of rise appear to be outside the expected range of natural variability and are broadly consistent with model-based predictions of climate change.

— Temperature increases indicate that the frequency of hot events is increasing relative to past frequencies and that the frequency of cold events is decreasing relative to past frequencies.

— Minimum temperatures have tended to rise at a greater rate than maximum temperatures, resulting in a reduction of the diurnal temperature range and larger changes in the extremes for minimum temperatures than in those for maximum temperatures.

— Several other trends have been detected (e.g., in stratospheric temperature) that are generally consistent with predictions of climate change.

• Factors for which there is a moderate to low degree of confidence:

— Regional changes in climate are likely to occur as a result of small changes in the patterns and intensities of major weather regimes (high pressure belts, monsoons, and so on) and other features of the circulation of the atmosphere, but the specific regional details cannot yet be defined with confidence.

— The hydrological cycle is expected to accelerate, with prospects for more severe droughts or floods in some places and less severe droughts or floods in other places. Some studies of historical data show evidence of increases in extreme rainfalls.

— Changes in the characteristics of tropical cyclones have been predicted by some models, particularly with indications of increases in the intensity of the strongest tropical cyclones, and possibly some changes in frequency at locations associated with small shifts in the zones of occurrence.

— Some alteration of the character of the ENSO phenomenon may occur. Shifts in the relative frequency of El Niño and La Niña events and of their intensities have been predicted by some models and some authors.

In estimating the possible impacts of climate change, relatively high confidence may be possible where the impact is directly and closely linked to a feature of predicted climate change for which there is relatively high confidence, such as rising global mean temperature. In other instances, however—especially those concerned with hydrological factors, multiple climatic factors, or local or regional situations—the size and direction of the predicted changes and resulting impact will be relatively uncertain. In such cases, knowledge necessarily will be confined to "sensitivities," where the size and direction of an impact is known only relative to a putative size and direction of a predicted climatic effect.

The above projections do not address another factor of considerable scientific interest and potential public concern, namely, the evidence of large and rapid climate changes in the distant past, long before the present era of industrialization. Paleoclimate studies have shown that temperature changes of several degrees Celsius have occurred within a matter of decades (Broecker 1997). A case has been made that the Little Ice Age (cooling documented in Europe in the seventeenth to the nineteenth centuries) is the most recent of a sequence of such events (Bond and others 2001). Speculation implicates such extreme climate changes in the collapse of several ancient civilizations in the Near East and the Americas (Fagan 1999).

Apparently, these sudden climate changes can be generated by the internal workings of the climate system, without external influence. At present, no accepted explanations exist. Mechanisms capable of producing such extreme events have not been identified, and even the most sophisticated climate models do not exhibit such large, abrupt changes. Thus, the possibility of significant climatic surprises in the future, of totally unforeseen climate shifts and changes, cannot be ruled out. They might arise from processes that are inadequately modeled (e.g., deep ocean circulation), processes that are currently unknown (compare the history of the ozone hole), or nonlinear environmental responses to human influence (e.g., the dramatic fires in Southeast Asia during the 1997–1998 El Niño). Nor can the possibility that anthropogenic influences on the climate system will trigger such large and rapid future changes be ruled out.

Regional Climate Change Scenarios

Overall, the IPCC has concluded that present climate models provide useful predictions at the global and continental scales but allow little confidence at subcontinental scales (Houghton et al. 1996; Watson, Zinyowera, and Moss 1998). (This conclusion is also indicated by the broad patterns of possible change illustrated in Plate 11-1, in which the regional scale is subsumed within continental-scale variation.) Furthermore, the predictions for particular regions can vary considerably between different models, between runs of the same model under different assumptions, and even between runs of the same model with the same set of assumptions but different initializing conditions. (For model output data sets and maps of model outputs, see the IPCC Data Distribution Centre website [http://ipcc-ddc.cru.uea.ac.uk/].) In a special annex to the IPCC regional impacts report (Watson, Zinyowera, and Moss 1998), a review of the status of regional climate modeling (Giorgi et al. 1999) concluded that "considering all models, at the 10^4–10^6 km^2 scale, temperature changes due to CO_2 doubling varied between 0.6 and 7 °C, and precipitation changes varied between –35% and 50% of control runs." In other words, the uncertainty of the projections is comparable to the average of the projections.

For the malaria research community, this conclusion means that current knowledge cannot reliably predict future climate conditions for the regions and subregions subject to or at risk of malaria occurrence. In this situation, one is therefore obliged to rely on the use of scenarios of possible climate change (which are based on an appraisal of climate model predictions and paleoclimatic evidence) for the region of interest. Such scenarios and analysis of local meteorological data provide a plausible and valuable starting point for analyzing possible impacts. Caution in their use is needed, and researchers must be careful to reflect the great uncertainties involved in scenarios by means of conditional language (i.e., *would*, not *will*). Unfortunately, the elaborate detail of many scenarios and of the estimated impacts based on them can convey an undue sense of confidence in the estimated impacts; it is all too easy to start treating scenarios as firm predictions.

Although the 1995 IPCC Second Assessment Report is the definitive source of information on impacts, the document is extremely difficult to use to obtain an overview for an individual country or region. Hundreds of pages of text in numerous sector chapters have to be scoured to identify the range and importance of likely impacts, and more often than not, no information is specific to the area of interest. Also, the available knowledge is very often generic to the globe, rather than specific to regions.

In response to such criticisms, in late 1996, the IPCC initiated steps to prepare region-specific information summaries on impacts and vulnerabilities. A division of the world into 10 geopolitical regions was agreed: Africa, Arctic and Antarctic, Australasia, Europe, Latin America, Middle East and Arid Asia, North America, Small Island States, Temperate Asia, and Tropical Asia. The resulting IPCC report, *The Regional Impacts of Climate Change* (Watson, Zinyowera, and Moss 1998), is largely based on the IPCC Second Assessment Report, but it also contains later results and additional local studies that meet normal IPCC criteria for inclusion. The report was completed under a very tight schedule for release immediately before the December 1997 Conference of the Parties to the U.N. Framework Convention on Climate Change in Kyoto, Japan. The IPCC Third Assessment Report, which was finalized in 2001, adopted a blended approach in its Working Group II volume on impacts to include regional assessments as well as the traditional sector-specific chapters.

As discussed above, given the state of the science of climate change prediction, models cannot produce acceptable regional scenarios. Even if they did, several factors would give rise to doubt about the utility of such scenarios:

- The range of uncertainty of each prediction would be high; hence, the predictions for the various predominantly tropical regions involved would not be significantly different from each other (e.g., might lie between 1 and 3 °C ± 3 °C).
- Some features of the role of climate in the malaria process, mainly related to the hydrological components and their dependence on the time distribution of rainfall (such as lying water characteristics), are not well known and are not predicted.
- The link between the climatic variable and the malaria risk factor is, in some cases, strongly affected by human behavior (e.g., with respect to water-related management), especially over the long time frame under consideration.
- The natural variations of climate on the seasonal, interannual, and decadal time scale are likely to be as great as if not greater than the changes caused by enhanced greenhouse gas concentrations alone (see Karl 1999).

Nevertheless, for the purposes of envisioning the impact of climate change on malaria risk at the regional scale over the next two decades, it would be reasonable to adopt a scenario in which

- temperature rises by 0.1 °C ± 0.1 °C per decade,
- the frequency of hot extremes increases and the frequency of cold extremes decreases (details depend on location and can be calculated from measured data), and
- hydrological factors—rainfall amount and frequency, drought and frequency—are somewhat more variable than they are today (again, plausible scenario estimates may be made using local data).

The Nature of ENSO

The most dramatic, most energetic, and best-defined pattern of interannual variability is the global set of climate anomalies referred to as ENSO. As recently as late 1982, even many knowledgeable observers were unaware that the largest El Niño in at least a century was already well under way. In 1985, the international Tropical Ocean–Global Atmosphere (TOGA) program was launched with the goal of predicting ENSO, if possible. To an unexpected degree, that goal has been met: ENSO events are now predicted well in advance with skill, although it is less than perfect.

Our understanding of ENSO identifies the tropical Pacific Ocean as the source region and interactions between the ocean and the atmosphere in that region as the generating mechanism. Other global aspects of the cycle are consequences of the changes in the tropical Pacific source region. Thus, ENSO climate prediction entails two predictions: of the core ENSO, per se, and of its global influence on climate. Less is understood about the other significant modes of variability in the climate system, especially about their predictability. Beyond the changes in the physical climate system, one would like to predict the impacts—on malaria, for example—and then develop response strategies on the basis of that knowledge. The mission of the newly formed International Research Institute for Climate Prediction (IRI; http://iri.columbia.edu) spans these issues from the prediction of climate system variations (SSTs in the tropical Pacific prominent among them) to the identification of social actions to mitigate the impacts of climate variations.

On the average, a "warm event" (El Niño) occurs about every four years, but the cycle is highly irregular. Sometimes only two years pass between events, sometimes almost a decade. Amplitude varies greatly. Although each episode has its own peculiarities, all follow the same general pattern. At an early stage, surface waters in the western equatorial Pacific Ocean become anomalously warm. Associated with the warmer surface temperatures are an increase in convective activity and, at a certain stage, a persistent slackening of the normally westward-flowing trade winds. A dramatic and expansive warming of the tropical Pacific Ocean from the international date line to the South American coast follows, and the trade winds are further disrupted. Very heavy rains fall in normally arid regions of Peru and Ecuador, droughts are experienced in Australia and southern Africa, and tropical cyclones occur anomalously in regions such as French Polynesia and Hawaii. Farther away, the Indian monsoon, the seasonal rains of northeast Brazil, and regional climates over parts of southeast Asia, North America, and eastern Africa are often disrupted.

The 1982–1983 ENSO event was the most extreme in at least a century. Equatorial waters from the South American coast to the international date line warmed by an average of 2 °C; the warming along the coast exceeded 6 °C. The trade winds actually reversed. The consequences of this event were often devastating. In Australia, the worst drought ever recorded spawned firestorms that incinerated whole towns; normally arid regions of Peru and Ecuador were inundated by as much as three meters of rain, the beaches of California were rearranged by the unusual winter storms, and drastic changes in the tropical Pacific Ocean resulted in mass mortality of fish and bird life. All in all, the 1982–1983 ENSO event caused an estimated $8 billion in damages and the loss of 2,000 lives.

Historically, El Niño has referred to a massive warming of the coastal waters off of Ecuador and Peru. This warming leads to widespread mortality of fish and guano birds, crippling the local economies. Heavy rainfall results in catastrophic flooding in coastal land areas. El Niño has been documented as far back as 1726, and El Niño rainfall more than a century earlier appears to have made it possible for the conquistadors to cross an otherwise impenetrable desert.

The atmospheric component of ENSO, the Southern Oscillation, is a more recent discovery. The seminal figure in its delineation was Sir Gilbert Walker, director-general of observatories in India. Walker assumed his post in 1904, shortly after the famine that resulted from the disrupted monsoon of 1899 (an El Niño year); he set out to predict the monsoon fluctuations, an activity begun by his predecessors after the disastrous monsoon of 1877 (also an El Niño year). Walker was aware of work indicating swings of sea-level pressure from South America to the Indian–Australian region and back over a period of several years. In the next 30 years, he added correlates from all over the globe to this primary manifestation of the Southern Oscillation. For example, he found that periods of low Southern Oscillation Index (SOI) are characterized by heavy rainfall in the central equatorial Pacific Ocean, drought in India, warm winters in southwestern Canada, and cold winters in the southeastern United States. No conceptual framework supported the patterns he found; Walker's methods were strictly empirical. Probably the very thoroughness of his search, together with the short duration of the records then available, made it easy for others to neglect his findings.

Recently, Walker's global correlations have been reexamined with decades of new, independent data and have been found to hold. Walker did not consider El Niño, even though both El Niño and the Southern Oscillation were known at the beginning of the twentieth century. Remarkably, the close connection between the two (Figure 11-1) was not appreciated until the 1960s, principally as a result of the work of Jacob Bjerknes.

Bjerknes (1969, 1972) did more than point out the empirical relationship between El Niño and the Southern Oscillation; he also proposed an explanation that depends on a two-way coupling between the atmosphere and the ocean. His ideas were prompted by observations of large-scale anomalies in the atmosphere and the tropical Pacific Ocean during the International Geophysical Year, 1957–1958. A major El Niño occurred during those years, bringing with it all the atmospheric changes connected to a low SOI. It is implausible that a warming confined to coastal waters off of South America alone could cause global changes in the atmosphere, but the 1957 data indicated that the rise in SST was not confined to the coast. Bjerknes suggested that this feature was common to all El Niño events; he was correct, and the term "El Niño" is now most often used to denote the entire set of basin-scale oceanic changes. In Bjerknes' account of the connection between the ocean and the atmosphere, the coastal events constituting El Niño are incidental to the important oceanic change, the warming of the tropical Pacific Ocean over one-quarter of Earth's circumference.

Bjerknes suggested a tropical coupling between El Niño and the Southern Oscillation; he also proposed that the changes in atmospheric heating associated with tropical Pacific SST anomalies cause changes in mid-latitude circulation patterns. This *teleconnection* idea is consistent with the global nature of Walker's concept of the Southern Oscillation. However, in Bjerknes' theory, the causes of ENSO are rooted solely in the coupling of the atmosphere and the ocean in the tropical Pacific Ocean. They are entirely internal to the climate system and not responses to volcanic eruptions, solar variations, or biological activity.

Modeling and Predicting the Core ENSO Phenomenon

Work over the past two decades, especially that under the auspices of the international TOGA program, has provided theoretical and observational support for Bjerknes' concept. Wyrtki (1975, 1979) introduced an essential addition, equatorial ocean dynamics, in the 1970s on the basis of data from a network of tide gauges in the Pacific Islands. The first model to successfully simulate ENSO (Zebiak and Cane 1987) was based explicitly on the Bjerknes–Wyrtki hypothesis. Since then, operational seasonal climate forecasting systems based on these approaches have become established at several centers.

The numerical ENSO model of Zebiak and Cane (1987) depicts in a simplified manner the evolution of the tropical Pacific Ocean and its overlying atmosphere. It is a dynamical model, rather than a statistical one; that is, it relies on the governing physical equations rather than simply a sequence of observations. Dynamical models also provide a means for a physical interpretation and understanding of whatever they simulate. One of the most significant results of the model simulations was the recurrence of ENSO at irregular intervals as a result of strictly internal processes, that is, without any imposed perturbations. Analysis of the model helped in developing a now widely accepted theory that treats ENSO as an internal mode of oscillation of the ocean–atmosphere system, perpetuated by a continuous imbalance between the tightly coupled sur-

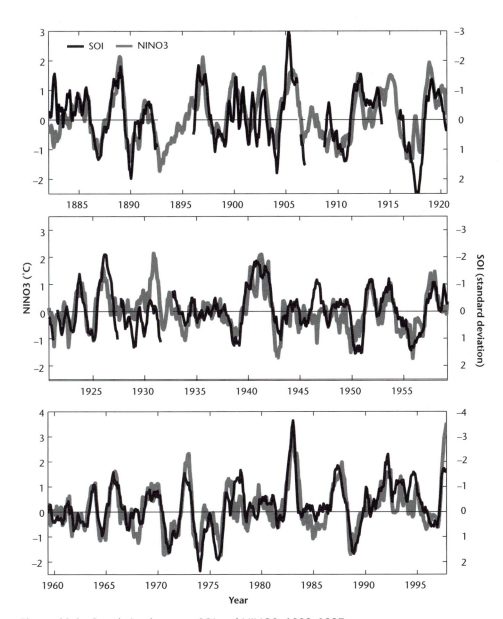

Figure 11-1. Correlation between SOI and NINO3, 1882–1997

Note: Notice the close relationship between the two indices. NINO3 = commonly used index (in °C) of El Niño, the SST anomaly in the NINO3 region of the eastern equatorial Pacific (90°W–150°W, 5°S–5°N); SOI = the most commonly used index (as a standard deviation) of the Southern Oscillation, the normalized sea-level pressure difference between Tahiti and Darwin, Australia.

face winds and temperatures on one hand and the more sluggish subsurface oceanic heat reservoir on the other.

This theory has several implications for the prediction of El Niño events. First, because the essential interactions take place in the tropical Pacific Ocean, data from that region alone may be sufficient for ENSO forecasting. Second, the memory of the coupled system resides in the ocean. Anomalies in the atmosphere are dissipated far too quickly to persist from one El Niño event to the next. The surface layers of the ocean are also too transitory. Hence, the memory must be in the thermal structure of the subsurface ocean. The crucial set of information for El Niño forecasts is the spatial variation of the depth of the thermocline (the thin region of rapid temperature change that separates the warm waters of the upper ocean from the cold waters of the abyssal ocean) in the tropical Pacific Ocean.

Starting with experimental studies in 1985, the Zebiak–Cane model has been used not only to simulate but also to predict El Niño (Cane, Zebiak, and Dolan 1986). As noted above, theory argued for a deterministic origin of ENSO, that is, a systematic evolution throughout the cycle rather than a sequence of random events. However, even deterministic systems that are chaotic have limited predictability, and in this case, the situation was made worse by a very poor observational base over vast regions of the tropical Pacific Ocean. Initially, the only observational data used in the forecasts were surface winds over the ocean. On the basis of these wind data, the ocean component of the model was run to generate currents, thermocline depths, and temperatures that served as initial conditions for forecasts—a necessary step because of the lack of direct observations of oceanic variables. Each forecast then consisted of choosing the conditions corresponding to a particular time and running the coupled model ahead to predict the evolution of the combined ocean–atmosphere system. By making predictions based on past periods, forecasts could be compared directly with reality. The results clearly demonstrated predictive skill at lead times longer than one year. They set the stage for the first predictions of the future, made in early 1986, which called unambiguously for an El Niño occurrence later that year. Figure 11-2 shows the SST anomalies for January 1987 as observed and as predicted in early 1986. The appearance of a moderate El Niño in both allow the forecast to be claimed as a success, although differences in timing and other details indicate that the prediction scheme was far from perfect.

Before the 1997 event, the model was generally successful in forecasting the major events (1972, 1976, 1982, 1986, and 1991) a year or more ahead but demonstrated little skill in predicting smaller fluctuations (some of which may influence climate elsewhere on the globe). Figure 11-3 illustrates the overall performance of these forecasts in terms of a widely used index of ENSO events, the SST anomaly in the NINO3 region of the eastern equatorial Pacific Ocean (90°W–150°W, 5°S–5°N). Forecasts are better in the 1980s than in the 1970s. Apparently, some periods are harder to predict than others.

In the 1980s, the Zebiak–Cane model was the only physical-based forecasting system with this level of skill, although there were (and are) comparably skillful statistical schemes. More recently, several other models have been developed for ENSO forecasting, many of which are based on the comprehensive physical models of the atmosphere and ocean known as general circulation models (GCMs). GCMs generally offer the greatest promise for accurate prediction because they simulate the climate system with the greatest verisimilitude. In addition, unlike models of the tropical Pacific Ocean alone, GCMs make it possible to predict the global impacts of ENSO. Their complexity, however, makes them less forgiving of errors and imperfections than the more simpli-

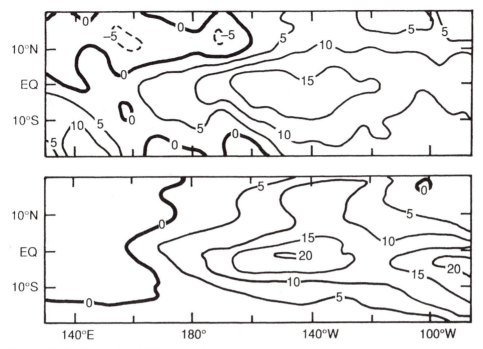

Figure 11-2. Forecasting SST Anomalies

Note: Observed SST anomaly field (0.1 °C) for January 1987 (*top*) is compared with that predicted by the Lamont atmosphere–ocean model for one year from January 1986 (*bottom*). This forecast, which was published in *Nature* in June 1986, was the first true forecast of El Niño with a dynamic model.

fied models are. It was thus a considerable achievement to bring them to the same general skill level as the Zebiak–Cane type of model and the schemes based on statistics.

Although the reaction to the first ENSO forecasts may have been surprise that they could be done at all, at this point the natural question to ask is why they are not being done better. The factors that limit current forecasting skill are inherent limits to predictability, flaws in the climate models, gaps in the observing system, and flaws in the data assimilation systems used to introduce the data into the models. Not enough is known to make a precise attribution of loss of skill factor by factor, and in any case, the effects are not simply additive; the different factors can combine in unpleasant ways. However, a rough assessment is possible.

The predictability of ENSO is unquestionably limited, but whether this limitation is due to chaos (Tziperman et al. 1994; Jin, Neelin, and Ghil 1994) or the effect of "noise" such as intraseasonal oscillations or weather disturbances intruding from mid-latitudes on the ENSO system (Penland and Sardeshmukh 1995) is the subject of continuing study. In either case, the ENSO system is so sensitive to initial conditions that small inaccuracies in the estimate of the initial state of the climate system can grow into substantial errors. Our best guess, based on numerical experimentation with models such as that of Zebiak and Cane (1987), is that the inherent limit to predictability is several years. On average, it takes several years for a small initial error to grow to a size comparable to that of a typical ENSO anomaly (Zebiak 1989; Goswami and Shukla 1991; Xue, Cane, and Zebiak 1997; Xue et al. 1997). Equivalently, only a small percentage of the forecasts at a lead time of less than one year will be substantially affected. At present, the primary problems lie elsewhere.

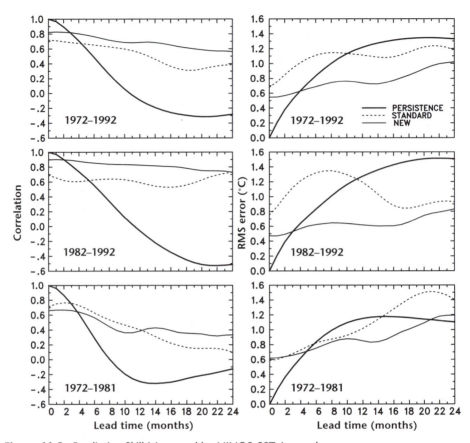

Figure 11-3. Predictive Skill Measured by NINO3 SST Anomaly

Note: Models' skill in predicting NINO3 SST anomalies is displayed in terms of how well predictions correlate with actual events (*left column*), and in terms of root-mean-square (RMS) errors in prediction (*right column*). Each figure compares three different models. The "persistence" model assumes that sea surface temperatures stay as they are. This is a poor predictor, with rapidly falling correlations and rising errors. The "standard" model performs far better, but the "new" model utilizing wind data performs best of all. Note, however, that the new model is almost uniformly best during the later decade (1982–92, *middle panel*) but not during the earlier one (1972–81, *bottom panel*).

Source: Chen et al. 1995.

Experience has shown that imperfections that seem acceptable when atmosphere models and ocean models are run independently become unacceptable when the two models are coupled together. Small flaws apparently reinforce each other. Even the most complete models necessarily include only approximate treatments of important physical processes. The most notable examples of inadequately represented processes are clouds and atmospheric convection, which are intimately tied to atmospheric heating. Variations in atmospheric heating are crucial in both the working of the ENSO cycle and generation of its global effects. Model shortcomings are surely a major limitation on forecast skill.

Although the observing system was certainly inadequate in the past, part of the legacy of the TOGA program is an array of highly instrumented buoys in the tropical Pacific Ocean. The experience of others (personal communication from A. Leetmaa, 1999) confirms our own estimates that the present observation system provides adequate initial conditions for the dominant Pacific Ocean. But maintenance of the observation system at an adequate level is not guaranteed, so interested parties must be vigilant. In addition, the roles of the tropical Atlantic and Indian Oceans in nearby regional climates, such as the Sahel and East Africa, indicate the need for better or new observations of the tropical Atlantic and Indian Oceans to support regional prediction schemes.

However, there are important shortcomings in the way the observational data are used. In the decades of experience with numerical weather prediction, data assimilation has been developed into a sophisticated and effective technology. Experience with coupled-model ENSO forecasting is only a decade old, and our understanding of data assimilation for this purpose is in its infancy. Figure 11-3 illustrates that even a fairly simple improvement in data assimilation methodology may improve forecasts noticeably (Chen et al. 1995). Work with coupled GCMs at the National Centers for Environmental Prediction (NCEP) in Washington, DC, also shows a substantial increase in skill from fairly small changes in the data assimilation system (Ji, Leetmaa, and Derber 1995).

ENSO forecasting certainly has room for improvement, and this analysis of its limits is hopeful. The inherent limits to predictability and the gaps in the observing systems are the most intractable and most expensive of the limiting factors, respectively. The best estimate is that they are not now the major limiting factors, but they will have to be faced if the other factors are reduced. The major problems at the moment are shortcomings in the simulation models and in the systems for introducing data into these models. Both should diminish in the face of concerted efforts by forecasting centers such as IRI and NCEP. The difficulty of the work is increased by the scarcity of data for past events, which restricts the time period suitable for evaluating putative improvements in the model and data assimilation system. Rapid gains in data assimilation should result by borrowing techniques developed for numerical weather prediction. Fixing the model flaws appears to be more difficult, but progress is expected.

The highly unusual warm event of 1997 holds useful lessons for ENSO forecasting. Figure 11-4 shows the strongest events of the period of instrumental data, approximately 10 years. Not only was the 1997 El Niño at least comparable to the strongest of these events; the rate at which the ocean warmed was also unprecedented. Many, perhaps most, of the models did a credible job of predicting the 1997 event. (The Zebiak–Cane model forecasts were an interesting exception; see Chen, Cane, and Zebiak 1999). Examples of some of the better forecasts, from the NCEP model, are illustrated in Figure 11-5. Forecasts from November 1996 and February 1997 indicate a warm event in mid-1997. Still, both underestimate the amplitude of the warming, especially the late-1996 forecast. In fact, few if any of the models predicted the outsized nature of the event to come (Barnston et al. 1999). Future analysis of this event should determine why the forecasts were inadequate and lead to improvements in models and forecasting procedures.

Impacts of ENSO on Climate

Figure 11-6 illustrates the global influence of an ENSO warm event. All of the relationships discussed in this section may be found in works by Ropelewski and Halpert (1987, 1996). As a first approximation, one may say that an ENSO cold event (La Niña) has effects opposite of those produced by El Niño, but there are significant exceptions. As a general rule, the effects of an ENSO event are strongest and most reliable in the tropical Pacific Ocean source region and the contiguous continents; a warm event usually means heavy rains in Peru and drought in Indonesia. Typical consequences are somewhat less reliable in the rest of the global tropics but still are highly likely. Thus, ENSO warm

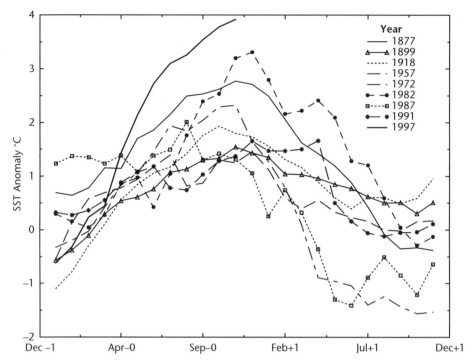

Figure 11-4. NINO3 SST Anomalies for the Strongest El Niño Events of the Past 120 Years

Notes: The rapidity of the rise in 1997 is unprecedented in the period for which instrumental data are available. Date is relative to an El Niño (year 0).

Source: International Research Institute for Climate Prediction.

events are often concurrent with a poor monsoon (less rainfall than anticipated) in India, low maize yield in Zimbabwe (Cane, Eshel, and Buckland 1994), drought in the Nordeste region of Brazil, and fewer hurricanes in the Atlantic Ocean. ENSO also has an influence in extratropical latitudes, but the extent of that influence is less certain than in the tropics. Other factors may intervene, and the extratropical climate system is characteristically more chaotic than in the tropics and thus less predictable.

Predictions of the global impacts of ENSO are currently made with physical models, statistical procedures, and other empirical methods. If the physical models are global coupled GCMs, then they predict global impacts along with core changes in the tropical Pacific Ocean. Alternately, a two-tiered approach is to predict tropical Pacific SSTs with a simple model and then use the predicted SSTs as boundary conditions to calculate global climate variations with a global atmospheric GCM (Barnett et al. 1994; Hunt, Zebiak, and Cane 1994). Empirical approaches may be two tiered, deriving forecasts by combining a predicted ENSO index such as the SOI or equatorial eastern Pacific SST (i.e., NINO3) with the historical relationship of a local climate variable (e.g., rainfall in Harare, Zimbabwe). They also may do the entire prediction at once, using recent observed values of an ENSO index to predict a future local condition. For example, Stone, Hammer, and Marcussen (1996) predicted global rainfall a season or more ahead based on the "phase" of the ENSO event using SOI values at two different times.

Physical models are not yet demonstrably better than statistical ones. However, there are sound reasons to believe that the physical models will ultimately prove superior at both understanding and predicting ENSO and thus that the greater effort needed

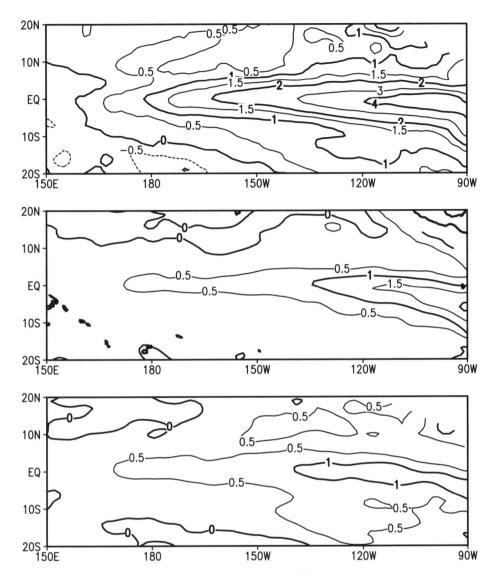

Figure 11-5. SST Anomalies Forecasts, June–August 1997

Note: Data are observed (*top*), forecast from data through February 1997 (*middle*), and forecast from data through November 1996 (*bottom*).

to develop them is justified. To begin with, empirical methods require an historical data set to train on, and such data sets are often too short or missing altogether. Because ENSO events occur about every 4 years, even a 50-year record will contain only a dozen or so examples of warm and cold extremes. Evidence also indicates that the statistical relationships are not entirely stable (they can change from decade to decade) and that climate change may lead to shifts in these relationships. Moreover, the response to ENSO events is often somewhat nonlinear, and the usual straightforward statistical methods may be inadequate. More sophisticated methods typically demand even more data to train on.

Not all ENSO connections are equally strong and reliable. More generally, each ENSO event is unique and has a distinctive pattern of global impacts. Furthermore, the

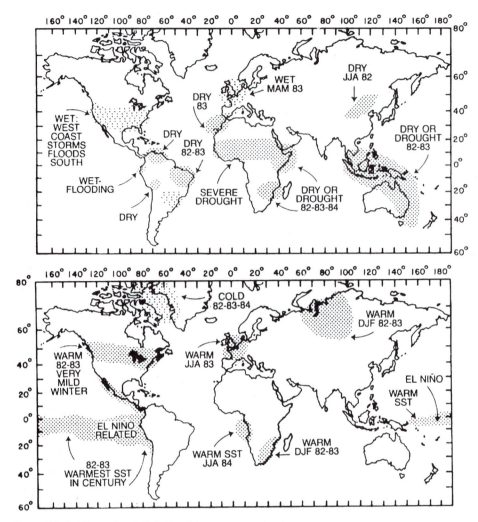

Figure 11-6. Warm Event Relationships

Note: ENSO extreme continental precipitation (*top*) and extreme temperature events (*bottom*) are shown. JJA = June–August; DJF = December–February; MAM = March–May.

Source: Adapted from Ropelewski and Halpert 1987.

magnitude of the variations that occur is not simply related to the strength of the El Niño event. Understanding of these differences is limited; they have hardly been classified satisfactorily, let alone explained in physical terms.

A corollary is that the differences between events are not well predicted at present. Several reasons might explain these poor predictions. Perhaps the prediction schemes fail to respond to the idiosyncrasies of each event such as the subtle (and not so subtle) differences in the pattern of its SST anomalies. It is not clear which features should be observed. The global response is known to be sensitive to the location and strength of the atmospheric heating in the tropics (Hoerling, Kumar, and Zhong 1997).

Because the atmosphere is a chaotic, dynamic system, small changes in boundary and initial conditions can be amplified to produce very large differences in the future state of the atmosphere. One result of this chaos is *weather*, that is, climate variability on a time scale much shorter than what we call "climate variations." Weather (and other short-term variability) may be thought of as random "noise" in the climate system that makes the system unpredictable. Whether one's conceptual view favors chaos or noise, the system is largely unpredictable; even with SST and other boundary conditions fixed, the atmosphere may evolve into very different states if started with only slight differences in its initial state.

Suppose, for example, one used an atmospheric model with correctly specified SST boundary conditions to make 10 simulations, each initialized with a best estimate of the state of the atmosphere in 1982 on successive days (say October 1, October 2, ..., October 10). The resulting outcomes for the 10 runs for a period six months later (April 1983) for a particular region would be very different (Barnett 1995). With a good model, one or more of the results might resemble the actual outcome, but nature runs this experiment only once, and it is not possible to say a priori which it will be. To be accurate, the prediction has to be stated as a probability distribution of the possible outcome states. This probabilistic character of the climate forecast is a consequence of the nature of the climate system and would still be true if the climate model were perfect: forecast skill is known to be limited by this intrinsic loss of predictability, especially in mid-latitudes and elsewhere.

ENSO is not the only mode of climate variability with large-scale impacts. The enormous current interest in the NAO is motivated by well-identified connections to climate anomalies in Europe, the Middle East, North Africa, and eastern North America (Hurrell 1995). SST variation in the tropical Atlantic has been related to droughts in the Sahel region (Folland, Palmer, and Parker 1986) and the Nordeste region of Brazil (Nobre and Shukla 1996). Climate anomalies in Australia have relationships to Indian Ocean SST anomalies that are independent of ENSO (Nicholls 1989). Perhaps these anomalies interact with ENSO, and our current inability to take account of the interactions limits our forecast skill. Moreover, we have yet to establish that any of the non-ENSO modes can be predicted several seasons ahead—or even that such a prediction is theoretically possible.

A brief global tour through the historical record and the 1997–1998 ENSO event illustrates the range of possibilities in impact forecasting (WMO 1999). In Indonesia and Papua New Guinea, for example, El Niño almost certainly brings drought and La Niña brings excess rain (Figure 11-7, left); the 1997 forest fires in Indonesia and famine-inducing drought in Papua New Guinea fit this pattern. In Australia, the expected rainfall anomalies are similar but not as reliable (Figure 11-7, right); the Australian drought of 1997–1998 was not nearly as severe as the size of the El Niño event would have suggested.

In Zimbabwe, ENSO is very strongly correlated with rainfall and even more strongly to the maize crop, which integrates rainfall and temperature effects (Cane, Eshel, and Buckland 1994). However, the relationship is not entirely reliable or straightforward. The most severe drought in at least the past 150 years in southern Africa was in 1992, despite only a moderate El Niño. On the other hand, 1997–1998 rainfall was close to normal over much of the region despite a very strong El Niño.

Although the Nordeste region of Brazil usually experiences drought in El Niño years, the relationship to tropical Atlantic SSTs is even stronger (Figure 11-8). Numerous atmospheric GCM experiments have shown that if the SSTs in the tropical oceans are known, then Nordeste rainfall is predictable. That is, our ability to forecast rainfall there is not limited by the intrinsic limits to predictability in the atmosphere. Unfortunately, the necessary tropical Atlantic SSTs cannot yet be predicted, and how predictable they are, in principle, is not known.

The Sahel is another region where rainfall is linked to tropical SSTs in both the Atlantic and Pacific Oceans, but the impact of the Atlantic is stronger than that of

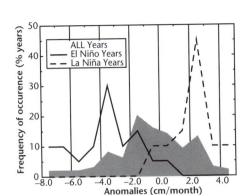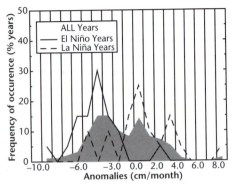

Figure 11-7. ENSO Impacts: Rainfall Anomalies, 1890–1989

Note: Climatological distribution (all years included) is shaded. *Left:* Indonesia (10°S–5°N, 105°E–150°E; June–November). *Right:* Australia (29°S–10°S, 138°E–154°E; November–February).

Source: International Research Institute for Climate Prediction.

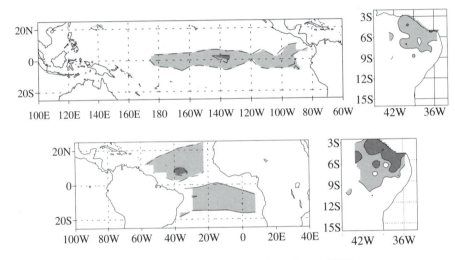

Figure 11-8. Rainfall in the Nordeste Region of Brazil vs. Tropical SSTs

Note: Singular value decomposition patterns for the rainy season months (February–May) are shown. *Top:* Relationship with tropical Pacific SST. *Bottom:* Relationship with tropical Atlantic SST. Light-shaded correlations are above 0.4; dark-shaded correlations are above 0.6.

Source: Data are from Y. Kushnir, Lamont-Doherty Earth Observatory, Columbia University.

ENSO. Moreover, Sahel rainfall is related to the NAO. Presumably, predictions of Sahel rainfall would be improved if one could know the future state of the Atlantic and the NAO. Because much of the NAO–Sahel connection is at interdecadal time scales, there is something to be gained by taking note of the present state of the NAO. Beyond that, the causes of the NAO are poorly understood, and its potential predictability is not known.

In India, poor monsoons are generally associated with El Niño events and excessive rains with La Niña events, but the connection is far from perfect. Sometimes El Niño year rainfall is average, and sometimes a monsoon is poor without an El Niño event. Based on this history, if one had been asked early in 1997 what sort of monsoon to expect for that year, the forecast would have to have been that a poor monsoon was likely. Indeed, the best of the atmospheric GCMs used for global prediction predicted rainfall significantly below average for June to September in India. In the event, the rainfall turned out to be indistinguishable from the climatological normal. The forecast of the Indian Meteorological Service was somewhat better, predicting a year only marginally below normal. (This forecast is issued only after a subjective evaluation but begins with a statistical prediction scheme that includes El Niño information and factors other than El Niño—factors seemingly included in the GCMs' initial and boundary conditions.)

Interestingly, the historic connection between ENSO and the monsoon has not held throughout the 1990s. Kumar, Rajagopalan, and Cane (1999) raise the possibility that the connection may have been severed by an alteration in the climate state (i.e., the warming of the Eurasian landmass), which may be attributable to the impact of anthropogenic greenhouse gases.

Future Prospects for Better Forecasts

Truly remarkable strides have been made in mobilizing efforts to develop climate prediction. Presently, many research groups are doing routine ENSO prediction using various methods. Regular observational updates for the tropical Pacific Ocean and summaries of forecast results are published monthly at the websites of IRI and of the U.S. National Oceanic and Atmospheric Administration's National Centers for Environmental Prediction and by a number of other organizations. This information has been used by groups in Australia, northeast Brazil, China, Ethiopia, India, Peru, the United States, and elsewhere to suggest actions to mitigate the effects of the local ENSO-associated climate variations. The 1997–1998 El Niño brought a high level of global awareness, creating a new context for the task of designing and implementing response strategies for ENSO impacts.

Demonstrating the possibility of long-range climate prediction is unquestionably a great advance. The forecasts are far from perfect, especially for the connections to local conditions with the greatest human consequences. The nature of the climate system does not allow unlimited predictability, so even a perfect forecasting system would not be able to deliver precise forecasts. To be correct, a forecast must be presented as a probabilistic statement. Some aspects of the climate are more predictable than others. For example, given an ENSO event, the probability distribution will differ greatly from the climatological expectation for some climatic features but not for others. For the former probability distribution, knowing that there is an ENSO event adds information. The forecast should be useful—all the more if the probability conditioned on ENSO is sharply peaked so that a rather specific outcome may be expected. Our current knowledge of the predictability of different features of the global climate is quite incomplete, but research over the next few years will add to it rapidly.

The task of exploiting our knowledge of ENSO connections is complicated by the increasing impact of anthropogenic influences in the atmosphere. Statistical prediction schemes, necessarily based on historical data, may become unreliable after the climate system changes appreciably. Perhaps, as the example of the Indian monsoon suggests, it has already happened.

Physical-based prediction schemes also may have new difficulties because different aspects of their physics are stressed by changing conditions. Moreover, the predictions of climate change and future climate variability are inextricably linked. To provide useful guidance for impact studies and policy use, the projected effects of global warming on climate must include estimates of future climate variability. Even projections of gross quantities such as global mean temperature are likely to be inaccurate if they do not properly account for variability. By the same token, prediction of climate variability such as ENSO must account for the effects of increasing greenhouse gas concentrations.

Conclusion

Although the predictions of future climate change are insufficient to accurately estimate the future regional impacts on malaria, a considerable amount of knowledge about climate is available to better understand and manage malaria in the near term. In this context, the target can shift from the assessment of long-term climate change impact alone to include adaptation to climate variability and change.

The impacts of a changed climate are largely variants of the impacts of the existing climate, acting through the same climatic processes and the same physical and biological sensitivities. Therefore, it is possible to respond to actual and potential changes by using the many adaptations to climate variability that already exist in the realm of climate information services, suitably adjusted for the small shifts in the climate.

Climate information services are used to help manage the impacts of existing climate variability and extremes. They include estimating the risks of climate extremes from historical data, developing probability distributions of climate elements, applying seasonal climate forecasts to interannual climate forecasts, deriving information such as soil moisture estimates, creating geographical summaries, and analyzing climate events. These services are underpinned by measurement networks, databases, advisory services, and real-time information provision.

Shifts in the frequency of extremes are likely to be the primary vehicles for major impacts of climate change. A necessary step toward effective adaptation is the ability to understand and manage existing impacts and beneficially apply existing climate information. The development of these applications for climate change purposes has immediate value and is thus a "no regrets" option. This intimate connection between climate change adaptation and traditional climate information services is not well recognized in either the adaptation or services communities.

Climate models cannot yet provide the full detailed predictions of future climate required for the study or use of adaptation options; this information has to be fleshed out from past data. Moreover, change has meaning only when measured against the past, and all climate predictions and trends must be referenced against historical data. For these various reasons, climate networks, measurement programs, and databases have an increasingly critical role to play in understanding climate variability and change and in managing and adapting to impacts. However, ironically, these foundations are increasingly under threat worldwide. This concern that has been recognized in the resolutions of the Conference of the Parties to the Framework Convention on Climate Change (see Basher 1999).

Existing public health measures can be adjusted on the basis of the measured and predicted shifts in climate, to the extent that the fundamental climate sensitivities of the diseases are known. A concept that should have value in the malaria field is the end-to-end approach being developed by IRI in which all factors relevant to the successful application of climate forecasts are studied and developed simultaneously—including decisionmaker needs, social and institutional context, the climatic sensitivity of the core system, the design of forecast product and dissemination methods, the forecast procedure, and the data requirements. By involving the users, forecasters, and other specialists in an integrated effort and facilitating interactions throughout the end-to-end chain (or web), everyone learns faster and the knowledge process embeds itself operationally more quickly.

Although the ability to predict climate both seasonally and in the very long term (i.e., climate change) has advanced markedly in the past two decades, climate prediction cannot provide all that the future health professional, researcher, and policymaker will want to know. This is a consequence of imperfect knowledge, but only in part; much is due to the intrinsic limits on the predictability of the climate system. Current skill often is not well matched to the space and time scales of interest. However, by considering the whole range of variability and predictability, short-term questions of immediate management interest as well as long-term questions regarding the future of the enhanced greenhouse world can be addressed simultaneously.

Acknowledgements

Mark Cane was supported by U.S. National Oceanographic and Atmospheric Administration Grant NA86GP0515. Thanks to Virginia DiBlasi-Morris and Larry Rosen for technical support.

References

Barnett, T.P. 1995. Monte Carlo climate forecasting. *Journal of Climate* 8: 1005–1022.

Barnett, T.P., L. Bengtsson, K. Arpe, M. Flugel, N. Graham, M. Latif, J. Ritchie, E. Roeckner, U. Schlese, U. Schulzweida, and M. Tyree. 1994. Forecasting global ENSO-related climate anomalies. *Tellus* 46A: 381–397.

Barnston, A.G., A. Leetmaa, V.E. Kousky, R.E. Levezey, E.A. O'Lenic, H.V. den Dool, A.J. Wagner, and D.A. Unger. 1999. NCEP forecasts of the El Niño of 1997–98 and its U.S. impacts. *Bulletin of the American Meteorological Society* 80(9): 1829–1852.

Basher, R.E. 1999. Data requirements for developing adaptations to climate variability and change. *Mitigation and Adaptation Strategies for Global Change* 4: 227–237.

Bjerknes, J. 1969. Atmospheric teleconnections from the equatorial Pacific. *Monthly Weather Review* 97: 163–172.

———. 1972. Large-scale atmospheric response to the 1964–65 Pacific equatorial warming. *Journal of Physical Oceanography* 2: 212–217.

Bond, G., B. Kromer, J. eer, R. Muscheler, M.N. Evans, W. Showers, S. Hoffmann, R. Lotti-Bond, I. Hajdas, and G. Bonani. 2001. Persistent solar influence on North Atlantic climate during the Holocene. *Science* 294:2130–2136.

Bouma, M.J., and J.J. van der Kayy. 1994. Epidemic malaria in India and the El Niño Southern Oscillation: Health and climate change. *Lancet* 344(1): 38–39.

———. 1996. The El Niño Southern Oscillation and the historic malaria epidemics on the Indian subcontinent and Sri Lanka: An early warning system for future epidemics? *Tropical Medicine and International Health* 1: 86–96.

Broecker, W. 1997. Thermohaline circulation, the Achilles heel of our climate system: Will manmade CO_2 upset the current balance? *Science* 278: 1582–1588.

Cane, M.A., G. Eshel, and R.W. Buckland. 1994. Forecasting Zimbabwean maize yield using eastern equatorial Pacific sea surface temperature. *Nature* 370(6486): 204–205.

Cane, M.A., S.E. Zebiak, and S.C. Dolan. 1986. Experimental forecasts of El Niño. *Nature* 321: 827–832.

Chen, D., M.A. Cane, and S.E. Zebiak. 1999. The impact of NSCAT winds on predicting the 1997/98 El Niño: A case study with the Lamont model. *Journal of Geophysical Research* 104: 11,321–11,327.

Chen, D., S.E. Zebiak, A.J. Busalacchi, and M.A. Cane. 1995. An improved procedure for El Niño forecasting: Implications for predictability. *Science* 269: 1699–1702.

Cullen, H.M., and P.B. deMenocal. 2000. North Atlantic influence on Tigris-Euphrates streamflow. *International Journal of Climatology* 20: 853–863.

Dilley, M., and B. Heymann. 1995. ENSO and disaster: Droughts, floods, and El Niño/Southern Oscillation warm events. *Disasters* 19: 181–193.

Fagan, B. 1999. *Floods, Farmers, and Emperors: El Niño and the Fate of Civilizations.* New York: Basic Books, 284.

Folland, C.K., T.N. Palmer, and D.E. Parker. 1986. Sahel rainfall and worldwide sea temperatures: 1901–85. *Nature* 320: 602–607.

Giorgi, F., G.A. Meehl, A. Kattenberg, H. Grassl, J.F.B. Mitchell, R.J Stouffer, T. Tokioka, A.J. Weaver, and T.M.L. Wigley. 1999. Simulation of regional climate change with global coupled models and regional modeling techniques. In *The Regional Impacts of Climate Change,* edited by R.T. Watson, M.C. Zinyowera, and R.H. Moss. Special Report of Intergovernmental Panel on Climate Change Working Group II. New York: Cambridge University Press, 425–437.

Goswami, B.N., and J. Shukla. 1991. Predictability of a coupled ocean-atmosphere model. *Journal of Climate* 4: 3–22.

Hoerling, M.P., A. Kumar, and M. Zhong. 1997. El Niño, La Niña, and the nonlinearity of their teleconnections. *Journal of Climate* 10: 1769–1786.

Houghton, J.T., L.G. Meira Filho, B.A. Callandar, N. Harris, A. Kattenberg, and K. Maskell. 1996. Summary for policy makers. In *Climate Change 1995: The Science of Climate Change.* Contribution of Working Group I to the Second Assessment Report of the Intergovernmental Panel on Climate Change. New York: Cambridge University Press, 1–7.

Hunt, B.G., S.E. Zebiak, and M.A. Cane. 1994. Experimental predictions of climatic variability for lead time of twelve months. *International Journal of Climatology* 14: 507–526.

Hurrell, J. 1995. Decadal trends in the North-Atlantic Oscillation: Regional temperatures and precipitation. *Science* 269: 676–679.

IPCC (Intergovernmental Panel on Climate Change). 1998. *The IPCC Third Assessment Report.* http://www.ipcc.ch (accessed October 2001).

Ji, M., A. Leetmaa, and J. Derber. 1995. An ocean analysis system for seasonal-to-interannual climate studies. *Monthly Weather Review* 123: 460–481.

Jin, F.-F., J.D. Neelin, and M. Ghil. 1994. El Niño on the devil's staircase: Annual subharmonic steps to chaos. *Science* 264: 70–72.

Karl, T.R. 1999. Regional trends and variations of temperature and precipitation. In *The Regional Impacts of Climate Change,* edited by R.T. Watson, M.C. Zinyowera, and R.H. Moss. Special report of Intergovernmental Panel on Climate Change Working Group II. New York: Cambridge University Press, 411–425.

Kumar, K.K., B. Rajagopalan, and M.A. Cane. 1999. On the weakening relationship between the Indian Monsoon and ENSO. *Science* 284: 2156–2159.

McMichael, A.J., M. Ando, R. Caracavallo, P. Epstein, A. Haines, G. Dendritsky, L. Kalkstein, R. Odongo, J. Patz, and W. Piver. 1996. Human population health. In *Climate Change 1995: Impacts, Adaptations, and Mitigation of Climate Change: Scientific-Technical Analysis,* edited by R.T. Watson, M.C. Zinyowera, and R.H. Moss. Contribution of Working Group II to the Second Assessment Report of the Intergovernmental Panel on Climate Change. New York: Cambridge University Press.

Nicholls, N. 1989. El Niño-Southern Oscillation impact prediction. *Bulletin of the American Meteorological Society* 69: 173–176.

Nobre, P., and J. Shukla. 1996. Variations of sea surface temperature, wind stress, and rainfall over the tropical Atlantic and South America. *Journal of Climate* 9: 2464–2479.

Palmer, T. 1993. A nonlinear dynamical perspective on climate change. *Weather* 48: 313–348.

Patz, J.A., K. Strzepek, S. Lele, M. Hedden, S. Greene, B. Noden, S.I. Hay, L. Kalkstein, and J.C. Beier. 1998. Predicting key malaria transmission factors, biting, and entomological inoculation rates using modelled soil moisture in Kenya. *Tropical Medicine and International Health* 3: 818–827.

Penland, C., and P.D. Sardeshmukh. 1995. The optimal-growth of tropical sea-surface temperature anomalies. *Journal of Climate* 8: 1999–2024.

Ropelewski, C.F., and M.S. Halpert. 1987. Global and regional scale precipitation patterns associated with the El Nino/Southern Oscillation. *Monthly Weather Review* 115: 1606–1626.

————. 1996. Quantifying Southern Oscillation-precipitation relationships. *Journal of Climate* 9: 1043–1059.

Stone, R.C., G.L. Hammer, and T. Marcussen. 1996. Prediction of global rainfall probabilities using phases of the Southern Oscillation Index. *Nature* 384: 252–255.

Timmermann, A., M. Latif, A. Bacher, J. Oberhuber, and E. Roeckner. 1999. Increased El Niño frequency in a climate model forced by future greenhouse warming. *Nature* 398: 694–696.

Tziperman, E., L. Stone, M.A. Cane, and H. Jarosh. 1994. El Niño chaos: Overlapping of resonances between the seasonal cycle and the Pacific ocean-atmosphere oscillator. *Science* 264: 72–74.

Watson, R.T., M.C. Zinyowera, and R.H. Moss (eds.). 1998. *The Regional Impacts of Climate Change.* Special report of Intergovernmental Panel on Climate Change Working Group II. New York: Cambridge University Press.

Whitcombe, E. 1993. Famine mortality. *Economic and Political Weekly* 28(23): 1169–1184.

WMO (World Meteorological Organization). 1999. *The 1997–1998 El Niño Event: A Scientific and Technical Retrospective.* WMO No. 905. Geneva, Switzerland: WMO.

Wyrtki, K. 1975. El Niño: The dynamic response of the equatorial Pacific Ocean to atmospheric forcing. *Journal of Physical Oceanography* 5: 572–584.

————. 1979. The response of sea surface topography to the 1976 El Niño. *Journal of Physical Oceanography* 9: 1223–1231.

Xue, Y., M.A. Cane, and S.E. Zebiak. 1997. Predictability of a coupled model of ENSO using singular vector analysis. Part I: Optimal growth in seasonal background and ENSO cycles. *Monthly Weather Review* 125: 2043–2056.

Xue, Y., M.A. Cane, S.E. Zebiak, and T. Palmer. 1997. Predictability of a coupled model of ENSO using singular vector analysis. Part II: Optimal growth and ENSO forecast skill. *Monthly Weather Review* 125: 2057–2073.

Zebiak, S.E. 1989. On the 30–60 day oscillation and the prediction of El Niño. *Journal of Climate* 2: 1381–1387.

Zebiak, S.E., and M.A. Cane. 1987. A model El Niño/Southern Oscillation. *Monthly Weather Review* 115: 2262–2278.

Chapter 12

Great Expectations
Malaria Vaccines and Antimalaria Drugs for the Next Century

Robert S. Desowitz

Cheap, effective, new malaria treatments could change the way we think about malaria. In this chapter, I review the past and present research developments related to malaria vaccines and antimalaria drugs.

History tells the story of a search for a malaria vaccine to immunize humans that is nearly a century long. Factors such as stage specificity, antigen variation, and the need for a safe-but-potent adjuvant have thwarted realization of that goal. Recent developments using recombinant technology of various antigens (including transmission blockers, DNA [deoxyribonucleic acid] vaccines, and new adjuvants) give promise that one or more vaccines will be available within the next 50 years.

Malariologists, researchers, and "field hands" alike now begin their addresses to public and professionals with the "malaria mantra": 3 billion at risk, 300 million infected, and 3 million dead each year. It is a sad statistic of despair, a fall from the exuberant expectation of the mid-1950s to mid-1960s, when it was prophesied that malaria would be not only brought under global control but also eradicated, that human malaria parasites would become as extinct as the dodo.

The prophet that had been anointed to lead the human race out of the malaria wilderness was the United Nations World Health Organization (WHO), whose staff and rod were DDT (a potent, cheap, nontoxic [to humans] residual insecticide) and chloroquine (a potent, cheap, nontoxic antimalaria drug). That war against malaria was willingly and generously funded by the industrialized nations; the United States is estimated to have contributed $1 billion.

However, by 1960, anopheline mosquito vectors had begun to develop physiological and behavioral resistance to DDT and other chlorinated hydrocarbon insecticides, and the malaria parasite species of greatest virulence, *Plasmodium falciparum*, had become insensitive to chloroquine and other antimalaria drugs. Resistance on the part of the mosquito and parasite progressed inexorably in degree and geographical expansion until 1968, when WHO threw in the towel and admitted that its army had been defeated by a brainless invertebrate and a single-celled protist.

Thus, at the turn of the twenty-first century, the malaria problem—particularly as it exists in its major repository of sub-Saharan Africa—persists in stark contrast to that of half a century ago. For all practical purposes, there are no new weapons in the antimalaria armamentarium to fight an African, let alone a global, war against malaria. Yet, for malaria researchers, funding during the past 25 years has been comparatively lavish. Moreover, malaria research has benefited greatly from the remarkable advances in genetics and immunology. The frustrating paradox is that as more and more is known about the malaria parasites' biology, less and less is known about how to control the malarial disease that these parasites cause. This current dissociation between research and reality makes it difficult to forecast malaria's future.

Malaria control essentially consists of two strategies:

- reducing or interrupting transmission through the mosquito and
- prevention or cure of infection in the human host.

Methods directed against the anopheline (e.g., engineering works [bonification], insecticides, repellents, microbial pathogens, and biological "engineering" by sterile male release or genetic control via transfection) are the topics of other researchers. In this chapter, I consider possible effective avenues to control malaria in the human host by 2050 through immunization with vaccines to prevent or ameliorate infection or through the widespread distribution of new, safe, inexpensive prophylactic and curative drugs that will not readily induce resistance.

On the Road to the Malaria Vaccine

To appreciate where we are today and where we might be 50 years hence, it is necessary to revisit the turn of the last century—1900, when the first attempts to vaccinate against malaria were carried out during a golden age of cross-fertilization among the emerging disciplines of microbiology, malariology, and immunology.

A Synoptic History

1910–1940. During the years leading to World War II, attempts were made to immunize humans and animals against their respective malarias. However, in the modern context, those attempts were limited and amorphous. Antigens were whatever material was available—sporozoites from mosquitoes, whole infected red blood cells (erythrocytes), or parasites from lysed infected erythrocytes. As in bacterial vaccines, whole parasites were used. However, unlike the bacteria, which could be isolated and washed to a pure, uncontaminated state, no such isolation techniques were then available for the intercellular or mosquito stages of the malaria parasites. Inevitably, these early vaccines contained extraneous blood cells or their stroma as well as bits and pieces of the mosquito host.

The host–parasite systems for immunization trials also were whatever happened to be available. Bird malarias were commonly used. The first-ever malaria vaccine that I could find in the literature was recorded in 1912 by Moldovan, who inoculated birds with *Plasmodium praecox* inactivated with serum from chronically infected birds. (There was no protective effect.)

Starting in 1917, when malariotherapy for neurosyphilis was introduced, humans became subjects for immunization experiments at special institutions in many parts of the world. The first of such vaccinations was in 1930 by Konstantsov, who inoculated *Plasmodium vivax* from lysed erythrocytes into paretics. It had as little effect on humans as Moldovan's vaccine had in birds. Primate malarias came into experimental use in the 1930s, notably with the 1932 discovery of *Plasmodium knowlesi* in the Malayan irus monkey and its experimental lethal infection in the rhesus. Birds, monkeys, or humans;

mosquito or vertebrate-stage vaccines—no significant successes were achieved in inducing immunity by vaccine.

There was, however, one exception to this unrelieved failure. Remarkably innovative research opened the way to all subsequent (including contemporary) attempts to afford immunity by a sporozoite vaccine. In 1940, an international (American, Indian, and Scottish) team of malariologists began experiments in immunizing chickens with living, ultraviolet radiation–inactivated *Plasmodium gallinaceum* sporozoites. In some chickens, a solid immunity to normal sporozoite challenge was induced. Those immune birds could be identified as having very high titers of sporozoite-agglutinating antibodies. However, the sporozoite-immune birds became infected when challenged with asexual stage–infected blood (Mulligan, Russell, and Mohan 1941; Russell and Mohan 1942; Russell, Mulligan, and Mohan 1942). These seminal experiments produced the knowledge from which malaria vaccinologists have continued to the present day:

- It is possible to induce immunity by vaccines of irradiation-inactivated living sporozoites.
- Immunity is stage-specific; it has to be absolutely "solid," because it will not protect if there is any breakthrough to asexual-stage parasitemia.
- A state of protective immunity might be identifiable by a serological test, in this case, the titer of a sporozoite-agglutination test. (This was the first—and the last—serological test to reliably predict the state of functional immunity.)

Dead sporozoites did not have the right stuff to induce protective immunity, and over the years, the living sporozoite vaccine, inactivated by more efficient sources of irradiation, became the benchmark of this "barrier" immunization. But there always was (or should have been) the realization that this was an all-or-nothing procedure; the immunity induced had to be absolutely solid. Moreover, there was the realization (or should have been) that a living sporozoite vaccine was logistically impossible to deliver to people of the tropical endemic zones.

For the most part, the avenue of inactivation successful for inducing immunity to sporozoites led up the garden path when applied to the asexual stages. Parasites, within the host erythrocytes, were incubated with immune sera or irradiated with X-rays in attempts to render them noninfectious but still immunogenic (Coffin 1951; Bennison and Coatney 1949). A few gave a slight immune protection, but none were significant successes, and this line of investigation fell into disfavor.

1941–1971. World War II opened without adequate antimalaria protection, chemotherapeutic or immunologic, to protect the Allied troops fighting in malaria-endemic areas. During the war years, the Americans continued to search for an effective vaccine. Killed asexual-stage parasites fared no better than sporozoites as vaccines. Infected erythrocytes treated with Formalin or phenol had little or no immunizing effect when inoculated into birds (Gingrich 1941) or monkeys (Eaton and Coggeshall 1939; Shortt and Menon 1940). Despite the unpromising results, researchers turned from experimental animals to experimental humans (Heidelberger et al. 1946a,b,c; Boyd and Kitchen 1936). The preparations were mainly Formalin-killed *P. vivax* within or extracted from the erythrocyte. The results were not promising in monkeys or in humans.

The major breakthrough came with the studies of Freund and colleagues, who were the first to demonstrate that immunization needed a vaccine helper—an adjuvant, the Freund's complete adjuvant (FCA) emulsion of mineral (paraffin) oil and *Mycobacterium* sp. In the first trial, two-month-old ducklings were inoculated with an adjuvant-containing vaccine of red blood cells infected with *Plasmodium lophurae* and killed with For-malin. A series of three intramuscular injections were given, one month apart. The ducklings were either completely protected at the time of the challenge or had only a low-grade parasitemia that went to self-cure (Freund, Sommer, and Walter 1945). There was, however, a problem: the ducks developed an adjuvant-induced *foie gras* (a fatty liver).

Despite the untoward side effects from Freund's adjuvant, it was the first successful nonliving vaccine of either a schizogonic- or sporogonic-stage antigen. Encouraged by these results, Freund et al. (1945, 1948) applied their immunization techniques to *P. knowlesi* in the rhesus monkey. Here was a model system of unrelenting pathogenicity; untreated, no rhesus survives the infection. Rhesus monkeys were given two to three injections of the adjuvant-containing, Formalin-treated infected erythrocytes 25–56 days apart and challenged one month after the last inoculation. All monkeys survived; one was completely protected, and the others developed a low-grade parasitemia that went rapidly to self-cure. But again, the adjuvant produced such severe side effects—suppurating lesions, fever, indurations—that there was no possibility of applying the Freund's adjuvant vaccines to human immunizations.

When the adjuvant was modified to produce fewer side effects (e.g., by replacing the *Mycobacterium* with lecithin), it lost its immune-boosting properties (Coffin 1951). Moreover, no other adjuvants, toxic or nontoxic, were available for human use. Experi-mental adjuvants such as a mixture of paraffin oil, BCG (bacillus Calmette Guerrin), and Tween 80 (Deschiens, Pick, and Sarauw 1956) and carboxymethyl cellulose (Desowitz 1967) gave partially protective results in avian and rodent malarias, but by 1970, the adjuvant-containing vaccines had reached another episodic dead end. Furthermore, there was little persuasive reason for pursuing this or any other malaria vaccine formula-tion. The war and its malaria problems had been successfully concluded. Chloroquine and DDT were here to stay. Colonial dependent populations had been liberated—the natives were on their own, and the best of luck to them.

1972–1977. By 1972, malarial matters had taken a distinct turn for the worse. Chloro-quine had come and gone; DDT had come and gone; the Global Eradication of Malaria Program had come and gone. The United States was again fighting a tropical war (in Vietnam this time), again without an adequate antimalaria armamentarium. The time was ripe for resurrecting research on the malaria vaccine. The agency and the agent to resurrect it came from an unexpected quarter.

The U.S. Agency for International Development (USAID) had undergone a succes-sion of name changes, but it had been, since its inception, a major conduit for American nonmilitary financial and technical largesse (especially for agriculture and health projects) to developing nations. However, USAID had never engaged or supported basic or applied research, even though antimalaria operations had long been on its agenda. From 1955 to 1970, the agency contributed approximately $1 billion to the WHO Glo-bal Eradication of Malaria Program and various national malaria eradication programs.

In 1965, Paul Silverman, a University of Illinois professor of parasitology who had experience in developing vaccines of helminths of veterinary importance, had met with Lee Howard, head of USAID's medical division. Silverman believed it was possible to make an effective malaria vaccine by combining multistage antigens, and he persuaded Howard to his point of view (Desowitz 1991). USAID called together an expert panel to advise on the vaccine's feasibility. The panel did not think much of the feasibility, but USAID decided to go ahead. The agency gave Silverman $2 million for the research and appointed an aging medical entomologist, soon to retire and without any expertise in immunology, as the project's administrative head.

Silverman and his group went to the classical *P. knowlesi*–rhesus model, although they soon dropped the sporozoite antigen component of the vaccine as too technologically difficult to be practicable. Their innovation was to produce a "cleaner" antigen by removing the parasite, intact, from the erythrocyte by means of a carefully regulated French pressure cell, followed by sucrose-gradient density concentration. This process removed most, but not all, of the adherent red blood cell stroma and, after Formalin treatment, gave a level of protection similar to that obtained almost 30 years previously by Freund's group—provided that they also incorporated FCA in their vaccine; without it, the vaccine provided no protection (Schenkel, Simpson, and Silverman 1973; Simpson, Schenkel, and Silverman 1974).

About the time Silverman's project was under way, a British group under Sydney Cohen of Guy's Hospital Medical School (London, U.K.) was pursuing the vaccine by a somewhat different approach. They rationalized that the key asexual-stage immunogen is the merozoite for two reasons: it is the only blood form that is completely free of erythrocyte components, and it is the crucial form in initiating invasion of the erythrocyte. They devised an elegant technique of isolating merozoites by passing short-term culture/merozoite-enriched blood through polycarbonate membrane sieves (Dennis et al. 1975). The Formalin-killed or lyophilized *P. knowlesi* merozoites made an effective vaccine in protecting rhesus monkeys—again, provided that it was incorporated in FCA (Mitchell 1977; Mitchell, Butcher, and Cohen 1974, 1975; Mitchell et al. 1977).

Finding an adjuvant acceptable for use in humans seemed, by 1980, an insurmountable barrier to the development of an asexual-stage malaria vaccine (reviewed in Miller 1977; Desowitz and Miller 1980). Other adjuvants had been screened in the *Plasmodium berghei*–rodent model, and some (e.g., carboxymethyl cellulose, saponin, and diethyldioctadecyl ammonium bromide) gave moderate to very good immune enhancement (Desowitz 1975; Desowitz and Barnwell 1980). But somehow, this critical line of research was not greatly pursued. By 1980, interest in the whole-parasite vaccine began to wane, and interest was later to be refocused on subunit, recombinant, and synthetic antigens or epitopes that were proposed to be better (more immunogenic) and safer malaria vaccines.

During this period, the first human immunizations with irradiated sporozoites were carried out. Fewer than half of the volunteers were solidly protected (Clyde et al. 1975), and in one trial in the Gambia, it was a complete failure (Bray 1976).

1977–1987. The late 1970s to late 1980s was a transitional and somewhat tawdry decade of malaria vaccine research. The breakthrough discovery of the method for the continuous culture of *P. falciparum* had been made in 1976 (Haynes et al. 1976; Trager and Jensen 1976), and the *Aotus* monkey had become available as an experimental host of *P. falciparum* a few years earlier (Geiman and Meagher 1967). The Cohen group departed the arena after successfully immunizing *Aotus* monkeys with their merozoite–FCA vaccine, but their parting words were, "The need for Freund's complete adjuvant remains a constraint on the formulation of a vaccine suitable for human use" (Mitchell et al. 1977).

Silverman also left the vaccine studies. The rest of his group moved to the University of New Mexico, where it was led by K.H. Rieckmann for a short time. The group's final study (Rieckmann et al. 1979) revealed that various asexual-stage *P. knowlesi* (schizont, merozoite, French press/lyophilized) vaccines gave only partial protection to the rhesus, even when incorporated with FCA.

Despite these unpromising results, USAID's commitment remained undiminished, and the agency embarked on a new administrative and strategic plan of action. The medical entomologist project administrator retired and was replaced with an agricultural entomologist project head, James Erickson. The vaccine research funding was essentially divided into three parts and awarded to Miodrag Ristic, a veterinarian at the University of Illinois (to produce a vaccine of *P. falciparum* culture-secreted exoantigens, similar to what he had devised for *Babesia* in cattle); Wasim Siddiqui of the University of Hawaii (to produce an asexual-stage antigen *P. falciparum* vaccine incorporating active, acceptable adjuvants to replace FCA); and Ruth Nussenzweig of New York University (to continue the development of a sporozoite vaccine).

The notorious disaster of the "Erickson regime" has been well publicized, but the dimension of criminal purloining of vaccine research monies by Erickson, Siddiqui, and Ristic was unprecedented (see details in Desowitz 1991). Remarkably, USAID was not shriven by these events and continued/continues to support malaria vaccine research, albeit at a reduced level.

Ristic's studies did not progress and will not be considered further here. Siddiqui, similar to the Cohen group, successfully immunized (survival with low parasitemia on homologous challenge) *Aotus* monkeys with a *P. falciparum* vaccine of mature segmenters emulsified in FCA (Siddiqui 1977). Attempts to replace FCA with a less side-reactive adjuvant, such as the muramyl dipeptide, gave some protection but not to the enhancement level of FCA (Siddiqui et al. 1978).

Because it was clearly impossible and impractical to devise and deliver a sporozoite vaccine of living, irradiated parasites, the logical step was to elucidate the major sporozoite immunogen and use it as a vaccine. In 1980, the Nussenzweig group, applying the recently developed hybridoma–monoclonal antibody (MAB) technology, discovered that this immunogen is a protein covering the sporozoite surface (circumsporozoite protein [CSP]) (Yoshida et al. 1980; Potocnjak et al. 1980). Additional analysis revealed that the immunogenic epitope of CSP was small and simple, a repetitive sequence of amino acids (each species of *Plasmodium* has its characteristic sequence), and that the sequence for *P. falciparum* CSP contained 40 Asn-Ala-Asn-Pro repeats. What made this immunogen particularly attractive was that its encoding gene could be inserted, by DNA recombinant technology, into a convenient microbial "factory" such as *Escherichia coli* (Dame et al. 1984). Even better, the simple epitope could be completely synthesized, eliminating the recombinant "middle man" (reviewed in Good, Berzofsky, and Miller 1988).

Unlike the asexual-stage vaccines, the "new" sporozoite vaccines were tested in humans. Preliminary studies had shown that both the synthetic construct (NANP) conjugated to the putative adjuvants, alum or tetanus toxoid, and a recombinant vaccine of the circumsporozoite epitope R32tet32/R48tet32 expressed in *E. coli* (Young et al. 1985) were immunogenic; that is, they elicited a specific antibody in experimental animals and human volunteers (summarized in WHO 1986). However, neither the synthetic *P. falciparum* sporozoite vaccine $(NANP)_3$_tetanus toxoid nor a recombinant DNA sporozoite vaccine afforded adequate protective immunity to human volunteers (Etlinger et al. 1988; Ballou et al. 1987).

With limited successes of the sporozoite and asexual-stage *P. falciparum* vaccines in humans and monkeys, USAID, WHO, and the researchers themselves began to promote and prophesize the vaccine for human use as just around the corner, a fulfilled hope just an experiment away. Beleaguered health authorities in malaria-endemic developing countries began to relax their expensive, imperfect antimalaria efforts and waited for the vaccine—which would never arrive.

1988–1999. Although the synthetic CSP vaccine (NANP)$_3$ gave disappointing results, synthetic vaccines still were a promising and attractive option (Zavala, Tam, and Hollingdale 1985). A Colombian researcher, Manuel Patarroyo, reasoned that if combined as a kind of chimeric multistage vaccine of asexual and sporozoite synthetic constructs, (NANP)$_3$ would be broadly effective. The synthetic *P. falciparum* vaccine that came to be known as SPf66 is a mixture of three synthetic asexual-stage peptides (one 83-kDa sequence derived from the merozoite surface protein, and two sequences from the 35- and 55-kDa intracellular schizont proteins) linked to the CSP (NANP) construct (Patarroyo et al. 1987, 1988). SPf66 is the only candidate vaccine to have undergone large-scale phase-III testing in humans. Thousands of adults and children in Africa, Asia, and South America have been vaccinated with it. The results, initially controversial in their statistical interpretation from the hypoendemic South American trials, were very disappointing when assessed under the holoendemic settings of Africa and Asia (reviewed in Targett 1992; White 1994; Maurice 1995; Ferreira 1996). A great deal of publicity has surrounded the SPf66 trials, and this experience is, in a way, an example of the overstatement of and the overdependency on shallow results.

Thus, to date, the whole, subunit, and synthetic antigen vaccines of each stage have not been able to artificially immunize humans against falciparum malaria, let alone the other malaria parasites of humans. This failure has variously been attributed to such factors as lack of a suitable adjuvant, parasite variation, human immune unresponsiveness, and different immune system pathways in stage-specific responses.

Recombinant technology, introduced during the 1980s, was quickly exploited by malaria vaccine researchers who recognized it as a way to "manufacture" large "pure" amounts of target antigens. Table 12-1, which is by no means a comprehensive account, gives a sense of the variety of recombinant antigens and the cells that transcribe them. The three main categories of malaria vaccines (asexual-stage antigens, sporozoite/preerythrocytic antigens, and transmission-blocking antigens) all have been expressed by means of recombinant technology. Although data are no longer being entered into the now-abandoned European Community Database of Antigens Used in Malaria Vaccination Experiments (http://ben.vub.ac.be/malaria/med.html), the database provides a remarkably comprehensive list and descriptions of the candidate antigens.

When used, these subunit/recombinant/synthetic antigens have proved to be no more immunogenic than the "native" whole parasite antigens. The Freundian principle continues to apply: without a suitable adjuvant, the new vaccine candidates are not protective. The search for an adjuvant (or adjuvants) that is safe for human use and that will render vaccine antigen candidates protectively immunogenic has received almost as much attention as the search for the vaccine antigens themselves. Table 12-2 summarizes some of the recent vaccine antigen–adjuvant formulations.

In 1997, an adjuvant-containing formulation of a recombinant *P. falciparum* sporozoite vaccine was produced by the pharmaceutical firm SmithKline Beecham Biologicals (Rixensart, Belgium). It was highly immunogenic and protected six of seven human volunteers against sporozoite challenge (Stoute et al. 1997). The vaccine, designated as RTS,S, consists of two CSP peptides of 207–395 amino acids recombinantly expressed in yeast and fused to a recombinant hepatitis B surface antigen of 226 amino acid residues. RTS,S was mixed with a combination of the adjuvants monophosphoryl lipid A and QS-21 (a saponin isolated by high-pressure liquid chromatography from the bark of the *Quillaja saponaria* tree of South America). Seven volunteers were inoculated intramuscularly in three divided doses over a period of 28 weeks with this adjuvant-containing vac-

Table 12-1. Recombinant and DNA Vaccines

Vaccine	Reference
Escherichia coli-Plasmodium falciparum major merozoite surface antigen	Holder, Freeman, and Nichols 1988
Vaccinia-*P. falciparum* RESA	Pye et al. 1991
P815 mastocytoma cells-*Plasmodium berghei* sporozoite surface protein 2	Khusmith et al. 1991
E. coli-P. falciparum Pfs48/45 transmission blocking	Milek et al. 1998
DNA *P. falciparum* encoding transmission-blocking antigens Pfs25-27	Lobo, Dhar, and Kumar 1999
Yeast-*Plasmodium vivax* MSP-1 plus copolymer P1005/tetanus toxoid/alum adjuvant	Yang et al. 1999
Baculovirus-expressed *Plasmodium cynomologi* MSP-1 (42- and 19-kDa fragments)	Perera et al. 1998
Vaccinia virus expressed MSP-1 *P. falciparum* signal and anchor region genes	Yang et al. 1997
Yeast *Pichia pastoris-P. vivax* apical membrane antigen plus SBAS2 adjuvant	Kocken et al. 1999
Plasmid DNA-preerythrocytic *P. berghei* antigen plus booster recombinant antigen in modified vaccinia virus Ankara	Schneider et al. 1998
DNA plastids-*P. falciparum* [preerythrocytic antigens] sporozoite surface protein 2/circumsporozoite protein/carboxyl terminus liver stage antigen 1/exported protein 1	Hedstrom et al. 1998
E. coli-Plasmodium yoelii PYPAg-1 gene for pAg-1 and pAg-1C	Burns, Adeeko, and Dunn 1999
Baculovirus-*P. falciparum* synthetic gene expressing a 41-kDa antigen (CDC/NIMALVAC-1, a multistage immunogen)	Shi et al. 1999
E. coli/CHO and HeLa cells-*P. falciparum* synthetic gene encoding MSP-1	Pan et al. 1999
E. coli-P. yoelii MSP-1, 82-kDa, 42-kDa, and 19-kDa protein fragments	Tian et al. 1997
Mycobacterium bovis BCG recombinant expressing *P. yoelii* MSP-1 15-kDa fragment: recombinant MSP-1 plus RIBI adjuvant	Matsumoto 1998
Yeast-expressed *P. vivax* MSP-1 yP2P30Pv200(19)	Collins et al. 1999
DNA plasmid encoding *P. falciparum* Pf155/RESA/M3 sequence plus plasmid or recombinant antigen-alum adjuvant booster	Haddad et al. 1999
DNA plasmid encoding *P. falciparum* serine repeat antigen	Belperron et al. 1999

Notes: RESA = ring-infected erythrocyte surface antigen; MSP-1 = merozoite surface protein 1 complex; kDa = kilodaltons.

cine. Protection was excellent, but after the second dose, about one-half the volunteers experienced moderate to severe constitutional side reactions—pain, fever, headache, malaise, and myalgia. It will be of considerable interest to follow the fate of this vaccine.

The most promising adjuvant is QS-21, a triterpene glycoside. It has high immune stimulatory activity and is in phase-I and -II trials with several antigens, including HIV-1 [human immunodeficiency virus-1], influenza, hepatitis B, and melanoma. It also is to be used as an adjuvant with a new formulation of SPf66. It is one of the very few known adjuvants that will enhance a T-cell–independent immune response. Although safe in the 1,600 individuals of the human trials carried out so far, QS-21 produces mild to

Table 12-2. Antigen–Adjuvant Preparations

Vaccine	Reference
Plasmodium falciparum Pf155/RESA-influenza virus fusion protein ISCOM/Quil A	Sjolander et al. 1991
P. falciparum sporozoite synthetic (NANP)$_3$-tetanus toxoid-recombinant human interferon	Sturchler et al. 1989
P. falciparum circumsporozoite synthetic (NANP)$_{3/4}$ or *Plasmodium knowlesi* PK26 peptide-TT plus preimmunization with TT	Lise et al. 1987
Plasmodium yoelii synthetic linear peptides from 17-kDa of hepatocyte erythrocyte protein plus TiterMax adjuvant	Charoenvit et al. 1999
P. yoelii and *Plasmodium berghei* multiple antigen constructs of circumsporozoite antigen plus P1005 copolymer/detoxified RaLPS in oil-in-water emulsion	Reed et al. 1997
P. yoelii whole blood-stage antigen plus P1005/RaLPS adjuvant	Patterson et al. 1999
P. falciparum preerythrocytic antigens LSA1, LSA3, SALSA, STARP, plus Montanide ISA-51 antigen	Perlaza et al. 1998
Seppic Montanide ISA-720 (oil metabolizable adjuvant) phase I human trial	Lawrence et al. 1997
P. falciparum synthetic preerythrocytic stage antigens to oxime bonds (polyoximes) plus tripalmitoyl-*S*-glyceryl cysteine adjuvant	Nardin et al. 1998
P. yoelii MSP-1 EGF-like modules of recombinant antigen plus SBAS-1 adjuvants	Ling et al. 1997
P. falciparum merozoite surface antigen 2 plus Montanide ISA-720, SAF-1/liposomes containing lipid A adjuvants	Pye et al. 1997
Plasmodium berghei synthetic CS protein 252-260 plus biodegradable polymer microspheres	Men et al. 1997

Notes: TT = tetanus toxoid.

moderate side effects (pain, fever, headache, malaise, and myalgia—similar to those experienced with the Stoute et al. malaria vaccine) in about 15% of those inoculated (Kensil and Kammer 1998). It is produced and being developed by Aquila Biopharmaceuticals (Framingham, Massachusetts) and is expected to become the first commercially available, potent adjuvant approved for human use.

Some malaria vaccinologists believe that the only method to circumvent such barriers as adjuvanticity and antigen immunogenicity is through manipulative DNA genetic technology. By this method, which has worked most successfully with experimental virus vaccines, a segment of the malaria parasite's genome encoding for the desired immunogenic antigen is actually inserted into a living carrier. One method is to insert the desired malaria parasite gene into a virus carrier, which, in turn, inserts itself into the human host gene. The other method is to inoculate naked *Plasmodium* DNA intramuscularly, where it would become incorporated into the myocyte genome—leading to more or less continuous antigenic stimulation. It is still too early to know the full impact of this form of vaccination. Safety remains a concern for DNA vaccines, because DNA may integrate inappropriately into the human genome, although no evidence of carcinogenic effects have yet been identified. Another concern is whether continuous antigenic elaboration will lead to immune complex disease (reviewed in Doolan and Hoffman 1997; Kwiatowski and Marsh 1997).

Transmission-Blocking Vaccines

The most separate facet of malaria vaccine research is the hunt for a transmission-blocking vaccine. I am especially in favor of its development. We members of the old school of malariology hold that the malarious sick are the charge of physicians and other health-care providers; the malariologist's pursuit is to interrupt transmission, to abate risk. Since the virtual demise of DDT, this goal has not been readily realizable, and vector control has been rather unsatisfactory and ad hoc. In contrast, the proffered alternative of transmission-blocking immunity is not to kill the vector but to kill the sexual-stage malaria organisms within it.

In 1976, Gwadz showed that immunizing chickens with Formalin-treated blood infected with both sexual and asexual *P. gallinaceum* reduced infectiousness to mosquitoes on subsequent challenge. Shortly thereafter, Carter and Chen (1976), using a more refined approach of immunizing chicken with extracellular gametes, obtained similar results in blocking transmission. Vaccination with the rodent malaria *Plasmodium yoelii* gametes gave similar effects (Mendis and Targett 1982).

The malaria vaccine zeitgeist of the 1980s required the elucidation and use of subunit proteins specific for the sexual stages. By 1985, three stage-specific polypeptides had been identified from the *P. falciparum* gamete surface: 25 kDa, 48/45 kDa, and 230 kDa (Kumar and Carter 1984; Carter et al. 1984; Vermeulen et al. 1985). The 25-kDa peptide appeared to be a particularly potent transmission-blocking immunogen; its encoding gametocyte gene has been cloned and its product sequenced (Alano et al. 1991). A monoclonal antibody to it has been produced (Vermeulen et al. 1985); its gene has been transfected in vaccinia (mice infected with the transfected virus elaborate transmission-blocking antibody [Kaslow 1990; Kaslow et al. 1991]) and recombinantly produced in yeast to give transmission-blocking antibodies in mice and monkeys (Barr et al. 1991).

Transmission-blocking antibodies circulating in the human host are inactive until ingested, together with gametocytes, by the mosquito vector. The main criticism leveled against the transmission-blocking vaccine is that it would have no direct effect on individual humans to relieve them of malaria disease. The transmission-blocking vaccine would have to be applied to entire populations for it to interrupt or even significantly reduce transmission. An act of altruism on the part of the global population would be required. Phase-III evaluation of the vaccine also would be extraordinarily expensive. Nevertheless, the use of an effective transmission-blocking vaccine would ultimately be so great that it, rather than the asexual-stage vaccines, could well be the answer to malaria. It could be given combined in a multistage preparation, or even with other common vaccines, such as the DPT [diphtheria, pertussis, tetanus] vaccine.

The biggest news about malaria vaccine research may not be of clinical success but rather of fiscal good fortune. In an act of philanthropic generosity rivaled only by the Rockefeller donations a century ago, Bill and Melinda Gates (of Microsoft) have given $750 million via their foundation, the Children's Vaccine Trust Fund, to develop and distribute vaccines for children in developing countries. This effort is expected to grow to $1.5 billion within five years, and the fund is expected to become the centerpiece of their foundation, which has an endowment of $17.1 billion.

The $50 million designated for malaria research may be "small potatoes" when viewed as part of the $750 million total, but still, it is a lot of money. The $50 million was given to a Seattle nonprofit organization, Program for Appropriate Technology in Health (PATH), to run the Malaria Vaccine Initiative (MVI) based in Rockville, Maryland.

The MVI appointed Regina Rabinovich, formerly of National Institutes of Health (NIH), National Institute of Allergy and Infectious Diseases (NIAID), as its director. The first act of the MVI was to sign an agreement with NIH/NIAID to support its long-range plan to

- carry out the preclinical and clinical testing of promising vaccine candidates,
- launch an Internet-based resource center for malaria research reagents, and
- publish a detailed genetic map of the malaria parasite.

I have learned that the money will be used primarily to fund phase-II and -III trials of candidate vaccines, a multitude of which wait in the wings (Table 12-2). But informants hesitate to say which of that multitude of candidates are actually safe enough and ready enough for human trials.

Even M.E. Patarroyo, the independent malaria vaccinologist, continues to have ample funds for his research. Fidel Castro and the king and queen of Spain remain his patrons, and the Spanish government has pledged about $60 million to provide to children, free of charge, a vaccine that Patarroyo believes to be of great promise.

Distinguished economists—notably, Jeffrey Sachs of Harvard—have assumed that the vaccine will become a reality within the next 5–10 years and have confronted the thorny problems of how much it will cost and who will pay for it. The industrial estimate is that it will cost $40 for an immunizing course. The international public health sector's estimate is that this cost can be reduced to $10 (but of course, there is no idea which, if any, vaccine will work; how many doses will be needed, or how often the immunizations will have to repeated to maintain protection; or how much the vaccine will cost to manufacture). Total foreign aid to Africa now totals about $16 billion, and the numbers work out to 1.5% of that total to immunize all African children with the $10 vaccine (Sachs 1999). In this profit-dominated era, interesting contests of proprietary patent rights will ultimately influence vaccine costs. A sign of the times is that the NIH Office of Technology Transfer was party to the MVI agreement, just in case any profitable patents might arise from this government–Gates research partnership. Patarroyo, on the other hand, assigned his patent rights on SPf66 to WHO (although it is not known whether the new formulation is similarly assigned) and has a football field ready to be converted into a factory for the profit-free manufacture of his vaccine.

Looking Ahead

In this short review, I have attempted to summarize the search for a malaria vaccine over the course of the past century. I cannot predict whether the vaccine will ever come to fruition. Many preparations are awaiting human trials, which will require anywhere from an estimated $300,000 to $1,200,000 to bring each candidate from phase-I to phase-III evaluation (double that for transmission-blocking vaccine trials) (Engers 1997). The Patarroyo SPf66 trials show that it can be done where there is a forceful will. Hopefully, that will has not been squandered on an ineffective vaccine.

Drugging Malaria into Submission

Predicting the role of drugs in abating malaria 50 years from now is, in some respects, even more problematic than predicting control by vaccination. When suitable antimalaria drugs were available, millions of lives were saved among native populations. Prophylactic antimalaria drugs prevented the sickness and death of military personnel, tourists, and visiting and resident businesspeople. (The economic benefit of antimalaria drugs for the tourism industry of many developing nations has not been adequately appreciated. Certainly, without available short-term prophylactic antimalaria drugs, tourists would not venture into malaria-endemic countries.) However, even during the 20- to 25-year utility of chloroquine, except for some pilot projects, there were no extensive mass chemotherapy strategies to eradicate malaria in the manner that DDT was intended to do in the Global Eradication of Malaria Program. When the program collapsed, a turn to primary health services (with their ad hoc distribution of chloroquine) was advocated. In some areas, such as Papua New Guinea, this approach remains the main national antimalaria effort.

Primary health care could be simple, conducted by village volunteers who have minimal basic training. In one such project in a holoendemic area of Kenya, volunteers gave chloroquine to villagers who complained of (self-diagnosed) malaria. Neither parasitologic rates (densities not measured) nor serologic titers were affected by the program, but after two years, mortality and morbidity had decreased significantly (Spencer et al. 1987).

More than 40 years ago, mass malaria prevention was attempted by distributing common table salt medicated with chloroquine or pyrimethamine (Clyde 1964). Pyrimethamine salt rapidly led to resistance in areas as widely separated as Cambodia and Irian Jaya (Indonesia). Chloroquine salt was more successful, but the drug tended to leach out when stored under conditions of high humidity, and the salt intake of young children—the population segment with the highest incidence of parasitemia—was limited. Nevertheless, we tend to forget today how effective the strategy was in some pilot trials. We should be mindful of this once-promising strategy and consider it again with newer antimalaria drugs less likely to give rapid rise to resistance. Combined with other strategies such as the use of pesticide-impregnated bed nets, an effective, economically possible program that leads to the interruption of transmission might be mounted.

Even so, in planning strategies for malaria control over the next several decades, it would be prudent to assume that a vaccine for widespread population use will not be available, or if available, not deployed. Therefore, prudence would dictate that antimalaria drugs will be needed, as they have been for more than 400 years, to cure illness and save lives. But which drug(s) fulfill this need today, and which drugs might be developed in the future?

As shown in Figure 12-1, *P. falciparum* is resistant to chloroquine throughout the world's endemic regions, except in a few areas. In vitro experiments have indicated that this resistance can be reversed by agents such as verapamil, a calcium-channel blocker (Martin, Oduola, and Milhous 1987), and in vivo experiments in the owl monkey have achieved the same results by using desipramine and other tricyclic antidepressant drugs (Bitonti et al. 1988). This line of research does not appear to be pursued, at present, in any major fashion. However, if a cheap, nontoxic synergistic resistance-reversing agent could be found, it would go a long way in solving the current control-by-treatment dilemma.

Despite the synthetic wizardry of modern pharmacology, the final therapeutic arbiter for severe malaria is a botanical derivative that has been in use for some 400 years: quinine. It may well be that the antimalaria drug to replace quinine in this new millennium will also be a botanical derivative, of an even more ancient lineage than quinine: artemisinin, the Chinese *qinghaosu* from sweet wormwood (*Artemesia annua*). More than 2,100 years ago, in 168 B.C., *qinghaosu* was mentioned in the Han dynasty's *Recipes for 52 Kinds*

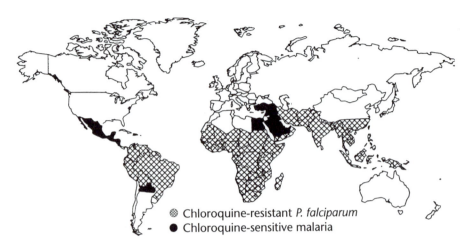

Figure 12-1. Distribution of Malaria and Chloroquine-Resistant *Plasmodium falciparum*

Source: Centers for Disease Control and Prevention, *Health Information for International Travel,* U.S. Department of Health and Human Services 1992–1999.

of Diseases as a sovereign remedy for hemorrhoids. About five hundred years later, in 340 A.D., Ge Hong advised its use for fever and chills in *Handbook of Prescriptions for Emergency Treatments.* From that time, *qinghaosu* has become a staple of Chinese traditional medicine for that purpose. In 1967, scientists in the People's Republic of China began a systematic search for new drugs from among traditional herbals and discovered artemisinin's striking activity against malaria parasites (Klayman 1985; Anonymous 1992).

The active principle of artemisinin, a sequestrene lactone peroxide, has been synthesized as artesunate for oral use and as artemether, an oil-soluble form, for intramuscular injection. Both agents have remarkable antiparasitic activity, reducing the parasitemia by about 10,000-fold within 24 hours (whereas this factor is about 10 for mefloquine). However, both agents also have a short half-life, necessitating a course of five to seven days. Nevertheless, the regimen is well tolerated, with few side effects. A course of artemether brings rapid parasitologic and clinical resolution in children with severe and cerebral falciparum malaria (White et al. 1992; Taylor et al. 1993). For uncomplicated hyperparasitemic falciparum malaria, a course of oral artesunate is effective, especially when accompanied by a single dose of mefloquine (Price et al. 1998) or three doses of pyrimethamine–sulfadoxine (von Seidlein et al. 2000).

The artemisinin antimalaria drugs are not approved by the U.S. Food and Drug Administration, but they are manufactured elsewhere, by Rhône-Poulenc and a Belgian company called Arenco. A product called Arsumax is produced in China by the Guillin Pharmaceutical Works for the French company Sanofi Winthrop. The artemisinins are excellent, almost ideal antimalaria drugs, but their cost, about $6 for the five-day course of treatment, may make it unavailable to the people who need it most (e.g., in sub-Saharan Africa, where the total malaria budget of a country usually does not exceed $0.50 to $1 per person).

It is expected that during the next several decades, new, unique classes of antimalaria drugs will be discovered. This search will be made possible and rational, the genetic oracles maintain, by the elaboration of the *P. falciparum* genome. A glimmer of things to come is revealed by the recent, curious finding of green alga DNA in Apicomplexa, the group of protozoans to which the malaria parasites belong.

Malaria researchers have returned to evolutionary fundamentals to discover metabolic pathways in the parasite that are completely lacking in humans so that drugs toxic to the parasite will not harm humans. The Apicomplexa have intricate subcellular structures (organelles) at their anterior end. In *Plasmodium* merozoites, two of the apical organelles contain protein ligands that, when expressed, are crucial in the invasion of the red blood cell.

Other organelles support the concept that eukaryotes not only evolved but also were assembled. It has been known for some years that the mitochondrion of a eukaryote, the laminated organelle that is the "battery" performing chemical energy-producing transactions, is actually a bacterium engulfed by some protist ancestor. That bacterium defied digestion and survived over hundreds of millions of years, dividing when its host cell divided. It became a permanent paying guest that has contributed, symbiotically, to its host's life process.

Thus, eukaryotes contain DNA in both the chromosomes within the nucleus and extranuclearly in the mitochondrion. In addition, *Plasmodium* and *Toxoplasma* (another Apicomplexan pathogen of humans) have a third kind of DNA within a membrane of an organelle called a plastid. Plastid DNA had been considered to be nothing more than a break-off fragment of mitochondrion DNA, but a recent study revealed it to be, astonishingly, a relic of a chloroplast DNA from a green alga incorporated, like the archaic mitochondrion bacterium, by some ancient Apicomplexan ancestor.

The analogous plastid DNA in plants and fungi encodes seven enzymes that mediate a biochemical process known as the shikimate pathway, which leads to the production of *p*-aminobenzoate (PABA) and folates, which then are converted into some of the amino acid building blocks of life. Human cells do not have a shikimate pathway and get their PABA and folates exogenously. That is why glyphosphate, a powerful herbicide that inhibits an enzyme in the shikimate pathway, will kill the weed and spare the gardener. In June 1998, Roberts et al. of the University of Chicago reported that *P. falciparum* and other apicomplexan parasites have a shikimate pathway, presumably mediated by the plastid. Moreover, the growth of the malaria and other apicomplexans was reportedly inhibited by the herbicide. Researchers see this as a possibility of attacking the parasite at its botanical side—a malarial herbicide, so to speak. Earlier, Fischera and Roos (1997) of the University of Pennsylvania's Department of Biology had reported that the fluroquinolone antibiotic Ciprofloxaxcin was a potent inhibitor of *Toxoplasma* replication by specifically attacking the plastid DNA.

It is encouraging that new classes (and new uses of old classes) of antimalaria drugs are becoming available. One showing exceptional promise is atovaquone, a hydroxy-naphthoquinone. The hydroxy-naphthoquinones' antimalarial activity was demonstrated during the empirical search of the World War II malaria drug program. Most of the naphthoquinones were considered too toxic and gave way to the safer, more easily synthesized 4-amino-quinolines, such as chloroquine. Atovaquone, synthesized during the 1970s, was the least toxic of the hydroxy-naphthoquinones and was resurrected to treat *Pneumocystis* infections associated with AIDS [acquired immune deficiency syndrome]. And here it is, after almost 60 years, back again as an antimalaria drug.

Atovaquone exerts the highest level of activity when it is combined with proguanil (the combined drug is known as Malarone), curing 99% of the cases of multiple-drug-resistant falciparum malaria (Looareesuwan et al. 1999). Atovaquone selectively inhibits mitochondrial electron transport of the parasite without damaging the mammalian host cell (Srivastava, Rottenberg, and Vaidya 1997). In Malorone, proguanil acts as a biguanide mitochondrion uncoupler in enhancing atovaquone's effect, even for strains resistant to proguanil alone (a dihydrofolate reductase inhibitor) (Srivastava and Vaidya 1999). Malarone is a blood schizonticide but probably acts on preerythrocytic stages as well. Malorone has been shown to be a highly effective prophylactic. One pill a week (250 mg atovaquone plus 100 mg proguanil hydrochloride) afforded >95% protection to adults and children in randomized clinical trials in Gabon (Lell et al. 1998), Kenya (Shanks et al. 1998), South Africa (van der Berg et al. 1999), and Zambia (Sukwa et al. 1999). Malorone may well be the twenty-first century's chloroquine—provided that the price is right and that resistance can be averted, or at least delayed.

If the future is anything like the past, a continuous succession of antimalaria drugs will be needed. As resistance to one drug develops, another should be available to take its place. Who will be responsible for the discovery of new antimalaria drugs (and for the treatment and prevention of other tropical diseases), their manufacture, their sale at affordable prices, and their distribution? Pharmaceutical companies of the industrialized nations have little economic incentive to pursue research and development on drugs for which there is little or no prospect of profit. If anything, there is a disincentive; a discovery, even a serendipitous one, of a new antimalaria drug would be followed by the uncomfortable moral pressure to carry out its costly five-year/$500 million development.

However, in an unprecedented, unique response to these needs, WHO—in partnership with the World Bank and the International Federation of Pharmaceutical Manufacturers Associations (FPMA)—has established a nonprofit foundation under Swiss law, the Medicines for Malaria Venture (MMV). The stated mission of the MMV is to discover, develop, and register affordable new drugs to treat malaria in countries where the disease is endemic and to make arrangements for the production and commercialization of products for which regulatory approvals are obtained. Its modus operandi is that of a small pharmaceutical company, but it conducts both its research and its development by using a virtual approach. Resources are provided jointly by various public-sector agencies and FPMA companies.

The yearly MMV budget is $30 million. Although this amount is not "big bucks" in terms of pharmaceutical R&D, it should be sufficient to fund an adequate number of screening projects. And certainly, $30 million has been of sufficient stimulus for all sorts of research groups, big and small, to come out of the drug development woodwork. Within a year of its formation, MMV received 101 letters of interest from 27 different countries. The Japanese pharmaceutical firms have agreed to donate some 25,000 items in their molecular library for screening of antimalarial activity. Three grants totaling $4 million have been awarded to date. Each grant has been to a major pharmaceutical firm linked to a university: Glaxo Wellcome with Bristol University (U.K.), SmithKline Beecham with the University of California, and Roche of Switzerland with the University of Nebraska.

Nevertheless, the ledger balance does not seem to reconcile; an estimated $150 million will be needed to develop a new drug from screen to popular use, and one successful antimalaria drug is expected to emerge every five years. That leaves a $120 million deficit every five years. Is this sum to be raised from (reluctant) pharmaceutical firms or from (reluctant) donor countries and charities?

Malaria never had it so good. WHO's Roll Back Malaria program intends to halve malaria mortality within 10 years. Bill Gates, via the Children's Vaccine Trust Fund, provides MVI with $50 million. With the private sector, WHO has created MMV to develop new antimalaria drugs. The Multilateral Initiative on Malaria, an alliance of organizations and researchers, is intent on applying the best of science to combat malaria in sub-

Saharan Africa. Initiatives, ventures, and alliances—all mobilized and all moneyed against malaria. Will it do any good, or will *Plasmodium* emerge triumphant once again?

Conclusion

Two major strategies proposed for the prevention and control of malaria, particularly regarding falciparum malaria in sub-Saharan Africa, are immunization by vaccine and chemotherapy. Although the search for an effective vaccine for human use has been pursued for more than 70 years, that goal has not been achieved. Impediments to malaria vaccine development include the stage specificity of the immune responses; the generally functional weakness of those responses; the still-imperfect understanding of the nature of those responses; and the need for a powerful, safe adjuvant to promote a functional immunity to nonliving malaria vaccines. New technologies such as synthetic and recombinant antigen production and DNA vaccines show promise but so far have not been sufficiently effective. Nor can it be predicted, with confidence, that a malaria vaccine ever will be available.

In contrast, effective antimalaria drug therapy has been available for more than 400 years in the west (quinine) and probably 2,000 years in the Orient (artemisinins). Although in many places malaria has developed resistance to chloroquine—the effective, safe, and inexpensive drug that had been, for many years, the antimalaria "sheet anchor"—new compounds are now in place. No one need die of malaria for treatment failure. The present problem is to get these new, very expensive drugs to people in developing countries who are at risk to endemic malaria. Another problem is promoting the continuance of antimalaria drug research and development by the reluctant, profit-motivated pharmaceutical industry so that new classes of antimalaria drugs will be ready to replace the present armamentarium when resistance to them develops.

References

Alano, P., W. Premwansa, M.C. Bruce, and R. Carter. 1991. A stage specific gene expressed at the onset of gametocytogenesis in *Plasmodium falciparum*. *Molecular and Biochemical Parasitology* 46: 81–88.

Anonymous. 1992. Editorial. *Lancet* 339: 649–651.

Ballou, W.P., S.L. Hoffman, J.A. Sherwood, F.A. Neva, D.M. Gordon, R.A. Wirtz, G.F. Wasserman, C.L. Diggs, M.R. Hollingdale, W.T. Hockmeyer, I. Schneider, J.F. Young, P. Reeve, and J.D. Chulay. 1987. Safety and efficacy of a recombinant DNA *Plasmodium falciparum* sporozoite vaccine. *Lancet* 1(8545, June 6): 1277–1281.

Barr, P.J., K.M. Green, H.L. Gibson, I.C. Bathurst, I.A. Quakyi, and D.C. Kaslow. 1991. Recombinant Pfs25 proteitn of *Plasmodium falciparum* elicits malaria transmission-blocking immunity in experimental animals. *Journal of Experimental Medicine* 174: 1203–1208.

Belperron, A.A., D. Feltquate, B.A. Fox, T. Horii, and D.J. Bzik. 1999. Immune responses induced by gene gun or intramuscular injection of DNA vaccines that express immunogenic regions of the serine repeat antigen from *Plasmodium falciparum*. *Infection and Immunity* 67: 5163–5169.

Bennison, B.E., and G.R. Coatney. 1949. Effects of X-irradiation on *Plasmodium gallinaceum* and *Plasmodium lophurae* in young chicks. *Journal of the National Malaria Society* 8: 280–289.

Bitonti, A.J., A. Sjoerdsma, P.P. McCann, D.E. Kyle, A.M.J. Oduola, R.N. Rossan, W.K. Milhous, and D.E. Davidson. 1988. Reversal of chloroquine resistance in malaria parasite *Plasmodium falciparum* by desipramine. *Science* 242: 1301–1303.

Boyd, M.F., and S.F. Kitchen. 1936. Is the acquired homologous immunity to *Plasmodium vivax* equally effective against sporozoites and trophozoites? *American Journal of Tropical Medicine* 16: 317–322.

Bray, R.S. 1976. Vaccination against *Plasmodium falciparum*: A negative result. *Transactions of the Royal Society of Tropical Medicine and Hygiene* 70: 258.

Burns, J.M., E.K. Adeeku, and P.D. Dunn. 1999. Protective immunization with a novel membrane protein of *Plasmodium yoelii*-infected erythrocytes. *Infection and Immunity* 67: 675–680.

Carter, R., and D.H. Chen. 1976. Malaria transmission blocked by immunisation with gametes of the malaria parasite. *Nature* 263: 57–60.

Carter, R., L.H. Miller, J. Rener, D.C. Kaushal, N. Kumar, P.M. Graves, C.A. Grotendorst, and R.W. Gwadz. 1984. Target antigens in malaria transmission blocking immunity. *Philosophical Transactions of the Royal Society of London Series B* 307: 95–115.

Charoenvit, Y., V.F. Majam, G. Corradin, J.B. Sacci, et al. 1999. CD4(+) T-cell- and gamma-interferon-dependent protection against murine malaria by immunization with linear synthetic peptides from a *Plasmodium yoelii* 17-kilodalton hepatocyte erythrocyte protein. *Infection and Immunity* 67: 5604–5614.

Clyde, D.F. 1964. *Suppression of Malaria in Tanganyika Using Medicated Salt.* World Health Organization document no. WHO/Mal/433.

Clyde, D.F., V.C. McCarthy, R.M. Miller, and W.E. Woodward. 1975. Immunization of man against falciparum and vivax malaria by use of attenuated sporozoites. *American Journal of Tropical Medicine and Hygiene* 24: 397–401.

Coffin, G.S. 1951. Active immunization of birds against malaria. *Journal of Infectious Diseases* 89: 1–7.

Collins, W.E., D.C. Kaslow, J.S. Sullivan, Morris, C.L. et al. 1999. Testing the efficacy of a recombinant surface protein (MSP-1) of *Plasmodium vivax* in *Saimiri boliviensis* monkeys. *American Journal of Tropical Medicine and Hygiene* 60: 350–356.

Dame, J.B., J.L. Williams, T.F. McCutchan, J.L. Weber, R.A. Wirtz, W.T. Hockmyer, W.L. Maloy, L. Schneider, D. Roberts, G.S. Sanders, E.P. Reddy, C.L. Diggs, and L.H. Miller. 1984. Structure of the gene encoding the immunodominant surface antigen on the sporozoite of the human malaria parasite *Plasmodium falciparum*. *Science* 225: 593–599.

Dennis, E.D., G.H. Mitchell, G.A. Butcher, and S. Cohen. 1975. In vitro isolation of *Plasmodium knowlesi* merozoites using polycarbonate sieves. *Parasitology* 71: 475–481.

Deschiens, R., F. Pick, and U. Sarauw. 1956. L'immunisation expérimentale de la poule domestique contre l'infestation à *Plasmodium gallinaceum*. *Bullétin de Pathologie Exotique* 49: 353–365.

Desowitz, R. 1967. Immunization of rats against *Plasmodium berghei* with plasmodial homogenate, carboxymethyl-cellulose (CMC bound) homogenate, and CMC followed by immune gamma globulin. *Protozoology* 2: 105–110.

———. 1975. *Plasmodium berghei*: Immunologic enhancement of antigen by adjuvant addition. *Experimental Parasitology* 38: 6–13.

———. 1991. *The Malaria Capers*. New York: W.W. Norton.

Desowitz, R.S., and J.W. Barnwell. 1980. Effect of selenium and dimethyl dioctadecyl ammonium bromide on the vaccine-induced immunity of Swiss-Webster mice against malaria (*Plasmodium berghei*). *Infection and Immunity* 22: 87–93.

Desowitz, R.S., and L.H. Miller. 1980. A perspective on malaria vaccines. *Bulletin of the World Health Organization* 58: 897–902.

Doolan, D.L., and S.L. Hoffman. 1997. Multi-gene vaccination against malaria: A multistage, multi-immune response approach. *Parasitology Today* 13: 171–177.

Eaton, M.D., and L.T. Coggeshall. 1939. Production in monkeys of complement-fixing antibodies without active immunity by infection of killed *Plasmodium knowlesi*. *Journal of Experimental Medicine* 70: 141–146.

Engers, H.D. 1997. Organization and Budgeting for Malaria Vaccine Trials. Working Paper. The African Vaccine Testing Network. http://www.amvtn.org/Meetings/Arusha/Arusha-papers/engers.htm.

Etlinger, H.M., A.M. Felix, D. Gillessen, E.P. Heimer, M. Just, J.R.L. Pink, F. Sinigaglia, D. Sturchler, B. Takas, A. Trzeciak, and H. Matile. 1988. Assessment in humans of a synthetic peptide-based vaccine against the sporozoite stage of the human malaria parasite, *Plasmodium falciparum*. *Journal of Immunology* 140: 626–633.

Ferreira, M.U. 1996. Malaria vaccine trials: The missing qualitative data. *Immunology and Cell Biology* 74: 301–305.

Fischera, M.E., and D.S. Roos. 1997. A plastid organelle as a drug target in apicomplexan parasites. *Nature* 390: 407–409.

Freund, J., H.E. Sommer, and A.W. Walter. 1945. Immunization against malaria: Vaccination of ducks with killed parasites incorporated with adjuvants. *Science* 102: 200–202.

Freund, J., K.J. Thomson, H.E. Sommer, A.J. Walter, and E.L. Shenken. 1945. Immunization of rhesus monkeys against malarial infection (*P. knowlesi*) with killed parasites and adjuvants. *Science* 102: 202–204.

Freund, J., K.J. Thomson, H.E. Sommer, A.W. Walter, and T.M. Pisani. 1948. Immunization of monkeys against malaria by means of killed parasites with adjuvants. *American Journal of Tropical Medicine and Hygiene* 28: 1–22.

Geiman, Q.M., and M.J. Meagher. 1967. Susceptibility of a New World monkey to *Plasmodium falciparum* from man. *Nature* 215: 437–439.

Gingrich, W.D. 1941. Immunization of birds to *Plasmodium cathemerium*. *Infectious Diseases* 68: 46–52.

Good, M.F., J.A. Berzofsky, and L.H. Miller. 1988. The T cell response to the malaria circumsporozoite protein: An immunological approach to vaccine development. *Annual Review of Immunology* 6: 663–688.

Gwadz, R.W. 1976. Successful immunization against the sexual stages of *Plasmodium gallinaceum*. *Science* 193: 1150–1151.

Haddad, D., S. Liljeqvist, S. Stahl, M. Hansson, et al. 1999. Characterization of antibody responses to a *Plasmodium falciparum* blood-stage antigen induced by a DNA prime/protein boost immunization protocol. *Scandinavian Journal of Immunology* 49: 506–514.

Haynes, J.D.C., C.L. Diggs, F.A. Hines, and R.E. Desjardins. 1976. Culture of human malaria parasites *Plasmodium falciparum*. *Nature* 265: 767–770.

Hedstrom, R.C., D.L. Doolan, R. Wang, A. Kumar, et al. 1998. In vitro expression and in vivo immunogenicity of *Plasmodium falciparum* pre-erythrocytic DNA vaccines. *Bioorganic and Medicinal Chemistry Letters* 2: 29–38.

Heidelberger, M., W.A. Coates, and M.M. Mayer. 1946a. Studies in human malaria. 2. An attempt to influence relapsing vivax malaria by treatment of patients with vaccine (*Pl-vivax*). *Journal of Immunology* 53(1): 101–107.

Heidelberger, M., M.M. Mayer, A. Alving, B. Craige, R. Jones, T.N. Pullman, and M. Whorton. 1946b. Studies in human malaria. 4. An attempt at vaccination of volunteers against mosquito-borne infection with Pl-vivax. *Journal of Immunology* 52: 113–118.

Heidelberger, M., C. Prout, J.A. Hindle, and A.S. Rose. 1946c. Studies in human malaria. 3. An attempt at vaccination of paretics against blood-borne infection with *Pl-vivax*. *Journal of Immunology* 52: 109–112.

Holder, A.A., R.R. Freeman, and S.C. Nichols. 1988. Immunization against *Plasmodium falciparum* with recombinant polypeptides produced in *Escherichia coli*. *Parasite Immunology* 10: 607–617.

Kaslow, D.C. 1990. Immunogenicity of *Plasmodium falciparum* sexual stage antigens: Implications for the design of a transmission blocking vaccine. *Immunology Letters* 25: 83–86.

Kaslow, D.C., S.N. Isaacs, L.A. Quakyi, R.W. Gwadz, B. Moss, and D.B. Keister. 1991. Induction of *Plasmodium falciparum* transmission-blocking antibodies by recombinant vaccinia virus. *Science* 252: 1310–1313.

Kensil, C.R., and R. Kammer. 1998. QS-21: A water soluble triterpene glycoside adjuvant. *Expert Opinion of Investigational Drugs* 7: 1475–1482.

Khusmith, S., Y. Charoenvit, S. Kumar, et al. 1991. Protection against malaria by vaccination with sporozoite surface protein 2 plus CS protein. *Science* 252: 715–718.

Klayman, D.L. 1985. Qinghaosu (artemisinin): An antimalarial drug from China. *Science* 228: 1049–1055.

Kocken, C.H., M.A. Dubbeld, A. Van der Wel, J.T. Pronk, et al. 1999. High-level expression of *Plasmodium vivax* apical membrane antigen 1 (AMA-1) in *Pichia pastoris*; strong immunogenicity in *Macaca mulatta* immunized with *P. vivax* and adjuvant SBAS2. *Infection and Immunity* 67: 43–49.

Konstansov, S.W. 1930. Malaria immunität, Malariavakzine und Vakzination. *Abteil Medizine-hygiene Virus und Parasite* 116: 241–256.

Kumar, N., and R. Carter. 1984. Biosynthesis of the target antigens of antibodies blocking transmission of *Plasmodium falciparum*. *Molecular and Biochemical Parasitology* 13: 333–342.

Kwiatkowski, D., and K. Marsh. 1997. Development of a malaria vaccine. *Lancet* 350: 1696–1701.

Lawrence, G.W., A. Saul, A.J. Giddy, R. Kemp, and D. Pye. 1997. Phase I trials in humans of an oil-based adjuvant SEPPIC MONTANIDE ISA 720. *Vaccine* 15: 176–178.

Lell, B., D. Luckner, M. Ndjave, T. Scott, and P.G. Kremsner. 1998. Randomised placebo-controlled study of atovaquone plus proguanil for malaria prophylaxis in children. *Lancet* 351: 709–713.

Ling, I.T., S.A. Ogun, P. Momin, R.L. Richards, et al. 1997. Immunization against the murine malaria parasite *Plasmodium yoelii* using a recombinant protein with adjuvants developed for clinical use. *Vaccine* 15: 1562–1567.

Lise, L.D., D. Mazier, M. Jolivet, et al. 1987. Enhanced epitopic response to a synthetic human malarial peptide by preimmunization with tetanus toxoid carrier. *Infection and Immunity* 55: 2658–2661.

Lobo, C.A., R. Dhar, and N. Kumar. 1999. Immunization of mice with DNA-based Pfs25 elicits potent malaria transmission-blocking antibodies. *Infection and Immunity* 67: 1688–1693.

Looareesuwan, S., J.D. Chulay, C.J. Canfield, and D.B. Hutchinson (Malarone Clinical Trials Study Group). 1999. Malarone (atovaquone and proguanil hydrochloride): A review of its clinical development for treatment of malaria. *American Journal of Tropical Medicine and Hygiene* 60: 533–541.

Martin, S.K., A.M.J. Oduola, and W.K. Milhous. 1987. Reversal of chloroquine resistance in *Plasmodium falciparum* by verapamil. *Science* 235: 899–901.

Matsumoto, S., H. Yukitake, H. Kanbara, and T. Yamada. 1998. Recombinant mycobacterium *Bovis bacillus* Calmette-Guerin secreting merozoite surface protein (MSP1) induces protection against malaria parasite infection depending on MSP1-stimulated interferon gamma and parasite-specific antibodies. *Journal of Experimental Medicine* 188: 845–854.

Maurice, J. 1995. Malaria vaccine raises a dilemma. *Science* 267: 320–323.

Men, Y., H. Tamber, R. Audran, B. Gander, and G. Corradin. 1997. Induction of a cytotoxic T lymphocyte response by immunization with a malaria specific CTL peptide entrapped in biodegradable polymer microspheres. *Vaccine* 15: 1405–1412.

Mendis, K.N., and G.A.T. Targett. 1982. Vaccination to prevent transmission of *Plasmodium yoelii* malaria. *Parasite Immunology* 4: 117–127.

Milek, R.L., W.F. Roeffen, C.H. Kocken, et al. 1998. Immunological properties of recombinant proteins of the transmission blocking vaccine candidate Pfs48/45, of the human malaria parasite *Plasmodium falciparum* produced in *Escherichia coli*. *Parasite Immunology* 20: 377–385.

Miller, L.H. 1977. *Immunity to Blood Parasites of Animals and Man*. New York: Plenum.

Mitchell, G.H. 1977. A review of metozoite vaccination against *Plasmodium knowlesi* malaria. *Transactions of the Royal Society of Tropical Medicine and Hygiene* 71: 281–282.

Mitchell, G.H., G.A. Butcher, and S. Cohen. 1974. A merozoite vaccine effective against *Plasmodium knowlesi* malaria. *Nature* 252: 311–313.

———. 1975. Merozoite vaccination against *Plasmodium knowlesi* malaria. *Immunology* 29: 397–407.

Mitchell, G.H., G.A. Butcher, W.H.G. Richards, and S. Cohen. 1977. Merozoite vaccination of douroucouli monkeys against falciparum malaria. *Lancet* 2: 1335–1338.

Moldovan, J. 1912. Ueber die Immunitatsverhastnisse bei der vogelmalaria. *Centralbllat fur Bakteriologie* 66: 105–110.

Mulligan, H.W., P.F. Russell, and B.N. Mohan. 1941. Active immunization of fowls against *Plasmodium gallinaceum* by injections of killed homologous sporozoites. *Journal of the Malaria Institute of India* 4: 25–34.

Nardin, E.H., J.M. Calvo-Calle, G.A. Oliveira, P. Clavijo, et al. 1998. *Plasmodium falciparum* polyoximes: Highly immunogenic synthetic vaccines constructed by chemoselective ligation of repeat B-cell epitopes and a universal T-cell epitope of CS protein. *Vaccine* 16: 590–600.

Pan, W., E. Ravot, R. Tolle, R. Mossbach, I. Turbachova, and H. Bujard. 1999. Vaccine candidate MSP-1 from *Plasmodium falciparum*: A redesigned 4917-bp polynucleotide enables synthesis and isolation of full-length protein from *Escherichia coli* and mammalian cells. *Nucleic Acids Research* 27: 1094–1103.

Patarroyo, M.E., P. Romero, M.L. Torres, P. Clavijo, A. Moreno, A. Martinez, R. Rodriguez, F. Guzman, and E. Cabezas. 1987. Induction of protective immunity against experimental infection with malaria using synthetic peptides. *Nature* 328: 629–632.

Patarroyo, M.E., R. Amador, P. Clavijo, A. Moreno, F. Guzman, P. Romero, R. Tascon, A. Franco, L.A. Murillo, G. Ponton, and G. Trujillo. 1988. A synthetic vaccine protects humans against challenge with asexual blood stages of *Plasmodium falciparum* malaria. *Nature* 332: 158–161.

Patterson, P.S., S.C. Bosshardt, V. Udhayukumar, L. Xiao, et al. 1999. Prolonged expression of IFN gamma induced by protective blood-stage immunization against *Plasmodium yoelii* malaria. *Vaccine* 18: 173–180.

Perera, K.L., S.M. Handunenetti, I. Holm, S. Longacre, and K. Mendis. 1998. Buculovirus merozoite surface protein 1 C-recombinant antigens are highly protective in a natural primate model for human *Plasmodium vivax* malaria. *Infection and Immunity* 66: 1500–1506.

Perlaza. B.L., Arevalo-Herrera, M., K. Brahimi, G. Quintero, et al. 1998. Immunogenicity of four *Plasmodium falciparum* preerythrocytic antigens in *Aotus lemurinus*. *Infection and Immunity* 66: 3423–3428.

Potocnjak, P., N. Yoshida, R.S. Nussenzeig, and V. Nussenzweig. 1980. Monovalent fragments (Fab) of monoclonal antibodies to a sporozoite surface antigen (Pb44) protect mice against malarial infection. *Journal of Experimental Medicine* 151: 1503–1504.

Price, R., C. Luxemburger, M. Vanvugt, F. Nosten, A. Kham, J. Simpson, S. Looareesuwan, T. Chongsuphajaisiddhi, and N.J. White. 1998. Artesunate and mefloquine in the treatment of uncomplicated multidrug-resistant hyperparasitaemic falciparum malaria. *Transactions of the Royal Society of Tropical Medicine and Hygiene* 92: 207–211.

Pye, D., S.J. Edwards, R.F. Anders, et al. 1991. Failure of recombinant vaccinia viruses expressing *Plasmodium falciparum* antigens to protect Saimiri monkeys against malaria. *Infection and Immunity* 59: 2403–2411.

Pye, D., K.L. Vandenberg, S.L. Dyer, et al. 1997. Selection of an adjuvant for vaccination with the malaria antigen MSA-2. *Vaccine* 15: 1017–1023.

Reed, R.C., V. Louis-Wileman, E.V. Cosmai, et al. 1997. Multiple antigen constructs (MACs): Induction of sterile immunity against sporozoite stage of rodent malaria parasites, *Plasmodium berghei* and *Plasmodium yoelii*. *Vaccine* 15: 482–488.

Rieckmann, K.H., E.J. Cabrera, G.H. Campbell, R.C. Jost, R. Miranda, and T.R. O'Leary. 1979. Immunization of rhesus monkeys with blood-stage antigens of *Plasmodium knowlesi*. *Bulletin of the World Health Organization* 57(Suppl. 1): 139–151.

Roberts, F., C.W. Roberts, J.J. Johnson, D.E. Kyle, T. Krell, J.R. Coggins, G.H. Coombs, W.K. Milhous, S. Tzipori, D.J.P. Ferguson, D. Chakrabarti, and R. McLeod. 1998. Evidence for the shikimate pathway in apicomplexan parasites. *Nature* 393: 801–806.

Russell, P.F., and B.N. Mohan. 1942. Immunization of fowls against moquito-borne *Plasmodium gallinaceum* by injections of serum and inactivated homologous sporozoites. *Journal of Experimental Medicine* 76: 477–495.

Russell, P.F., H.W. Mulligan, and B.N. Mohan. 1942. Active immunization of fowls against sporozoites but not trophozoites of *Plasmodium gallinaceum* by injections of homologous sporozoites. *Journal of the Malaria Institute of India* 4: 311–319.

Sachs, Jeffrey. 1999. *Financial Times*. May 5.

Schenkel, R.H., G.L. Simpson, and P.H. Silverman. 1973. Vaccination of Rhesus monkeys (*Macaca mulatta*) against *Plasmodium knowlesi* by the use of nonviable antigen, *Bulletin of the World Health Organization* 48: 597–604.

Schneider, J., S.C. Gilbert, T.J. Blanchard, T. Hanke, et al. 1998. Enhanced immunogenicity for CD8+ T cell induction and complete protective efficacy of malaria DNA vaccination by boosting with modified vaccinia virus *Ankara*. *Nature Medicine* 4: 397–402.

Shanks, G.D., D.M. Gordon, F.W. Klotz, G.M. Aleman, A.J. Oloo, and D. Sadie. 1998. Efficacy and safety of atovaquone/proguanil as suppressive prophylaxis for *Plasmodium falciparum* malariaclin. *Infectious Diseases* 27: 494–499.

Shi, Y.P., S.E. Hasnain, J.B. Sacci, B.P. Holloway, et al. 1999. Immunogenicity and in vitro protective efficacy of a recombinant multistage *Plasmodium falciparum* candidate vaccine. *Proceedings of the National Academy of Sciences USA* 96: 1167–1169.

Shortt, H.E., and K.P. Menon. 1940. Attempts to produce active immunity to malaria in monkeys by vaccination with parasitic substances. *Journal of the Malaria Institute of India* 3: 191–193.

Siddiqui, W.A. 1977. An effective immunization of experimental monkeys against a human malaria parasite, *Plasmodium falciparum*. *Science* 198: 338–339.

Siddiqui, W.A., D.W. Taylor, S.-C. Kan, K. Kramer, S.M. Richmond-Crum, S. Kotani, T. Shiba, and S. Kusumoto. 1978. Vaccination of experimental monkeys against *Plasmodium falciparum*: A possible safe adjuvant. *Science* 201: 1237–1239.

Simpson, G.L., R.H. Schenkel, and P.H. Silverman. 1974. Vaccination of rhesus monkeys against malaria by use of sucrose density gradient fractions of *Plasmodium knowlesi* antigens. *Nature* 247: 304–305.

Sjolander, A., K. Lovgren, S. Stahl, et al. 1991. High antibody responses in rabbits immunized with influenza virus ISCOMs containing repeated sequence of the *Plasmodium falciparum* antigen Pf155/RESA. *Vaccine* 9: 443–450.

Spencer, H.C., D.C.O. Kaseje, W.E. Collins, M.G. Shehata, A. Turner, P.S. Stanfill, A.Y. Huong, J.M. Roberts, M. Villinski, and D.K. Koech. 1987. Community-based malaria control in Saradidi, Kenya: Description of the programme and impact on parasitaemia rates and antimalarial antibodies. *Annals of Tropical Medicine and Parasitology* 81(Suppl.): 13–23.

Srivastava, I.K., and A.B. Vaidya. 1999. A mechanism for the synergistic antimalarial action of atovaquone and proguanil. *Antimicrobial Agents and Chemotherapy* 43: 1334–1339.

Srivastava, I.K., H. Rottenberg, and A.B. Vaidya. 1997. Atovaquone, a broad spectrum antiparasitic drug, collapses mitochondrial membrane potential in a malarial parasite. *Journal of Biological Chemistry* 14: 3961–3966.

Stoute, J.A., M. Slaoui, D.G. Heppner, P. Momin, K.E. Kester, P. Desmons, B.T. Wellde, N. Garcon, U. Krzych, M. Marchand, W.P. Ballou, and J.D. Cohen for the RTS,S Malaria Vaccine Evaluation Group. 1997. A preliminary evaluation of a recombinant circumsporozoite protein vaccine against *Plasmodium falciparum* malaria. *New England Journal of Medicine* 336: 86–91.

Sturchler, D., R. Berger, H. Etlinger, et al. 1989. Effects of interferons on immune response to a synthetic peptide malaria sporozoite vaccine in non-immune adults. *Vaccine* 7: 457–461.

Sukwa, T.Y., M. Mulenga, N. Chisdaka, N.S. Roskell, and T.R. Scott. 1999. A randomized, double-blind, placebo-controlled field trial to determine the efficacy and safety of Malarone (atovaquone/proguanil) for the prophylaxis of malaria in Zambia. *American Journal of Tropical Medicine and Hygiene* 60: 521–525.

Targett, G.A.T. 1992. SPF66, A candidate synthetic malaria vaccine: Immunogenicity versus protection. *Parasitology Today* 8: 354–355.

Taylor, T.E., B.A. Wells, P. Kazembe, M. Chisale, J.J. Wirima, E.Y.E.C. Ratsma, and M.E. Molyneux. 1993. Rapid coma resolution with artemether in Malawian children with cerebral malaria. *Lancet* 341: 661–662.

Tian, J.H., S. Kumar, D.C. Kaslow, and L.H. Miller. 1997. Comparison of protection induced by immnization with recombinant proteins from different regions of merozoite surface protein 1 of *Plasmodium yoelii*. *Infection and Immunity* 65: 3032–3036.

Trager, W., and J.B. Jensen. 1976. Human malaria parasites in continuous culture, *Science* 193: 673–676.

van der Berg, J.D., C.S. Duvenage, N.S. Roskell, and T.R. Scott. 1999. Safety and efficacy of atovaquone and proguanil hydrochloride for the prophylaxis of *Plasmodium falciparum* malaria in South Africa. *Clinical Therapeutics* 21: 741–749.

Vermeulen, A.N., T. Ponnudurai, P.J.A. Beckers, J.P. Verhave, M.A. Smits, and J.H.E.T. Meuwissen. 1985. Sequential expression of antigens on sexual stages of *Plasmodium falciparum* accessible to transmission-blocking antibodies in the mosquito. *Journal of Experimental Medicine* 162: 1460–1476.

von Seidlein, L., P. Milligan, M. Pinder, K. Bojang, C. Anyalbechi, R. Gosling, R. Coleman, J.I. Ude, A. Sadiq, M. Duraisingh, D. Warhurst, A. Alloueche, G. Targett, K. McAdam, B. Greenwood, G. Walraven, P. Olliaro, and T. Doherty. 2000. Efficacy of artesunate plus pyrimethamine-sulphadoxine for uncomplicated malaria in Gambian children: A double-blind, randomised, controlled trial. *Lancet* 355: 1–9.

White, N.J. 1994. Tough test for malaria vaccine. *Lancet* 334: 1172–1173.

White, N.J., D. Waller, J. Crawley, F. Nosten, D. Chapman, D. Brewster, and B.M. Greenwood. 1992. Comparison of artemether and chloroquine for severe malaria in Gambian children. *Lancet* 339: 317–321.

WHO (World Health Organization). 1986. WHO,TDR/IMAL/SWG (9)/86.3. Geneva, Switzerland: WHO.

Yang, C., M.W. Carroll, A.P. Torres-Duarte, B. Moss, and E.A. Davidson. 1997. Addition of MSA1 signal and anchor sequences to the malaria merozoite surface antigen 1 C- terminal region enhances immunogenicity when expressed by recombinant vaccinia virus. *Vaccine* 15: 1303–1313.

Yang, C., W.E. Collins, J.S. Sullivan, D.C. Kaslow, L. Xiao, and A.A. Lal. 1999. Partial protection against *Plasmodium vivax* blood-stage infection in Saimiri monkeys by immunization with a recombinant C-terminal fragment of merozoite surface protein 1 in block copolymenr adjuvant. *Infection and Immunity* 67: 342–349.

Yoshida, N., R.S. Nussenzweig, P. Potocnjak, N. Yoshida, V. Nussenzweig, and M. Aikawa. 1980. Hybridoma produces protective antibodies directed against the sporozoite stage of malaria parasite. *Science* 207: 71–73.

Young, J.F., W.T. Hockmyer, M. Cross, W.R. Ballou, R.A. Wirtz, J.H. Trosper, R.L. Beaudoin, M.R. Hollingdale, L.H. Miller, C.L. Diggs, and M. Rosenburg. 1985. Expression of *Plasmodium falciparum* circumsporozoite proteins in *Escherichia coli* for potential use in a human malaria vaccine. *Science* 228: 968–962.

Zavala, F., J.P. Tam, and M.R. Hollingdale. 1985. Rationale for development of a synthetic vaccine against *Plasmodium falciparum* malaria. *Science* 228: 1436–1440.

Chapter 13

Impacts of Global Population Trends

Wolfgang Lutz

Changes in population size, density, and age distribution may impact malaria directly, by affecting the susceptible people who live in malaria-endemic areas, and indirectly, by influencing other determinants of malaria, such as population movement and socioeconomic status. In this chapter, I describe demographic trends, the uncertainties associated with them, and the role of the population variable in climate change.

Population tends to be a rather emotional topic because it deals with "hot" topics—birth, death, sex, marriage, gender roles, and international migration—and thus touches the foundations of cultural, religious, and national identities. It also is a highly political topic, at both national and international levels. This aspect is illustrated by the series of decennial U.N. International Conferences on Population and Development, the most recent of which was held in Cairo, Egypt, in 1994. This conference was characterized by a change in paradigm, away from the preoccupation with population control to an emphasis on reproductive rights and health. In this context, this series of population conferences appears conspicuously detached from the series of U.N. environmental conferences. At the political level, the interactions between the human population and its natural environment are not yet sufficiently appreciated.

Population studies combine elements of the natural sciences (biological aspects of reproduction and longevity, population dynamics) with the social sciences (socially, culturally, and economically determined fertility behavior; effects of lifestyle on health and migration). *Demography* is the quantitative and analytical core of this established field of studies, which is complemented by the analysis of the determinants and consequences of demographic trends. Demography reaches out to many other disciplines. Although the tradition of collaboration among demography, epidemiology, and health research is long and distinguished, the interactions between population and environmental change have received attention only recently. The effects of this interaction must be studied in both directions: as population parameters that drive environmental change, and as the effect of environmental change on population (mostly in terms of migration and health issues). I attempt to present both issues.

Demographic patterns have changed dramatically over the past several decades, particularly in less-developed countries (LDCs). First mortality rates, then fertility rates fell much more quickly than in more-developed (or industrialized) countries (MDCs).

The demographic transition from high to low fertility and mortality rates is not yet complete in many LDCs, as it is in MDCs, but its progress is reflected in the declining rates of global population growth.

Three predictions appear almost certain for the coming decades. The world population will

- rise significantly from its present level of around 6 billion, although it may start to decline during the second half of the next century;
- persist in tilting the distribution from MDCs to LDCs; and
- continue to age.

Probabilistic projections from the International Institute for Applied Systems Analysis (IIASA) indicate that global population is unlikely to double from its present size; in contrast, the population older than 60 years will almost certainly increase severalfold. The over-60 age group, measured as a proportion of total population, almost certainly will double and probably will triple over the next century.

After a short discussion of the relevance of population to malaria, I consider the factors that underlie long-term population trends and the uncertainties involved. Then, I give special attention to the issues of urbanization and climate change.

Human Population and Malaria Transmission

Human population trends and patterns are linked with malaria in several ways. Most important, humans are the victims of malaria; this aspect concerns us the most. The degree to which people suffer from malaria strongly depends on the size, structure, and distribution of the population. The number and distribution of infected people also play important roles in transmitting disease to other still-uninfected people. Of the three basic components of human population change (migration, fertility, and mortality), human migration is closely related to malaria transmission, as discussed extensively in Chapter 15. And finally, human population dynamics is one of the important determinants of global climate change, which in turn is assumed to have implications for malaria transmission.

Figure 13-1 depicts the links between population trends and malaria transmission. In this chapter, I focus primarily on population dynamics and on the possible effects of population growth and population aging on climate change. It is meant to complement other chapters that deal predominantly with the process of malaria transmission.

Long-Term Population Trends

The most important source of uncertainty in population projections is the future path of fertility rates, although the impacts of alternative trends in mortality and migration also are significant. In this section, I discuss the assumptions for each of these three demographic components that underlie IIASA's projections. Variations in the paths of these variables can give rise to large differences in the projected future population size and age structure. For example, in 2100, the 95% confidence interval for global population is 5.7 billion to 17.3 billion. Although this level of uncertainty might be considered high, relative to other components driving global environmental change, population is one of the more robust factors to be considered. At the same time, this range has the potential to significantly change the outlook for future greenhouse gas emissions and climate change.

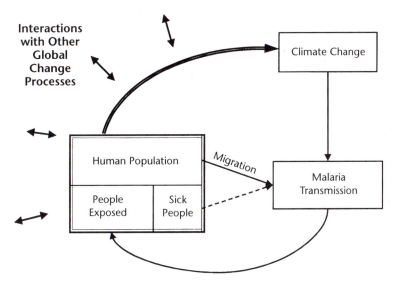

Figure 13-1. Links between Human Population Dynamics, Climate Change, and Malaria Transmission

The broad outlines of the history of global population growth are by now familiar. At the dawn of the agricultural revolution (8,000 years before present), total population was about 250,000 (Cook 1962). It took all of human history (until 1800) for global population to reach 1 billion—roughly today's population of Europe and North America combined. It took 130 years (until 1930) to reach 2 billion. In only 60 more years (1960), the total was 3 billion. The fourth billion was reached between 1960 and 1975, the 5 billion mark was passed in 1987, and the 6 billion mark was reached in 1999.

Less well appreciated are the facts that both the annual growth rate and the annual absolute number of people added to the world population have peaked and are expected to continue to decline. The growth rate peaked at 2.1% per year in the late 1960s and fell to about 1.5% by 1995 (Table 13-1); the annual absolute increment of world population peaked at about 87 million per year in the late 1980s and was about 81 million at the end of the twentieth century. This does not mean, of course, that little additional population growth is to be expected; most midrange population projections foresee future population rising to 8 to 12 billion by the end of the twenth-first century. However, the statistics are indicative of the tremendous changes that have taken place over the past four decades.

As shown in Table 13-1, the total fertility rate (TFR; average number of children per woman) declined modestly in most parts of the world from 1950–1955 to 1970–1975, then declined over the subsequent 20 years with a rapidity that was unimaginable in the 1960s. This second period of decline was especially pronounced in Asia, where TFR fell by more than two children per woman (a statistic that is, however, heavily influenced by a dramatic decline in Chinese fertility rates during the 1970s). One exception has been in Africa, where fertility rates remained well above six children per woman, on average, through the late 1980s; since then, fertility rates have begun to decline. Meanwhile, in regions such as Europe and North America (which had already achieved very low fertility rates by 1970–1975), rates were maintained or continued to fall.

During the 1950s and 1960s, reductions in mortality rates that resulted from the spread of modern hygiene and medicine were even more significant than declining

Table 13-1. Demographic Trends in the World since 1950

Region	Year		
	1950	*1970*	*1995*
	Total population (millions)		
World	2,524	3,702	5,687
MDCs	813	1,008	1,171
LDCs	1,711	2,694	4,516
Africa	224	364	719
Asia	1,402	2,147	3,438
Europe	547	656	728
Latin America and Caribbean	166	284	477
North America	172	232	297
Oceania	13	19	28
Growth rate (%)	*1950–1955*	*1970–1975*	*1990–1995*
World	1.78	1.95	1.48
MDCs	1.21	0.79	0.40
LDCs	2.05	2.37	1.77
Africa	2.23	2.56	2.68
Asia	1.91	2.27	1.53
Europe	1.00	0.60	0.16
Latin America and Caribbean	2.65	2.43	1.70
North America	1.70	1.01	1.01
Oceania	2.21	2.09	1.37
Life expectancy, both sexes (years)	*1950–1955*	*1970–1975*	*1990–1995*
World	46.5	57.9	64.3
MDCs	66.5	71.2	74.2
LDCs	40.9	54.7	62.1
Africa	37.8	46.0	51.8
Asia	41.3	56.3	64.5
Europe	66.1	70.8	72.7
Latin America and Caribbean	51.4	61.1	68.5
North America	69.0	71.5	76.2
Oceania	60.9	66.6	72.9
TFR (no. of children per woman)	*1950–1955*	*1970–1975*	*1990–1995*
World	5.00	4.48	2.96
MDCs	2.77	2.11	1.68
LDCs	6.17	5.42	3.30
Africa	6.64	6.57	5.71
Asia	5.90	5.09	2.84
Europe	2.56	2.14	1.57
Latin America and Caribbean	5.88	5.01	2.93
North America	3.47	2.01	2.02
Oceania	3.84	3.21	2.51

Note: Data for Growth rate, Life expectancy, and TFR (total fertility rate) are given over a five-year period starting in the year given at the top of the column.
Source: United Nations 1997a.

fertility rates. From 1950 to 1955, the first period for which estimates are available, life expectancy was lowest in Africa (38 years) and Asia (41 years), whereas it already had improved significantly in Latin America (51 years). Over the subsequent 20 years, life expectancy increased impressively worldwide. In Asia, by far the most populous continent, it increased by 15 years over this short period, and in Africa, it improved by 8 years. Improvements continued over the next 20 years to 1990–1995, but at a somewhat slower speed; Asia, Latin America, and Africa all experienced substantial improvements.

These rapid increases in life expectancy were mostly due to strongly falling child mortality rates, so more children survived to adulthood. Because fertility rates also remained high (or even increased somewhat due to better maternal health), population growth rates soared in the 1950s and 1960s. As shown in Table 13-1, growth rates in 1950–1955 were highest in Latin America and the Caribbean because high fertility rates in the region were associated with already lower child mortality rates. By 1970–1975, however, the population growth rate in Africa surpassed that in Latin America as Africa's mortality rates fell and fertility rates hovered at about 6.5 children per woman, on average. Because fertility rates have remained relatively high in this region, population growth accelerated to almost 2.7% in 1990–1995; if this growth rate were to remain constant, population would double in 26 years.

These trends in fertility and mortality rates resulted in different patterns of population growth in different parts of the world. In fact, the dominant feature of the global demographic landscape has been the contrast between the well-off populations of Europe, Japan, and North America and the poorer populations of Africa, Asia, Latin America, and the Middle East. As shown in Table 13-1, the population of MDCs is relatively small (about 1.2 billion in 1995) and expanding very slowly (0.4% per year) after a 44% increase since 1950. That of LDCs is large (about 4.5 billion in 1995) and expanding rapidly (almost 1.8% per year) after increasing by a factor of 2.6 since 1950. As a consequence, the share of today's industrialized countries in the world population decreased from 32% in 1950 to 21% in 1995 and probably will decrease much more in the future. In addition, despite the rapid changes in most LDCs, inhabitants of MDCs on average live significantly longer (life expectancy at birth for both sexes combined is about 74 years, versus 62 years in LDCs) and have fewer children (TFR is almost 1.7 children per woman, versus 3.3 children per woman in LDCs).

Population Aging

The widely varying historical experiences of the different regions of the world have left strong imprints on the age structures of their populations. Age structures are often depicted in "age pyramids" that show the number of males and females in five-year age groups. Figure 13-2 shows age pyramids for the two most extreme cases, sub-Saharan Africa and western Europe. In Africa, the pyramid is typical of a rapidly growing population, showing larger and larger cohorts at the bottom, in the young age groups. There are more than twice as many children under 5 years old than adults aged 20–25, four times as many as those aged 40–45, and 10 times as many as elderly (aged 65–70). In western Europe, the pattern is completely different: the number of women aged 60–65 approximately equals the number of children under age 5, and the largest age groups are those between 30 and 40. The pyramid is narrower at the bottom because of the very low fertility rates since the 1970s; at the same time, declining mortality rates have widened the top by increasing the size of older-age cohorts.

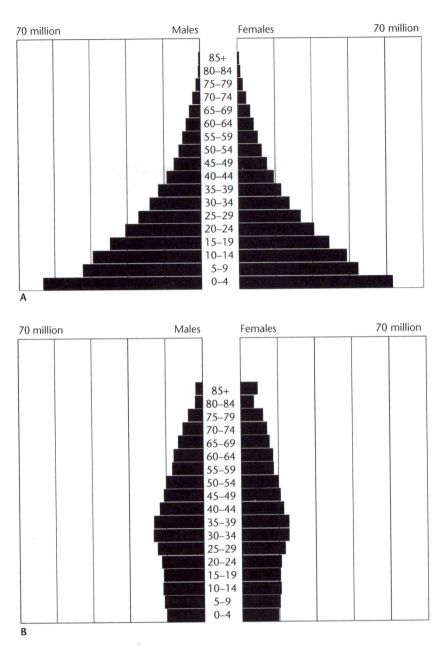

Figure 13-2. Age Pyramids of Sub-Saharan Africa (*A*) and Western Europe (*B*), 2000

Source: O'Neill, MacKellar, and Lutz 2001 (p. 43).

The narrowing of population pyramids at the bottom (from low fertility rates) and fattening at the top (due to extended longevity) is called *population aging*. The two components are referred to as aging "from the bottom" and "from the top." Population aging is an enormously important social phenomenon, especially in relation to the uncertain future of pension and health-care systems. Aging will continue in MDCs and has already started in LDCs. Just as the speed of improving mortality rates accentuated the implications of demographic transition for population growth rates, the speed of declining fertility rates in LDCs will accentuate the aging phenomenon.

Population aging probably will become a dominating feature of social change worldwide, posing several serious challenges—from the financial security of the elderly to increasing needs for health care, changing consumer behavior, and possible changes in productivity. It also raises the issue of intergenerational equity, which probably will receive increased attention, in addition to more prevalent concerns about social equity and gender equity. These aging-related questions are very likely to gain importance in today's countries with low fertility rates and in an increasing number of LDCs as they make the demographic transition.

The Concept of Demographic Transition

The *demographic transition* began in MDCs in the late eighteenth century and spread to LDCs in the last half of the twentieth (Notestein 1945; Davis 1954; Davis 1991; Coale 1973) The conventional theory of demographic transition predicts that, as living standards rise and health conditions improve, first mortality rates decline and then, somewhat later, fertility rates decline. Demographic transition "theory" has evolved as a generalization of the typical sequence of events in what are now MDCs, where mortality rates declined comparatively gradually beginning in the late 1700s and then more rapidly in the late 1800s and where, after a lag of 75–100 years, fertility rates declined as well. Societies experienced transition in different ways, and today, various regions of the world are following distinctive paths (Tabah 1989). Nonetheless, the broad result was, and is, a gradual transition from a small, slowly growing population with high mortality and fertility rates to a large, slowly growing population with low mortality and fertility rates. During the transition itself, population growth accelerates because the decline in death rates precedes the decline in birth rates.

On the theoretical level, demographic transition can be explained in two ways. One views the decline in fertility rates as a direct response to the decline in mortality rates. This so-called homeostasis argument stresses that societies tend to find an equilibrium between births and deaths. When death rates decline due to progress in medicine and better living conditions, the equilibrium is disturbed and the population grows unless birth rates adjust to the new mortality rates and also start to decline. The fact that fertility rates tend to decline many years after mortality rates may be explained by a perception lag. The other view assumes that modernization of society acts as a joint driving force of declining mortality and fertility rates. According to this view, the decline in fertility rates lags the decline in mortality rates because fertility is more strongly embedded in the system of cultural norms and therefore changes more slowly than mortality-relevant behavior. The historical record of Europe—where fertility and mortality rates sometimes declined simultaneously, and population growth was generally much lower than in today's countries with high fertility rates—gives more support to the second explanation. But the two arguments are not necessarily mutually exclusive.

Figure 13-3 illustrates demographic transition in Mauritius, a developing country that has had good records of births and deaths for more than a century. Up to around World War II (mid-1940s), birth and death rates show a pattern of strong annual fluctuations, mostly as a result of diseases and changing weather conditions, which are typical for "premodern" societies. Whenever birth rates are consistently above death rates, the population grows, as was the case in Mauritius during the late nineteenth century. After World War II, death rates on Mauritius declined precipitously because of the eradication of malaria and the introduction of European medical technology. Birth rates, on the other hand, remained high or even increased somewhat due to the better health status

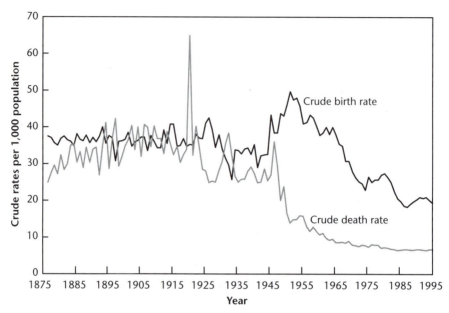

Figure 13-3. Birth and Death Rates for Mauritius, 1875–1995

Source: Mauritius Central Statistical Office.

of women (a typical phenomenon in the early phase of demographic transition). By 1950, the high birth rate had resulted in a population growth rate of more than 3% per year, one of the highest at that time. Later, birth rates declined, mostly during the late 1960s and early 1970s, when TFR fell from more than six to less than three children per woman in only seven years, probably the world's most rapid national decline in fertility rates. This occurred on a strictly voluntary basis and was a result of increased education for females and successful family-planning programs (Lutz 1994). Because of the still very young age structure of the Mauritian population, birth rates are still higher than death rates, and the population is growing by about 1% per year despite fertility rates around replacement level (i.e., two surviving children, or TFR somewhat more than 2.0 children per woman, depending on mortality conditions).

Empirically observed trends in all parts of the world have overwhelmingly confirmed the relevance of the concept of demographic transition to LDCs. With the exception of pockets where religious or cultural beliefs are strongly pro-natalist (i.e., actively trying to increase the birth rate), fertility rates are declining in all regions except sub-Saharan Africa, and even in that region, many signs of a fertility-related transition can be perceived. In Southeast Asia and many Latin American countries, fertility rates are on par with those in MDCs only several decades ago; in countries including China, Korea, and Taiwan, fertility rates are below replacement levels.

The biggest difference between the demographic transition process in what are now MDCs and LDCs has been the speed of declining mortality rates. In Europe, Japan, and North America, mortality rates declined over the course of about two centuries as a result of reduced variability in the food supply, better housing, improved sanitation, and progress in preventive and curative medicine. In contrast, in LDCs, mortality rates declined very quickly after World War II as a result of the application of Western medical and public health technology to infectious, parasitic, and diarrheal diseases. Life expectancy in Europe rose gradually from about 35 years in 1800 to about 50 years in 1900, 66.5 years at the end of World War II, and 74.4 years in 1995. In LDCs, life expectancy shot up from 40.9 years at the end of World War II to 62.1 years in 1995. The increase that took MDCs about one and a half centuries to achieve came to pass in LDCs in less than half a century. As a result of the quick decline in mortality rates, populations in LDCs are growing three times faster today than did the populations of the present MDCs at comparable stages of demographic transition.

Studies of the factors influencing changes in fertility rates must begin with the proximate determinants of fertility: age at marriage (or beginning of sexual activity), prevalence and effectiveness of contraception, prevalence of induced abortion, and duration of the infertile period after giving birth, especially due to breastfeeding (Bongaarts and Potter 1983). Fertility rates must decline through changes in one or more of the four proximate determinants.

The adoption of contraception has been the principal source of declining fertility rates in LDCs. Coale (1973) lists three "preconditions" required for a decline in fertility rates:

- Fertility must be regarded as being within the realm of conscious choice.
- Lower fertility must offer objective advantages.
- Acceptable means of reducing fertility must be at hand.

These three preconditions for a lasting decline in fertility rates suggest three parallel strategies for fostering the transition from high fertility rates to low fertility rates:

- Emphasize universal basic education to bring fertility increasingly into the realm of conscious choice. Modern mass media also may exert an important influence. These strategies also are likely to bring about changes in attitude and culture.
- Pursue changes in socioeconomic variables, mostly neoclassical economic costs and benefits that arise from variables such as child labor, female participation in the modern-sector labor force, and support in old age. Changes in the "value" of children also affect couples' desired family size.
- Invest in reproductive health and the availability of family-planning services, including maternal and child health programs that reduce infant mortality rates. Help women match their desired and actual number of children by focusing on the unmet need for family planning.

This framework suggests that if two of the three preconditions are already met, the introduction of the third may trigger a rapid decline in fertility rates. In the case of the rapid decline in Mauritian fertility rates (Figure 13-3), the young female population was already literate, and large families were increasingly perceived as an economic burden. The strong and strictly voluntary family-planning campaign strengthened the negative perception of high fertility and provided efficient family-planning services that were even supported by the influential Roman Catholic church (which supported only the "natural" ones) and then triggered the precipitous decline in fertility rates. In some other countries, huge investments in family planning were almost without effect because one of the other two preconditions was not met.

This view of the three necessary preconditions offers a solution to the fundamental "chicken and egg" ambiguity regarding causation: does the provision of family planning through national programs lead to lower fertility rates via increased adoption of contraception, or do couples' desires for declining fertility, translated into demand for contraception, induce a supply response in the form of a national family-planning program? The difference between the positions was well captured by the rallying cries of

MDC and LDC delegates to the 1974 Population Conference held in Bucharest, Romania: "Contraception is the best contraceptive" on the one hand, and "Development is the best contraceptive" on the other. A new position, which emerged forcefully at the 1994 International Conference on Population and Development in Cairo, might be expressed as "Empowerment of women is the best contraceptive."

The first point of view was supported, generally speaking, by members of the international family planning community; the second point of view by neoclassical economists; and the third point of view by women's advocates. Each point of view—the first emphasizing the role of national family-planning programs, the second emphasizing costs and benefits of childbearing, and the third emphasizing the status of women—has insights to offer. Putting emphasis on basic education, especially of women, may offer a synthesis of these views because it positively affects all three factors.

Clearly, there is a synergism among the various factors: national family-planning programs, combined with socioeconomic development and empowerment of women, lower fertility rates. Investing in basic education for females has positive effects on all three factors, in addition to its direct strong link to lower fertility rates. And it is hard to see any negative effect of more education. It is a win–win strategy in this context and the best candidate for priority action.

One question that is still completely unresolved in the context of the demographic transition is when and at what level the fertility rate stops declining. Previously, scholars have assumed that fertility rates will reach replacement-level fertility rates (two surviving children per woman, or a TFR of slightly above 2.0 children per woman) and then fluctuate around this level. But empirical data show that in most countries, declines in fertility rates have not stopped at the replacement level. Especially in Europe, several countries have been significantly below the replacement level for more than two decades, and there is no indication that fertility rates will increase to that level in the foreseeable future. In modern society, especially in the European and Asian context, many social forces tend to keep fertility rates very low.

The question of posttransition fertility rates also makes a big difference for the world population outlook, as described in the next section. In the case of assumed long-term fertility rates below replacement level, the speed of the declining fertility rates over the coming years will have a greater impact on the population size in 2050–2100 than previously thought (Lutz, Sanderson, and Scherbov 1998). The following probabilistic world population projections already take into account possible long-term fertility rates below replacement levels.

World Population Outlook

The conventional approach to projecting population, as practiced by the U.N. Population Division and many national statistical offices, is to produce a medium set of projections based on assumptions regarding fertility, mortality, and migration rates, plus high and low variants based on certain assumptions about high and low fertility rates combined with medium mortality and migration rates. This standard practice is useful for getting information about the most likely future population path but is not appropriate for assessing the uncertainty in future population trends and for considering the impact of possible future surprises, for example, in the case of possible mortality crises or international migration streams. These issues can be captured only by fully probabilistic world population projections, first published by IIASA in 1996 (Lutz, Sanderson, and Scherbov 1996).

There is no one simple way to apply probabilistic methods to population projections (Lutz, Goldstein, and Prinz 1996; Lee 1998). Assumptions about the future variance of the distributions of the three components traditionally have been based on time series analysis or ex post analysis of projection errors. Both approaches have methodological problems, but the most important flaw for a global projection is the lack of appropriate time series data for large parts of the world population. For this reason, the approach chosen for the IIASA projections was more intensively based on expert judgement. The procedure fits a normal distribution to the three values (high, middle, and low) that resulted from the expert discussions; 90% of the cases were between the high and low values. Results were derived through a set of 4,000 simulations that randomly combined fertility, mortality, and migration rates from the three normal distributions for the 13 world regions. These simulations also considered the possibility that trends in fertility and mortality rates may be correlated within regions (e.g., a high fertility rate in sub-Saharan Africa is more likely to go hand in hand with a high mortality rate than a low mortality rate) and that regional trends may be either independent of each other or correlated.

The assumptions made for future trends in fertility, mortality, and migration rates in all 13 world regions are extensively described and substantively justified elsewhere (Lutz 1996) and therefore are not described here. In brief, the greatest sources of uncertainty in future trends are related to the future course of acquired immune deficiency syndrome (AIDS) mortality in Africa and South Asia, the upper limit of the human life span, the speed of declining fertility rates in countries that are still in the midst of demographic transition, the long-term level of posttransition fertility rates, and the future volume of international migration.

Figure 13-4 shows the distribution of future population sizes derived from the full set of 4,000 projections at five-year intervals, from 1995 to 2100. The possibility of almost linear population growth between 1995 and 2100 is unlikely. The possibility is equally unlikely that the world's population will peak in the middle of the twenty-first century and fall thereafter to below 6 billion by 2100. The much more probable range of future paths (between the 0.2 and 0.8 fractiles, covering 60% of all cases) is remarkably small. By 2050, this uncertainty range is fewer than 1.5 billion people, and by 2100, it doubles to about 3 billion people.

Figure 13-4 also shows that in more than 60% of all cases, the growth of the total world population levels off during the second half of the next century or even starts to decline. Given that the world population in mid-1996 was estimated at 5.8 billion, the probability of a doubling—that is, reaching or surpassing the 11.6 billion mark at any point during the next century—is only 33%. In other words, there is a two-thirds probability that world population will not double during the twenty-first century (Lutz, Sanderson, and Scherbov 1996, 1997).

Regional results for uncorrelated trends in fertility and mortality rates are listed in Table 13-2. Sub-Saharan Africa displays the largest range of uncertainty in future population size, with a 95% confidence interval in 2100 ranging from 578 million to 4.345 billion, around a mean of 1.9 billion. This large range results from the unusually large uncertainty surrounding trends in fertility and mortality rates in the region in addition to the assumption that the two trends will be uncorrelated. On the other hand, if fertility and mortality rates are assumed to be positively correlated within the region, the range of uncertainty narrows significantly (Lutz, Sanderson, and Scherbov 1996).

The distribution of the percentage of the global population above age 60 is shown in Figure 13-5. All the lines are rising, indicating confidence that the percentage of older

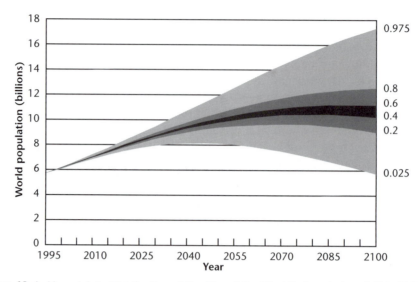

Figure 13-4. Uncertainty Distribution of the Size of the World's Population, 1995–2100

Note: Shading indicates three probability ranges into which cases fall: light, 95% interval; medium, 60% interval; dark, 20% interval. Numbers on the right give the fractiles of the distribution.

Source: Lutz, Sanderson, and Scherbov 1996.

people in the population will rise over time. In 2050, the mean global over-60 population is projected to be 20% of the total global population, compared with 9.5% in 1995, with a 95% uncertainty interval between 15 and 26%. By 2100, the mean is projected to increase to 27%, with a 95% uncertainty interval between 19 and 41%. In other words, there is a 95% chance that the proportion of elderly will at least double over the next century. In the most likely case, it will almost triple and may even more than quadruple. The uncertainty in the percentage above age 60 grows significantly during the second half of the twenty-first century, mainly as a result of the uncertainty in future old-age mortality rates when combined with uncertainty in fertility rates.

Three near certainties emerge from the range of scenarios and from the probabilistic projections:

- World population will increase substantially from its current level. Even in the lowest-growth scenario, population increases by close to 2 billion before commencing its decline. However, a doubling of the current world population is considered unlikely.
- The distribution of world population will continue to shift toward LDCs. Even assuming rapid decline in fertility rates and little improvement in mortality rates, LDCs still account for a rising share of world population.
- The world population will continue to age. Probabilistic projections show that a doubling of the proportion of the population over age 60 is a near certainty.

World Urbanization Trends

Although it is highly unlikely that the world population will double over the next century (or ever), the number of people living in urban areas probably will double by 2030. According to 1996 U.N. population estimates and projections, the total global urban population will increase from 2.58 billion in 1995 to 5.12 billion in 2030 (Table 13-3). This significant increase in absolute numbers will result from a combination of popula-

Table 13-2. Human Population Size by Region for Probabilistic Projections, 2020, 2050, and 2100

Region	Population (millions)				
	1995	Mean	Median	2.5%	97.5%
2020					
North Africa	162	277	277	254	300
Sub-Saharan Africa	558	1,059	1,058	965	1,159
China region[a]	1,362	1,670	1,670	1,526	1,826
Pacific Asia	447	629	629	576	678
Pacific OECD	147	155	155	145	167
Central Asia	54	87	87	76	100
Middle East	151	300	300	279	324
South Asia	1,240	1,845	1,845	1,737	1,949
Eastern Europe	122	124	124	116	133
European FSU	238	224	224	209	240
Western Europe	447	479	479	446	512
Latin America	477	697	696	646	746
North America	297	356	356	320	400
2050					
North Africa	162	440	439	309	583
Sub-Saharan Africa	558	1,625	1,605	1,085	2,316
China region[a]	1,362	1,888	1,865	1,351	2,574
Pacific Asia	447	802	796	579	1,047
Pacific OECD	147	146	146	117	182
Central Asia	54	139	137	88	206
Middle East	151	520	515	380	692
South Asia	1,240	2,380	2,368	1,833	2,970
Eastern Europe	122	111	110	86	141
European FSU	238	189	188	144	241
Western Europe	447	472	471	370	584
Latin America	477	930	925	707	1,177
North America	297	405	403	303	534
2100					
North Africa	162	630	598	228	1,202
Sub-Saharan Africa	558	1,909	1,738	578	4,345
China region[a]	1,362	2,051	1,873	709	4,428
Pacific Asia	447	876	829	322	1,696
Pacific OECD	147	125	120	59	221
Central Asia	54	212	194	65	477
Middle East	151	786	738	320	1,516
South Asia	1,240	2,365	2,246	1,014	4,327
Eastern Europe	122	83	78	31	168
European FSU	238	147	138	53	290
Western Europe	447	430	416	196	769
Latin America	477	1,163	1,106	489	2,142
North America	297	482	467	229	865

Notes: Columns labeled 2.5% and 97.5% provide data on the lower and upper bounds, respectively, of the 95% confidence interval; 2.5% of all observations lie below the lower bound and 97.5% of all observations lie below the upper bound. All figures are based on 1,000 simulations and were produced using DIALOG, the multistate population projection model. Fertility and mortality are assumed to be uncorrelated within regions. FSU = former Soviet Union.

[a]"China region" includes Cambodia, Hong Kong, Mongolia, North Korea, Taiwan, and Vietnam.

Source: Lutz, Sanderson, and Scherbov 1996.

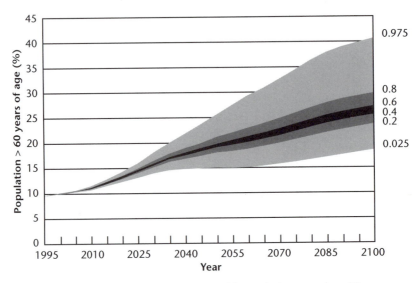

Figure 13-5. Uncertainty Distribution of the World Population over Age 60

Note: Shading indicates three probability ranges into which cases fall: light, 95% interval; medium, 60% interval; dark, 20% interval. Numbers on the right give the fractiles of the distribution. *Source:* Lutz, Sanderson, and Scherbov 1996.

tion growth and an expected increase in the urban proportion of population (from 45% in 1995 to 61% in 2030).

Table 13-3 lists the estimated urban populations (1995) and projected urban populations (2030) for 5 main regions and 20 subregions according to the United Nations (1997a). It shows that presently, the lowest proportion of urban population is found in Africa and Asia, where about one-third of the population lives in areas classified as urban. In sharp contrast, in Europe and the Americas (North America plus Latin America and the Caribbean), roughly three-quarters of the population live in urban areas. These data reveal a rather strong dichotomy in the world. They also indicate that the bulk of the world's rural population is in Asia.

The most highly urbanized regions (more than 80% urban) at present are Australia and New Zealand, northern Europe, and western Europe. Surprisingly, South America— which has experienced rapid urbanization, from 43% in 1950 to 77% in 1995—is already more urbanized than North America.

The comparison between more-developed (75% urban), less-developed (38% urban), and least-developed (23% urban) regions (Table 13-3) supports the general view that urbanization tends to go along with development. This picture is only very rough, however, and many significant deviations are related to historical settlement patterns, culture, and environmental conditions.

The projections produced by the U.N. Population Division are based on assumed future urban proportions superimposed on the usual population projections for each country. They do not present true multistate projections in which natural growth (births minus deaths) and migration are projected separately for each subpopulation. Because fertility rates tend to be universally lower in urban areas than in rural areas, much of the future urban growth probably will result from rural–urban migration rather than from high fertility rates in cities. Evidence indicates that even in African cities, fer-

Table 13-3. Total Urban Population and Urban Proportions by World Regions, 1995 (Estimated) and 2030 (Projected)

| | Urban population | | | |
| | (millions) | | (%) | |
Region	1995	2030	1995	2030
Africa	251	864	34.9	51.7
Eastern Africa	50	225	22.4	39.5
Middle Africa	27	111	32.7	53.2
Northern Africa	76	182	48.0	67.2
Southern Africa	23	56	47.8	64.1
Western Africa	76	288	36.3	58.8
Asia	1,192	2,736	34.7	55.2
Eastern Asia	524	1,012	36.9	56.4
South Central Asia	393	1,067	28.7	48.5
Southeastern Asia	162	398	33.5	52.2
Western Asia	113	260	67.6	80.4
Europe	535	572	73.5	82.9
Eastern Europe	218	226	70.2	81.3
Northern Europe	78	85	83.5	88.8
Southern Europe	92	101	64.1	75.2
Western Europe	148	160	81.5	87.8
Latin America and Caribbean	350	599	73.4	83.2
Caribbean	22	37	61.7	73.7
Central America	82	152	66.3	76.1
South America	246	410	77.4	87.2
North America	226	316	76.2	84.4
Oceania	20	31	70.1	74.5
Australia and New Zealand	18	26	84.9	88.9
Melanesia	1	4	20.9	37.6
Micronesia	0.2	0.6	42.7	60.5
Polynesia	0.2	0.5	41.5	57.6
MDCs	877	1,015	74.9	82.6
LDCs	1,697	4,102	37.6	57.3
Least-developed countries	132	558	22.7	40.9
World total	2,574	5,117	45.3	61.1

Source: United Nations 1997b.

tility rates have strongly declined (e.g., in Addis Ababa, Ethiopia, it is said to be already below replacement levels). AIDS mortality rates in Africa tend to be higher in the cities than in the countryside, which will also tends to slow African urban growth.

In recent urbanization projections, the speed of urbanization often has been conspicuously overestimated, especially for certain megacities. Only one decade ago, Mexico City was projected to reach 24 million inhabitants by 2000 and become the world's largest city, with far more than 30 million inhabitants in 2030. But the growth of Mexico City has stagnated; now, its population is not expected to surpass the 20 million mark even in 2015—which would make it only the world's seventh-largest agglomeration at that point, (United Nations 1997b). The United Nations now estimates that in 2015, the largest urban agglomeration will still be Tokyo, Japan (28.9 million); followed by Mumbai (Bombay), India (26.2 million); Lagos, Nigeria (24.6); São Paolo, Brazil (20.3); Dhaka, Bangladesh (19.5); Karachi, Pakistan (19.4); Mexico City, Mexico (19.2); Shanghai, China (18.0); and New York (city), U.S.A. (17.6).

In Mexico City, the sudden change in trends seems to have several causes, most prominently, the movement of several industries out of the city area, economic development in other parts of the country, and the high level of air pollution and crime in Mexico City. Aside from the undisputed leadership of Tokyo, the above predictions for 2015 should be treated with caution. Mechanisms similar to those in Mexico City may well operate in Mumbai or Lagos, and estimates for other cites are very close to each other.

For the study of the population exposed to malaria, more detailed projections concerning future places of residence would be desirable. However, such projections do not exist at a global level. For specific case studies, such detailed information can be produced and would deserve further elaboration.

Population and Climate Change

Climate change and population growth are among a select group of issues that will have global implications for generations. Yet, while recent international agreements on population and global environmental issues have recognized relationships between the two, none has made specific recommendations based on analyses of particular linkages. On the environment side, Agenda 21 (signed at the Earth Summit in 1992 and intended as a blueprint for sustainable development) recommends only that nations take demographic factors into account in the policymaking process. On the population side, the Program of Action (agreed to at the International Conference on Population and Development in Cairo in 1994) also discusses links between population and environment but does little more than repeat the language of Agenda 21.

One logical arena for the analysis of relationships between population and climate change is the Intergovernmental Panel on Climate Change (IPCC), which is charged with assessing the science of climate change and its potential impacts, as well as formulating response strategies. Yet, it has paid little attention to population. For example, the IPCC's 1996 reports on mitigation and adaptation options evaluate a wide array of strategies but not policies to slow population growth (Watson, Zinyowera, and Moss 1996; Bruce, Lee, and Haites 1996). Several reasons for this omission are likely (Bongaarts, O'Neill, and Gaffin 1997), not least the North–South tension over the relative roles of population and consumption in environmental degradation. Yet, IPCC leaves unexamined a potentially important link between two of what likely will be grand themes of the twenty-first century.

Humans consume natural resources through their consumption of goods and services; pollution, including the emissions of CO_2 and other greenhouse gases, arises because the production (and often consumption) of goods and services gives rise to residual pollutants. This production depends ultimately on consumer demand—even government and military expenditures ultimately depend on households' demand for public services and security. Some goods are consumed directly, such as fresh fruits and vegetables; *intermediate goods* are used to produce goods and services that are subsequently consumed directly (for example, steel used in automobile manufacture or electricity used to light office buildings); and *investment goods* are used to build up the capital stock necessary to produce intermediate goods and consumption.

Therefore, human consumption of goods and services as well as human choices about consumption are directly related to concentrations of greenhouse gases. The role of consumption as prime mover, sometimes called the assumption of "consumer sovereignty," is crucial to the neoclassical economic model of the environment, because it permits economists to argue that consumers make intelligent trade-offs between the consumption of goods and the quality of the environment.

Production is driven by the kinds of choices made by consumers as well as by the scale of consumer demand, determined in part by population size. If fertility is also subject to human choice, and if there are inverse relationships between the number of people and the quality of the environment and between the number of people and the material standard of living, then an implicit neoclassical population/environment/consumption trade-off is defined. Even if the methodologically individualistic neoclassical model of human choice is rejected in favor of a more complex model (say, based more closely on cultural values), and despite the fact that social scientists, philosophers, and humanists may differ on how choices are defined and made, the crucial element of choice remains.

When confronted with such a complex reality, the normal scientific response is to search for simple models that broadly summarize the impact of population on availability of natural resources and the quality of the environment. A logical first step in this direction is assessing the scale effect of population, that is, the impact of population independent of possible feedback effects on other relevant variables. Keyfitz (1992) called this the "direct" effect of population growth on the environment and, citing ambiguities and disputes regarding the nature of indirect effects, argued that it should be the focus of attention. Downplaying the direct linear-scale effects of population while stressing its less-well-understood indirect nonlinear effects, Keyfitz argues, can result in defining "the population problem" out of existence. This direct effect underlies the concerns expressed by ecologists (Daily and Ehrlich 1992) and ecological economists (Daly 1991).

Indeed, the literature on indirect effects fails to present particularly strong conclusions. Research findings can be summarized in three points:

- The relationship between population and the level of per capita income is ambiguous or, more accurately, depends on a broad range of contextual variables. Two opposing views—one that demographic growth mires populations in poverty, another that demographic growth stimulates improvements in technology and organization—can be traced back as far as the eighteenth century. A large postwar literature on population and development has failed to reach strong conclusions one way or the other.

- Population growth often increases the share of production accounted for by agriculture and the proportion of the land base devoted to food production. In this sense, demographic increase has the effect of concentrating output into a heavily polluting sector. The theme of virtuous and vicious adjustments to population pressure against the natural resource base was derived for the most part from research on population and food. Frustratingly, we find no strong grounds for either optimism or pessimism regarding the role of population.

- Most deforestation in mid-latitude tropical forests occurs in a few "hot spots" and can be traced ultimately to the expansion of agriculture. Largely because of its link to agriculture, rapid population growth has long been correlated with rapid loss of forest cover. The correlation says nothing about the more complex underlying causal relationship. For example, commercial logging is a significant factor, because it leads the way for shifting cultivators and often is closely tied to government policies in the area of export subsidies. Also, whereas micro-level evidence that the combination of rapid population growth, poverty, and inadequate access to good land (and renewable resources of all kinds) leads to deterioration of the renewable resource base is abundant, it tends to be anecdotal.

In addition to direct and indirect effects, there is a set of effects that might be called "induced effects": changes in the way social institutions cope with ecological stress, including changes in the institutions themselves, as a result of shifts in demographic regime. Where social science research on indirect effects is abundant and equivocal, research on induced effects is sparse and, with some notable exceptions (McNicoll 1990; Tiffen and Mortimore 1992), speculative. Under some circumstances, rapid population growth appears to give rise to social and institutional changes that promote environmentally sound adaptation; under others, to institutional and social gridlock, with ensuing environmental degradation. Because institutions—hence, social solidarities—are at the heart of induced effects, it is not surprising that they may be highly nonlinear and discontinuous.

Conclusion

Because slowing population growth probably will reduce greenhouse gas emissions in the long run and improve the resiliency of vulnerable populations to climate-related impacts, climate change strengthens the case for voluntary family-planning programs by increasing the returns on investment. It also strengthens the case for indirect population policies, particularly investments in the education of females, which are appealing because they increase individual welfare but also tend to lower fertility rates. Both types of programs qualify as no-regrets climate change policies.

Climate change, which is exacerbated by high birth rates, also adds to the costs side in the weighing of external costs and benefits to fertility. Economic costs and, even more so, benefits of childbearing are inherently difficult to estimate comprehensively. Possibly more important, humans are perhaps innately reluctant to view fertility decisions as purely economic in nature. As a result, although these kinds of studies are useful in shedding light on the consequences of childbearing and can serve as a guide to policymaking, they never have been accepted as a principal basis for policy decisions. However, the fairly conclusive results on externalities through greenhouse gas emissions support the general notion that population growth imposes external environmental costs on society. It also suggests that population growth may be just one of a class of largely unmeasured environmental externalities. This concept strengthens the case for programs to lower fertility rates.

The threat of climate change may strengthen equity-based reasoning for population policies in that its consequences will fall most heavily on the least-well-off societies. However, equity-based justifications for population policy are not cut and dried. On the one hand, we can argue that climate change impacts will fall most heavily on the shoulders of the least-well-off societies and, thus, that we should pursue population planning to reduce the number of those who are likely to be the least well off in the future. On the other hand, if we assume that socioeconomic development will occur, the current generation will be the least well off, so we should not be sacrificing now for future (wealthier) generations. We can argue that population policy is advisable as it would mean that fewer people would be at risk in the future. We can also argue that if development provides suitable substitutes for amenities that climate now provides, we will be able to pursue sustainability even if climate changes dramatically.

Overall, it is difficult to assess how climate change relates to justifications for population policies. Current dominant thinking in population policymaking gives little weight to its demographic consequences, even though those provide the main link to the climate change issue.

The empowerment of women and securing of reproductive rights and health are the primary justifications for the recommendations stemming from the 1994 International Conference on Population and development (known as the Cairo Programme of Action). Most current population policies probably are win–win with respect to climate change. Policies such as providing reproductive health services (including family planning), investing in education (especially for women), reducing infant and child mortality rates, and equalizing gender relations not only will increase the welfare of individuals directly (*and hence reduce their vulnerability*), but also probably reduce future environmental stress (*through lower fertility rates*).

This conclusion need not seem suspiciously optimistic. Because fertility is generally understood to be embedded in a web of bidirectional links to poverty, low status of women, and environmental degradation, improvement in any of these factors probably will lead to lower fertility rates. Therefore, any policy that produces such an improvement will be justifiable, most directly through its effect on welfare and secondarily through its effect on fertility rates (Birdsall 1994). On the other hand, this conclusion must be tempered by the realization that such vicious-circle reasoning applies to only the roughly 40% of the global population who live in poverty. Although this fraction also has the highest fertility rates, the ultimate effect on global population growth would be less than one might otherwise expect.

The limitations of slowing population growth as a means of addressing climate change must be kept clearly in sight. Population is subject to considerable inertia, so reducing fertility rates over the next few decades will not significantly reduce population size until the second half of the twenty-second century. Therefore, emissions reductions in the short term can be achieved only through reductions in per capita emissions (although to realize long-term reductions in population size, fertility rates also must be reduced in the short term). Even in the long term, slowing population growth is no panacea. Although it certainly can make stabilizing greenhouse gas concentrations easier, displace more expensive energy-related emissions reductions, and make societies more resilient to climate change impacts, slowing population growth is less efficient than many other more direct policies to achieve the same goals.

Alone, slowing population growth will not by any means solve the climate problem. However, population policies (direct programs, such as the provision of family-planning services, as well as indirect measures, such as investments in female education) should be considered as potential elements of a portfolio of options for mitigating and adapting to climate change—something the climate community has yet to do.

Acknowledgement

This chapter draws heavily on O'Neill, MacKellar, and Lutz 2001.

References

Birdsall, N. 1994. Another look at population and global warming. In *Population, Environment, and Development*. New York: United Nations, 39–54.

Bongaarts, J., and R. Potter. 1983. *Fertility, Biology, and Behavior*. New York: Academic Press.

Bongaarts, J., B.C. O'Neill, and S.R. Gaffin. 1997. Climate change policy: Population left out in the cold. *Environment* 39(9): 40–41.

Bruce, J.P., H. Lee, and E.F. Haites (eds.). 1996. *Climate Change 1995: Economic and Social Dimensions of Climate Change*. Contribution of Working Group III to the Second Assessment of Report of the Intergovernmental Panel on Climate Change. New York: Cambridge University Press.

Coale, A.J. 1973. The demographic transition. In *Proceedings of the International Population Conference* (volume 1). Liège, Belgium: International Union for the Scientific Study of Population.

Cook, R.C. 1962. How many people have ever lived on earth? *Population Bulletin* 18(1).

Daily, G.C., and P.R. Ehrlich. 1992. Population, sustainability and the earth's carrying capacity. *BioScience* 42(10): 761–771.

Daly, H.E. 1991. Elements of environmental macroeconomics. In *Ecological Economics: The Science and Management of Sustainability*, edited by R. Costanza. New York: Columbia University Press, 32–46.

Davis, K. 1954. The world demographic transition. *Annals of the American Academy of Political and Social Science* 237: 1–11.

———. 1991. Population and resources: Fact and interpretation. In *Resources, Environment and Population: Present Knowledge*, edited by K. Davis and M.S. Bernstam. Oxford, U.K.: Oxford University Press, 1–21.

Keyfitz, N. 1992. Seven ways of making the less developed countries' population problem to disappear—in theory. *European Journal of Population* 8: 149–167.

Lee, R.D. 1998. Probabilistic approaches to population forecasting. *Population and Development Review* 24(Supplement: Frontiers of Population Forecasting, edited by W. Lutz, J.W. Vaupel, and D.A. Ahlburg): 156–190.

Lutz, W. (ed.). 1994. *Population-Development-Environment: Understanding their Interactions in Mauritius*. Berlin, Germany: Springer-Verlag.

———. 1996. *The Future Population of the World: What Can We Assume Today?* (revised edition). London, U.K.: Earthscan.

Lutz, W., J.R. Goldstein, and C. Prinz. 1996. Alternative approaches to population projection. In *The Future Population of the World: What Can We Assume Today?* (revised edition), edited by W. Lutz. London, U.K.: Earthscan, 14–44.

Lutz, W., W. Sanderson, and S. Scherbov. 1996. Probabilistic population projections based on expert opinion. In *The Future Population of the World: What Can We Assume Today?* (revised edition), edited by W. Lutz. London, U.K.: Earthscan, 397–428.

———. 1997. Doubling of world population unlikely. *Nature* 387: 803–805.

———. 1998. Expert-based probabilistic population projections. In *Frontiers of Population Forecasting*, supplement to *Population and Development Review* (volume 24), edited by W. Lutz, J.W. Vaupel, and D.A. Ahlburg. New York: Population Council, 139–155.

McNicoll, G. 1990. Social organization and ecological stability under demographic stress. In *Rural Development and Population: Institutions and Policy*, edited by G. McNicoll and M. Cain. New York: Oxford University Press, 147–160.

Notestein, F.W. 1945. Population: The long view. In *Food for the World*, edited by T.W. Schultz. Chicago, IL: University of Chicago Press, 36–57.

O'Neill, B.C., F.L. MacKellar, and W. Lutz. 2001. *Population and Climate Change*. Cambridge, U.K.: Cambridge University Press.

Tabah, L. 1989. From one demographic transition to another. *Population Bulletin of the United Nations* 28: 1–24.

Tiffen, M., and M. Mortimore. 1992. Environment, population growth and productivity in Kenya. *Development Policy Review* 10(4): 359–387.

United Nations. 1997a. *World Population Prospects: The 1996 Revision.* New York: United Nations.

——. 1997b. *World Urbanization Prospects: The 1996 Revision.* New York: United Nations, Department of Economic and Social Affairs, Population Division.

Watson, R.T., M.C. Zinyowera, and R.H. Moss. (eds.). 1996. *Climate Change 1995: Impacts, Adaptations, and Mitigation of Climate Change: Scientific-Technical Analyses.* New York: Cambridge University Press.

Chapter 14

Reading the Tea Leaves
Economic Scenarios for the Twenty-First Century

Lester B. Lave and Hadi Dowlatabadi

World population and per capita income will be important, directly and indirectly, to the future well-being of Earth's environment and of human beings. Population and income are the principal determinants of greenhouse gas emissions and hence of global warming.* Both are uncertain, especially for the developing countries. Although population and income affect global warming, there also is a feedback effect in which global warming affects population and income. However, the effect of population and income on greenhouse gas emissions and hence on global warning is much greater than the feedback effect. Furthermore, the feedback effect is tempered by human reactions to climate change, which depend on the level of technology and the effectiveness of research and development in abatement technologies.

In this chapter, our focus is the effect of climate change on the incidence of malaria and other tropical diseases. We argue that climate is not destiny; a warmer climate may not necessarily result in a greater incidence of malaria. Climate is a necessary condition but not a sufficient condition for the existence of infectious tropical diseases. A warmer climate would expand the area where these disease vectors are viable; however, whether disease actually occurs is a much more complicated issue. Public health measures, access to personal health services, nutrition status, population density, and location modify the effect of climate.

If climate were the only important factor in determining the incidence of vector-borne disease, incidence would follow the climatic gradients on Earth's surface. Endemicity would decrease gradually from areas where the climate is optimal for vector and parasite development to areas where climate is less conducive to disease. However, the incidence of malaria does not follow such a smooth pattern geographically. Instead, we find sharp transitions from geopolitical areas of pestilence to areas where malaria (and many other vector-borne diseases) are rarely seen. The areas have similar climates, but disease incidence is related to differences in socioeconomic conditions. This reality leads

---

Greenhouse gases inhibit the reflection of heat into space, warming Earth and its atmosphere. The most important greenhouse gas is water vapor; however, in terms of emissions, greenhouse gases refer to the anthropogenic (human-made) release of other gases, such as carbon dioxide and methane. *Global warming* is an increase in the Earth's average temperature, which is predicted to accelerate as a result of the accumulation of anthropogenic greenhouse gases in the atmosphere.

us to assert that, although climate conditions determine whether malaria can be present, actual incidence of disease is determined by the prevailing socioeconomic conditions.

For example, in the past, malaria was endemic in the eastern United States, southern Canada, England, and much of southern Europe. The disease is no longer endemic in these areas, even though the climate is about as hospitable to the vector as it was in the past. These areas have experienced increased income, which brought with it improvements in public health, health care, and nutrition. In areas of southern Louisiana and Florida, malaria was eradicated in the 1940s and 1950s by pesticides in addition to the benefits of lifestyle changes brought about by higher incomes.

Little global warming is expected before 2050; even in 2100, no dramatic warming is expected. Thus, any change in malaria incidence before 2050 is unlikely to be due to global warming. Indeed, only by about 2100 will warming be sufficient to cause much change in malaria incidence. To predict the incidence of tropical infectious disease for an area in 2050 and 2100, we need to know that area's future climate, income level, state of medical knowledge, population, and aspects of social organization (e.g., level of public health expenditures). We agree that the world will be generally warmer in the future, increasing the potential for vector-borne disease. But based on past experience, per capita income in each region will be more influential than climate on the future incidence of tropical infectious disease.

Accuracy of Social and Economic Event Predictions

Can anyone predict events 100 or even 50 years from now? Readers can gain some perspective on this question by guessing which nation has the following characteristics:

- Average life expectancy is 47 years.
- Fourteen percent of homes have a bathtub.
- The five leading causes of death are pneumonia and influenza, tuberculosis, diarrhea, heart disease, and stroke.
- Ninety percent of adults can read, but only 6% graduate from high school.
- The average wage is 22 cents an hour; the average worker makes $200–400 per year.
- Marijuana, heroin, and morphine are available over the counter at corner drugstores.
- Ninety percent of "physicians" have no college education.

These statistics describe the United States in 1900. Could a knowledgeable analyst in 1900 have predicted what the next 100 years would bring? We assert that predicting the future a century hence is impossible.

The usual way of forecasting the future is trend extrapolation, as described by Meadows et al. (1974). Population, economic activity, and resource use are assumed to grow at historical rates—until the system crashes. Extrapolating future economic conditions based on current trends is a poor method of prediction. Such an extrapolation on U.S. trends a century ago would have fallen far from the mark today, because the United States produces few of the goods and services that it produced 100 years ago, and the two economies bear little resemblance. The futurists of 1900 had little idea of what the world would be like in 2000, aside from predicting improvements in income, mobility, and communication. They could not imagine the new technologies, because they could only extrapolate from the technologies that were familiar. Even less were they able to imagine the indirect effects of these inventions, that is, the way that they have shaped society and influenced the epidemiology of infectious disease.

We humbly confess our inability to forecast the economic world of 2100 or even of 2050. Furthermore, we urge you not to give credence to futurists who are less humble than we are. The brightest people using the best models might be able to predict a new technology, political regime, or economic organization. However, predicting the cascading effects as society adjusts to these changes is impossible.

Lessons from the Recent Past

Growth Rates

Predicting per capita income levels is most important in predicting the future incidence of malaria. Over more than a century, the United States led the world in the growth of income and productivity, averaging 2% per year. Gross domestic product (GDP) per capita was 7.2 times higher in 1969 than in 1870. Over shorter time periods, other nations have done much better. From 1950 to 1969, Japanese GDP per capita rose 8.6% per year, multiplying 4.8 times! In 20 years, the Japanese economy did what it took the U.S. economy 78 years to accomplish. However, during the past decade, the Japanese economy has stagnated.

The economies of several Southeast Asian countries also have grown rapidly. Whether nations such as Indonesia and Malaysia can sustain these growth rates, or even current income levels, is uncertain. Some autocratic governments accomplish economic miracles only to stumble, losing their drive and even most of their past gains. For example, from post–World War II through the 1980s, the Soviet Union experienced rapid growth, followed by political dissolution and disastrous drops in income.

As *Limits to Growth* (Meadows et al. 1974) reminds us, exponential growth is incompatible, eventually, with a finite world. Technological change, globalization, international liberalization of trade, and higher incomes force the economy to reinvent itself continually. The per capita income of most people has changed little in the past century or half-century. The most likely prediction is that these incomes will change little over the next 100 years. If income does grow, then slow and steady growth is more likely.

Urbanization and Infrastructure Development

In today's world, rich societies are organized around large urban centers with high population densities. Rural areas in rich nations are populated with people who earn their living from the land (agriculture and tourism), serve other rural dwellers, or can market their services remotely. The present spatial distribution of humans across the landscape of rich nations evolved over centuries from a much smaller population centered around agricultural activities in rural areas. Mechanization of agriculture and the advent of industrial manufacturing led to a push–pull dynamic, driving people from the rural areas to urban centers. Early urban centers were heavily polluted and ridden with disease. Their expansions were unplanned, and basic services (such as waste disposal and the provision of potable water) were absent or provided haphazardly. During this era, vector-borne disease was still common.

As time passed, two events played out over and over in various cities: sewer systems were developed to cope with the run-off of animal waste from newly paved roads, and the roads were paved to accommodate heavy omnibuses. (Omnibus transportation was needed to bring workers to factories in city centers because the city centers could no longer house the necessary workers within walking distance of the factories [McShane

1994].) Neither of these steps was directly motivated by a desire to reduce mosquito habitat. Nor were they directly demanded by people growing wealthier and seeking a better environmental condition. In fact, city residents who lived along the route strongly resisted the transformation of open roads into thoroughfares for workers and goods. However, well-functioning urban communities and their transit systems brought improved surface water management as well as wealth from manufacturing jobs.

Today, many of the largest population centers in the world are in poor countries. These population centers have not evolved along the same path as those described above. Unplanned expansion of modern metropolises has led to large populations in shanty towns—with no potable water, sewer systems, surface water management, or waste disposal services—situated around the cities. These developing-world megacities are breeding grounds for infectious disease.

From 1980 to 1995, the population of urban areas around the world grew from 1.7 billion to 2.7 billion. This rapid growth necessitated the delivery of basic services on an unprecedented scale by many impoverished governments. In areas for which information is available, we know that over this 15-year period, about 440 million additional urban dwellers were provided with basic sanitation services and potable water. Regrettably, at least 600 million urban dwellers continued to live without basic sanitation services in 1995 (calculated using data from The World Bank Group 2000, Table 3.10).

The expected trend in urbanization points toward even larger fractions of the population being located in large urban centers (Figure 14-1). One can ask, "if conditions are so dire in these cities, what is driving the rush to urbanization in the poorer nations of the world?" The ready answer appears to be "a search for economic opportunities."

Income, Equity, and Social Organization

Per capita income is an inadequate indicator of public health in areas where societies have different distributions of income and access to resources. Malaria is absent in the countries with the highest incomes (e.g., Singapore). It also is absent in areas where social organizations have devoted a greater share of available resources to provision of public goods, such as education and health (e.g., Cuba, where 8.2% of GDP is devoted to public health services). Any projections of future socioeconomic conditions must be made in the context of both the level of income and the nature of social organization in each country or region. In the absence of strong social contracts, governments spend less on the creation and maintenance of public goods such as sanitation, public health, and environmental quality.

The recent reemergence of malaria in the states that emerged from the breakup of the Soviet Union is a sad reminder that persistent vigilance in detection, treatment, and vector control is critical to reducing the incidence of malaria. In much of the former Soviet Union, malaria was all but absent for decades. The previous regime allocated significant resources to health services, which were institutionally stable and run with military zeal. The fall of the Soviet Union was followed by a large fall in income for the populations of many newly independent states. However, even in nations where incomes have not fallen dramatically, the difference in governmental provision of public goods has led to precipitous declines in social services and public health.

Scenarios vs. Predictions

Although no one can predict future population or income levels, insights can be obtained by investigating the implications of assumptions concerning the most impor-

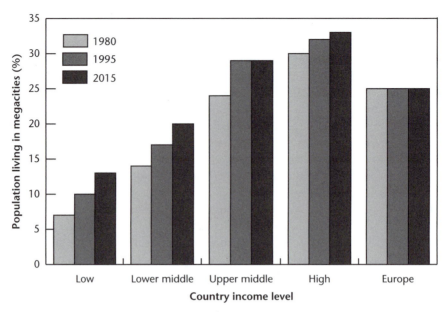

Figure 14-1. Growing Population in Megacities

Note: The World Bank projects growth in cities with more than 1 million inhabitants in all regions and income groups except for European cities in the upper-middle-income category.

tant determinants of the future. These "scenarios" or "contingent forecasts" can be simple stories or the results of quantitative, causal models (Table 14-1).

The most important factor for predicting the incidence of malaria in 2050 or 2100 is the level of per capita income, which in most nations acts as a surrogate for education, nutrition, public health expenditures, personal health care, and fertility rates. Collapsing all the dimensions into income is simplistic, but we judge the simplification to generate insights. For example, countries with the highest incomes have the lowest birth rates. Rapid population growth makes it almost impossible to raise income levels, because there is too little social capital to educate children and to provide potable water, sanitation, and other public health necessities. An uneducated, sickly population is unlikely to earn high incomes. But if income can grow faster than population for an extended period, high income will tend to diminish fertility rates and slow population growth.

We present three scenarios that explore future levels of income. In the first, "Woe is us," income levels fall across all nations. Such income decreases might be precipitated by war, criminal behavior, or running out of natural resources.

The second scenario, "Business as usual," is one in which the rich nations get richer, a few poor nations graduate to the ranks of the rich, and the other nations stay relatively poor. It reflects the experience of sub-Saharan Africa and parts of Asia in the twentieth century. Despite foreign aid, private charity, and the efforts of institutions such as the World Bank, many poor nations have seen little increase in per capita income levels. Their lack of growth has not hampered the growth of the rich nations.

"Nirvana," the third scenario, is a happy one in which incomes grow more rapidly in the poor nations than in the rich nations, and all nations get richer over time. This scenario might be encouraged by the rich nations opening their economies to the poor ones and implicitly or explicitly subsidizing their development. For example, the United

Table 14-1. Three Economic Development Scenarios

Feature	Scenario		
	"Woe is us"	*"Business as usual"*	*"Nirvana"*
Population	Growth far beyond locally sustainable levels leads to mal-nutrition and migra-tion on massive scales.	Growth stabilizes at close to 12 billion.	Women enter the work force, fertility drops, incomes rise, and population stabilizes below the 10 billion mark.
Income and equity	Social discord or unstable, corrupt government leads to collapse of economic systems in the rich countries. Poorer nations fare no better.	With few exceptions, rich nations and poor nations retain their current income and social inequalities.	Incomes rise, especially in poorer nations. Social contracts are strengthened through a commitment to equality and social justice.
Urban areas	Larger population densities create ideal habitats for urban malaria in poor and formerly rich nations.	Megacities abound in low- and middle-income countries. Peri-urban dwellers in poor countries have minimal to nonexistent sanitation.	Well-managed urban conditions reduce many disease risks for city dwellers.
Rural areas	Frontier areas are occupied in some instances, creating new habitats suitable for malaria; in others, the habitat grows less hospitable for malaria. Health needs of rural populations are neglected.	Rural population densities decline through migration to megacities. Settlement of marginal lands for agricultural production increases.	Medical progress and high incomes permit widespread high standard of living and universal access to quality health care.

States opened its economy to exports from Japan and the "Asian tigers" (e.g., Hong Kong, Korea, Singapore, and Taiwan), enabling them to develop rapidly. However, as discussed below, much more effort is needed to make the poor nations richer.

"Woe Is Us"

The "Woe is us" scenario signals a breakdown in the rich nations as well as the poor ones. The breakdown might be caused by running out of a crucial resource (unlikely) or by a deteriorating social structure. A good deal of research has been done on how consumers behave when their incomes drop below expectations. They try to maintain private consumption and cut back on public goods such as environmental quality and their subsidies for sustainability. They use the cheapest source of energy, despite greenhouse gas emissions.

Eventually, the drop in income would decrease energy use and lower consumers' ability to damage the climate, if incomes dropped enough. Resource use and environmental discharges are roughly proportional to GDP. However, rich nations have increased the efficiency with which they use energy and other resources, lowering environmental discharges per dollar of GDP. As incomes fall, they might be expected to lose this efficiency and environmental advantage. With falling incomes, charity toward poor countries would likely stop.

The "Woe is us" scenario portrays a thoroughly unpleasant world, desired by no one except misanthropes. Although falling incomes would lead to increased pollution and greenhouse gas emissions initially, if incomes fell far enough, fossil fuel use would also fall, resulting in lower greenhouse gas emissions. Humanity would eventually lose its ability to generate enough greenhouse gases to damage the climate. Still, even if this scenario mitigated climate change, it would portend other terrible consequences for the environment, sustainability, public health, and philanthropy.

"Business as Usual"

If the productivity and per capita income of the poorest nations grow at 2% per year for a century, these nations will pass the $2,000 per capita income mark within that time. An income of $10,000 per year for a family of five is not a U.S. suburban lifestyle, but it is far beyond the current income levels of the poorest nations. Tol and Dowlatabadi (2001) estimate that malaria can be conquered when income reaches $3,100 per capita, which would occur soon after 2100 for the poorest nations.

In the "Business as usual" scenario, the rich nations stay rich and continue to care for environmental quality and sustainability. Poor nations either grow rich or remain impoverished. Nations with high incomes based on their mineral resources lose wealth. Nations without the foundations for development either quickly adopt them or slip backward.

In the peaceful variant of the "Business as usual" scenario, the expectations of the poor adjust to their fate. The rich nations give aid in the form of food during famines and some aid for infrastructure, which eases the consciences of the rich and helps the poor but does not break the cycle of poverty. The best and brightest students of the poor nations go to the rich nations for education. Those idealistic enough to return to help their home countries quickly realize the impossibility of the task, so they return to the rich nations. The rich nations welcome these migrants, whose added energy and vitality compensate for declining populations. Those who remain in the poor nations are envious of the rich nations but are not inclined to make trouble. If they do, and civil war or threats against rich nations result, then the rich nations can dampen the threat of war by cutting off aid to rebels, imposing economic embargoes, or even encouraging other nations to attack the rebels in return for more foreign aid.

In the antagonistic version of "Business as usual," poor-nation leaders educated in the rich nations see their fellow citizens as victims of the rich. They foment revolution and attack the rich nations with terrorists. Their goal is to increase aid, but the increased aid tends to disappear into Swiss bank accounts and the nations never manage to get onto a growth trajectory. Civil wars, launched with noble intent, drive poor nations into deeper poverty, and prolonged civil unrest intensifies their public health problems. Terrorism and danger to tourists threaten rich nations.

In both "Business as usual" variants, the rich nations regulate themselves by their concerns for the environment and sustainability. Poor nations that are capable of doing so quickly join the ranks of the rich nations and, after a few decades, imitate them. Many poor nations stay poor, using little energy and so contributing little toward global warming. During an unpleasant interim period, populations in the poor nations are higher than the poor nations can support, even with foreign aid. Eventually, the "Business as usual" scenario settles down to a point where resource use and environmental discharges are not very different from the "Nirvana" scenario, even though most of the world's population lives in poverty.

"Nirvana"

The "Nirvana" scenario could be much more aggressive with a sevenfold growth of income in 30 years, based on the experience of Japan and the Asian tigers. Part of the advantage of Japan and the Asian tigers was that they had had access to advanced technology from the rich nations. Japan's economic growth rested on a base of giving high priority to education, public health, and social infrastructure, together with a stable government; people were willing to sacrifice current consumption for a rich future. Korea and Singapore adopted the same model. Indonesia, Malaysia, and Thailand (often referred to as the "little tigers") thought they were pursuing a similar model but did not make the same investments in education and public health and with more corrupt governments. These nations managed rapid growth for some time.

Universal and high-quality education, public health, and infrastructure, together with a stable, uncorrupt government, are not typical of the poorest nations today. Changing a nation's culture to adopt these values is far from easy. Without them, the poorest nations are unlikely to develop. Poor nations with extensive mineral resources, such as Angola and the Democratic Republic of the Congo, seem perhaps more disadvantaged; their mineral wealth brings exploitative outsiders and fosters civil war that victimizes the population, prevents growth, and seems to benefit only a few individuals.

Cultural obstacles to paid work for women also hinder development. The western pattern has been that, as economic activity increases, women are recruited to the paid work force, boosting family income. When families see the trade-off between increased family income and having more children, many choose the higher income. Economies with surplus labor and high actual or disguised unemployment keep women out of the work force, whereas a growing, prospering economy draws women into the work force while providing the resources for education, public health, and investment in both the workplace and the infrastructure.

The "Nirvana" scenario makes everyone smile. The poor nations develop economically. As a necessary condition of or along with development, women enter the paid labor force. High incomes lead to greater concern for the environment and sustainability. Higher income leads citizens of the poor nations to focus on services, as do consumers in the rich nations.

Summary

1. No one can predict with confidence the state of the economy or society in 2100 or even 2050. However, scenarios can provide insight.
2. Per capita income is the principal driving force for the next century. Income will be the primary influence on the future world population, access to health care, level of public health, quality of the environment, and human welfare.
3. The foundation for economic growth in a nation is twofold: (a) giving a high priority to education, public health, and savings, and (b) having a stable, uncorrupt government. Nations with these foundations stand a good chance of making it to the

circle of rich nations; those without these attributes may grow for a few years or may exploit natural resources (such as petroleum) and grow for a few decades, but eventually will be at a subsistence level.

4. Three scenarios offer insight for the world of 2100:

    —   The "Woe is us" scenario assumes that incomes decline in all nations, increasing the threat of civil unrest and even civil war. Lower incomes will likely motivate people to seek the cheapest sources of energy—fossil fuels—and to curtail "discretionary" expenditures, such as those related to pollution controls and environmental sustainability. This scenario presents the greatest threat to Earth's environment and human welfare, both of which are likely to suffer substantially.

    —   In the "Business as usual" scenario, the rich nations stay rich and the poor nations stay poor, but perhaps an occasional poor nation advances to the rich circle. The rich nations are motivated to subsidize the poor ones, but the social climate in the poor nations prevents economic development. The best and brightest from the poor nations are educated in the rich nations and remain there, welcome as the populations in the rich nations continue to decline. Subsidies from the rich nations help to stem civil unrest and civil war in the poor nations and to halt terrorism against the rich nations.

    —   In the "Nirvana" scenario, all nations become richer. Within 100 years or so, income levels in even the poorest nations reach a level at which malaria is controlled, fertility rates fall, and people desire environmental improvements and sustainability. Increasing income cures many social and medical ills by the end of the century or shortly thereafter.

Conclusion

What are the implications of these economic scenarios for malaria?

*   Human welfare depends on per capita income and the associated levels of education, public health, health services, and environmental concern. Broadly distributed, high incomes enable people to demand a clean, high-quality environment. However, population pressure also makes resources scarce, making it more difficult to achieve a quality environment. Depending on the scenario, in response to the level of resources committed to public health activities, malaria could either disappear or become more widespread.

*   Distributional inequalities drive population movement (whether in search of new economic opportunities or simply flight from starvation, tyranny, or war). Such population movement can destroy wilderness areas and create habitats where malaria flourishes. It also can introduce malaria into new populations or lead to unplanned urbanization where high population density and poor living conditions combine to create incubators of public health disasters. As long as large numbers of mobile people remain infected with malaria, this disease will remain a constant threat worldwide.

*   Once locally eliminated, malaria requires constant attention to case detection, treatment, and vector control. A successful program of this kind requires adequate resources and permanent effort. Scarce resource futures do not allow this kind of sustainability.

Whatever path economic development takes, these principles probably will remain valid and influence the success or failure of malaria control programs. Similarly, the ability and will to deploy yet-to-be developed antimalaria technologies will depend on economic and social progress.

References

McShane, C. 1994. *Down the Asphalt Path: The Automobile and the American City.* New York: Columbia University Press.

Meadows, Donella H., and others. 1974. *Limits to Growth: A Report for the Club of Rome's Project on the Predicament of Mankind.* Universe Books: New York.

Tol, R.S.J., and H. Dowlatabadi. 2001. Vector-Borne Diseases, Development and Climate Change. *Integrated Assessment* 2: 173–181.

The World Bank Group. 2000. *World Development Indicators 2000.* Washington, DC: The World Bank Group.

Chapter 15

Population Migration and Malaria

Janice Longstreth and Anatole Kondrachine

Population movement has long been recognized as an important factor in the distribution of diseases, and it seems likely that the next 50 years—like the past 50 years—will only confirm that importance for malaria. The movement of rural populations into cities, migrant workers onto agricultural holdings, and settlers and workers into developing areas over the past half-century has been associated with changes in the epidemiology of malaria. At the same time, changes in vector and parasite characteristics have added yet another layer of complexity to the task of developing approaches that will finally conquer this disease.

Three factors interact to produce the complexity associated with migration and malaria:

- the parasite, vector, and immune status of the sending location and population;
- the parasite, vector, and immune status of the receiving location and population; and
- factors that operate independently of population movement to affect the growth and development of the vectors and parasites (e.g., global warming).

In this chapter, we first review each of these factors individually, then evaluate several real-world examples of how these factors have interacted to change the epidemiology of malaria. We close with our best estimates of how these factors will interact in the future to affect the status of malaria in developing and developed nations.

Migration and population movement in the developing world, particularly the origins and outcomes of rural-to-urban movement, have received much attention from demographers, planners, and policymakers, but the consequences of such movement in terms of public health have not yet been fully elucidated (Service 1989). Although changes in the incidence of an imported disease such as malaria in developed nations such as the United States often can be traced to population movement (Figure 15-1) (CDC 1996), such connections are more difficult to document in less-developed countries, particularly where malaria is endemic, because the changes are much greater and the resources for surveillance much fewer.

Indeed, any attempt to project the implications of population movement on the global malaria situation over the next 50 years necessitates a fair degree of guessing. Many

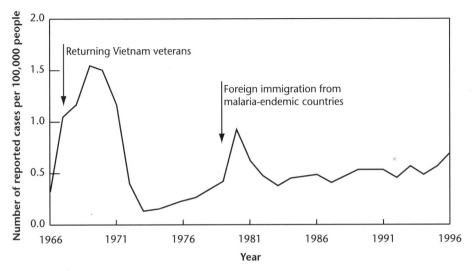

Figure 15-1. Malaria Cases by Year in the United States, 1966–1996

Note: Since 1985, approximately 1,000 cases of malaria have been reported annually in the United States; recent immigrants and visitors accounted for 50% of these cases.

Source: CDC 1996.

details must be considered, and they can interact in so many complex and frequently unforeseen ways that the best one can hope to develop is a reasonable guesstimate.

Three key factors must be evaluated in any assessment of the likely impact of population movement on malaria over the next five decades:

- the form, origin, and likely extent of population movement;
- the consequences of movement for receiving locations and populations; and
- any factors that may modify parasite and vector development and spread independent of populations.

In this chapter, we examine these factors, first discussing each factor in general, then illustrating with examples how these factors interact to produce the current consequences of population movement on malaria development, and finally integrating this information into a qualitative assessment of the likely changes in malaria distribution and importance in developing and developed nations over the next 50 years.

Background

Form, Origin, and Extent of Population Movement

In general, the two basic forms of population movement that affect the geographical spread of malaria are unidirectional and circular. Two examples of unidirectional movement include that by individuals or families who seek economic or social opportunity (e.g., settlers, transmigrants, rural-to-urban migrants, and retirees) and movement by individuals for whom migration is driven by war or environmental disaster of such magnitude that return is not possible. Examples of circular movement include seasonal migration (e.g., pastoral nomads and agricultural labor), movement for regional trade and marketing, tourism and pilgrimage, and occupation-related nonseasonal migration (e.g., returning military personnel, students, or employees).

It also is important to consider several characteristics of a particular migrant population's originating location: the degree of malaria risk, the vectors and parasites that confer that malaria risk, and the quality of and accessibility to health-care resources. Clearly, the greater the incidence of malaria in a sending location, the more likely it is that population movement from that location will change the epidemiology of malaria in the receiving location, particularly if the receiving location is relatively malaria-free. Furthermore, if the population of the sending location has some access to health-care services or vector-control programs, then it is more likely that drug-resistant forms of the parasite or pesticide-resistant vectors will be introduced or increased.

Malaria is endemic in about 100 mostly tropical and subtropical countries; it occurs in Africa, Asia, the Caribbean, Central and South America, parts of the Commonwealth of Independent States, and islands of the South Pacific (NAS 1992). High transmission areas include the border forests in South America (e.g., Brazil), Southeast Asia (e.g., Thailand and Indonesia), and most of sub-Saharan Africa (APHA 1995). Indeed, Africa is the area most threatened by malaria, partly because it has the most efficient mosquito vectors, the *Anopheles gambiae* complex (Miller 1995), and partly because it has the greatest number of poor people in remote rural areas with low population densities and poor to nonexistent health-care services—characteristics that define high-risk populations on every continent (Trigg and Wernsdorfer 1999). Indeed, 90% of the 300–500 million clinical cases and the one to three million deaths that occur yearly due to malaria occur in Africa south of the Sahara.

In terms of the extent of population movement, the world's migrant populations will very probably continue to grow, both within countries and internationally. In the mid-1990s, about 2% of the global population (125 million people) lived outside their country of birth or citizenship (Martin and Widgren 1996). The major sending regions at that time were eastern Africa, eastern and southern parts of central Asia, Southeast Asia, and Central America. Because only 20 million of these individuals, at most, were refugees and asylum seekers (Martin and Widgren 1996), the remaining more than 100 million people probably were seeking economic opportunities or were involved in business ventures—and these people are only those migrating internationally; those migrating internally are likely to represent a much larger group.

In the context of continued world population growth and development, there is every reason to believe that unidirectional movement to seek economic opportunities and circular movement due to trade, religion, education, and defense will increase over the next five decades. All of these forms of migration are directly linked to economic development or an increase in the standard of living. As the standard of living increases, more of the rural poor will move to the cities to take advantage of the resources there, and more retirees will have the resources to travel or move to locations suited to leisure pursuits (and there will be more retirees because of the graying of the population). Expansion and globalization of the world economy will bring about an increase in trade- and business-related travel (although such travel may also be somewhat reduced as a result of advances in telecommunication), and religious (e.g., pilgrimages, visits to "the promised land") and recreational travel will become affordable to a larger proportion of the population. As Keyfitz (1991) points out, "People in the middle class or higher, whether they live in developed or less developed countries … are on the move incessantly, as commuters, as vacationers, for business or for pleasure, by car, bus, and plane." Of course, increases in some of these kinds of movement are more likely than others to change the epidemiology of malaria, just as travel from some locations and under certain conditions presents greater risks.

The likely status of population movement associated with wars and environmental disasters is difficult to predict. From 1976 to 1995, the number of world refugees (often individuals displaced by wars and disasters) grew from 3 million to about 15 million. Also in 1995, the total number of "internal refugees" (who were forced from their homes and communities but still resided in their own countries) was reportedly about 12 million. In the coming decades, one hopes that rationality would prevail and the number of armed conflicts would decrease, thereby reducing the number of refugees. However, with a growing global population comes increased competition for resources, which in the past has often been equated with armed conflicts. Furthermore, weather-related natural disasters may increase, either in severity or in frequency, as a result of climate warming. As more energy is put into the system, storm surges will grow larger. This factor, coupled with an increase in the global population that tends to concentrate along waterfronts, raises the specter of ever larger storm-related disasters.

It is difficult to predict whether seasonal migrations will increase or decrease. In the case of agricultural migrants, given an expanding world population and the need for more food, one might predict an increase. However, increased automation and more productive crops may be offsetting factors if they are available at costs competitive with migrant labor and traditional crops.

Consequences for the Receiving Population

During the mid-1990s, the regions that received the most international migrants were western Europe, North America, and parts of Oceania (Australia and New Zealand)—all very developed regions without malaria. Figure 15-2 is a map that illustrates the major and minor population flows that occurred during the 1990s, with the malaria status of each receiving country and sending country identified.

The impact of population movement on the malaria epidemiology of receiving populations is likely to be quite different depending on whether those populations are in developing countries or developed countries. The developed countries have managed to eradicate malaria. Consequently, international rather than domestic travel places the developed countries at risk. However, if malaria is introduced, it is generally done at such a level that it can be managed by the surveillance, vector control, and other prevention strategies already in place. It seems unlikely that the disease would go undetected long enough to reach epidemic proportions or become established endemically.

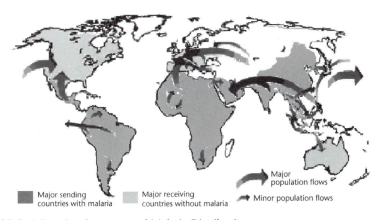

Figure 15-2. Migration Patterns and Malaria Distribution

Source: Adapted from Martin and Widgren 1996.

This last conclusion has at least one possible flaw. It relates to the housing and health-care situations for many immigrants in developed countries. As a general rule, housing for low-income foreign workers is substandard (Frey and Mammey 1996). Such populations often are very densely housed in dwellings with inadequate access to water and sanitation (NAS 1992; Turner, Swezy, and Longstreth 1992) and in locations that may contain large numbers of homeless people who sleep outdoors in warm weather, thereby providing opportunities for nighttime exposure to mosquitoes. In addition, such immigrant populations frequently have inadequate access to health care (NAS 1992) and are reluctant to seek and receive care for reasons ranging from a language barrier to fear of deportation. Furthermore, such populations are frequently served by unlicensed health-care facilities that use obsolete techniques and medicines; this factor, coupled with delays in seeking attention (Turner, Swezy, and Longstreth 1992), may contribute to the development of drug-resistant disease.

Such immigrant populations could conceivably harbor an outbreak of malaria for an extended period before it came to the attention of public health-care providers. In fact, the three most recent U.S. outbreaks occurred in such populations. Furthermore, the delay in detecting these cases was sufficient to interfere with the identification of anopheline breeding sites and adult anopheles (Zucker 1996), thus increasing the difficulty of vector-control activities and increasing the likelihood that the infection could be maintained in a particular location.

In developing countries, the effects of internal and international population movement on the epidemiology of malaria in receiving populations are likely to be quite different from those in developed nations. If the migrating population brings with it a malaria parasite not present at the receiving location, then several consequences are possible. Possible outcomes of introducing a different parasite include more severe infections (e.g., cerebral malaria), drug-resistant infections, and infections with multiple organisms (Luxemburger et al. 1996).

Interactions of Migration with Land Use Change

The development of former forests (i.e., deforestation) to provide for a growing population can both destroy and create habitat. In such cases, development may also be the factor that attracts nonimmune populations into the sphere of malaria-carrying mosquitoes. Furthermore, urban development (e.g., the building of housing developments and roads) can increase vector habitat, at least during the early stages, because excavation pits and other depressions catch water and provide breeding areas for mosquitoes.

Migration as a Contributor to Major Malaria Paradigms

Below, we present several examples of how the factors discussed above (i.e., development, poverty, population movement, and the introduction of new parasites) have interacted in the past. All the examples are taken from the developing world. Although similar instances probably occurred in the developed world before World War II, documentation of such occurrences is sparse.

Urban Malaria

The phenomenon of urban malaria is an excellent example of the manifold ways in which the epidemiology of malaria can be changed by the interaction of population movement with other factors, such as increased vector habitats and the introduction of additional vectors. In developed and developing countries, people come to cities with hopes of employment and improved standards of living. The global urban population has increased exponentially over the past 50 years. In 1950, 28% of the total population lived in cities; this percentage rose to 36–39% in 1970 and 41.6% in 1985. It was estimated that about half of the world population was living in cities as of 1989 (Service 1989); today the percentage is undoubtedly greater.

India. In India, where urban malaria has been a very important public health problem for quite some time (Kondrashin and Orlov 1985; Reuben 1989), the urban population has increased by 141.6% since 1975. At present, nearly one-third of India's population resides in cities and shanty towns. The population of Mumbai (formerly Bombay) is increasing by 350,000 people per year. As a result, every night, more than 1 million of its inhabitants sleep in the street—easy prey to malaria-bearing mosquitoes. It is not surprising, therefore, that all of India's major cities are affected by malaria.

Urban malaria in India has a different pattern than in any other part of the world. Indian urban malaria, carried by *Anopheles stephensi*, which breeds in cisterns and pits, is restricted to towns and cities, but nearby rural areas are malaria-free. Inadequate water supplies in small towns requires water storage, and in states such as Haryana, small towns have reported many malaria cases (Kondrashin 1992). The city of Chennai (formerly Madras) alone now accounts for more than half of the total malaria cases in the state of Tamil Nadu. Building sites, in which temporary cisterns are constructed by the seasonal workers who come from various parts of the country, are well-known sources of vector breeding (Reuben 1989). Urban malaria epidemics entirely due to this cause regularly occur in Mumbai, Kolkata (formerly Calcutta), and the entire state of Goa (Kondrachine 1998).

Africa. Urbanization also is accelerating very rapidly in Africa. The growth of African cities is proceeding faster than elsewhere (Service 1989). Migration is one of the main factors responsible for the urban growth. In West Africa, for example, migration may account for 40–50% of urban growth; moreover, as many as 10–20% of the people may come from neighboring countries. In Kenya, only 16.7% of population lived in towns in the 1980s, but it was expected that those living in towns would constitute 26.2% of the Kenyan population by 2000. Brazzaville, Congo, accounts for more than 500,000 people, which is about one-third of the country's population. Twenty percent of the Senegalese population is concentrated in Dakar.

At present, roughly 36% of the total African population resides in urban areas. With the growth rate of African towns averaging 6–8% a year, within two or three decades, the urban population in Africa probably will reach the level of that of South America, where more than 70% of the population lives in cities (Service 1989). Although urban malaria transmission is less well documented in Africa than in South Asia, it undoubtedly occurs in many urban centers, such as Kinshasa (Democratic Republic of the Congo), Lagos (Nigeria), Freetown (Sierra Leone), Mombasa (Kenya), Dar es Salaam (Tanzania), Ouagadougou (Burkina Faso), and Khartoum (Sudan). That said, it should be noted that urbanization generally decreases malaria transmission in large African cities relative to rural surroundings. Comparative studies in Burkina Faso in urban and rural areas indicated that inoculation rates (i.e., bites that transfer parasite) were 1–10 per person per year in urban areas and 50–200 in rural zones (Rossi et al. 1986; Esposito et al. 1988; Modiano et al. 1999). Typically, the urban center of an African town in a region of stable malaria has one-hundredth the incidence of malaria of the suburbs and periphery (personal communication from J. Mouchet, May 17, 2000).

One of the main characteristics of the transmission pattern of urban malaria in Africa is its diversity in terms of intensity of the transmission in various parts of the city. For example, in Kinshasa, at the end of the rainy season, the malaria infection rate was much higher in the more recently developed parts of the town than anywhere else because extensive excavation work at the construction sites created additional breeding places for malaria vectors (Service 1989). In Accra (Ghana), there is a well-defined distinction between malaria in people who live in slums and malaria in people who live in modern housing (Gardiner et al. 1984).

Resettlement and Development Projects

Globally, every year, more and more people are being moved and resettled. Many of them are refugees fleeing political or economic pressures. Very often, population resettlement is associated with resource development, particularly irrigation projects. Before the permanent resident population arrives, the area may be populated by construction workers, and these temporary residents may introduce malaria. A labor force also attracts other, often unexpected, people such as traders and squatters. This situation can lead to overcrowding and a deterioration in the overall health of the population.

Resettlement may involve sociocultural and economic factors as well as environmental ones. For example, bringing together people from different social, religious, and ethnic backgrounds may hinder social cohesion in settlements (Service 1989), rendering the implementation of malaria prevention and control strategies among the settlers very difficult.

Resettlement projects and occupational migration may increase in Africa over the next few decades. The probable scenario of association of that kind of population migration with the malaria problem might follow the pattern that was recently observed in Ethiopia. Various types of occupational migration in Ethiopia have occurred since the 1960s, when people from overpopulated but relatively salubrious highlands started moving toward sparsely populated lowlands, largely because of land pressure, soil exhaustion, population growth, and recurrent droughts. This pattern is consistent with the situation elsewhere in Africa, where the main motivation for migration is economic. The large highland area of Ethiopia, which constitutes 50% of all land above 2,000 meters in Africa, is associated with a highly varied topography and climate. As a rule, malaria had not occurred at this altitude by the mid-1970s (Meskal and Kloss 1989).

By 1974, 27 irrigation schemes were operated by Ethiopian and expatriate concessionaires in the Awash River valley. The scarcity of indigenous laborers and the inexperience of the local pastoral nomads as well as their reluctance to completely abandon their herding way of life for sedentary agriculture required farmers to obtain laborers from the highlands. In 1974, about 100,000 of the 250,000 people inhabiting this valley were migrant farm laborers from the highlands. In all the irrigation schemes except one, the migrants outnumbered the indigenous pastoralists. The extension of the road network into the Awash valley and provision of public transportation facilitated the movement of migrant laborers. More than 75% of all migrants were males aged 15–30 years, including married males whose families remained in the home areas, thus ensuring their return—often with malaria parasites.

Despite the intensive malaria control measures applied in the labor camps, malaria still ranked among the 10 most prevalent diseases in the valley (Demissie et al. 1977).

Malaria prevalence rates were significantly higher in all irrigation projects in the valley than in surrounding savannas, which is consistent with the findings at similar African locations (Gebre Mariam 1988; Roundy 1985; Packard 1986). Furthermore, the local pastoral nomads maintained the transmission cycle by their seasonal movement because malaria is difficult to control among highly mobile groups (Packard 1986).

Population growth in developing countries has led to government development projects that increase the lands for cultivation at the expense of the tropical forests. In Latin American countries, the area of cultivated land increased from 98 million hectares to 117 million hectares between 1970 and 1980, and it had increased to 128 million hectares by 1989. In parallel, deforestation also increased dramatically; the area of tropical forests was reduced from 998 million hectares in 1970 to 913 million hectares in 1994.

The magnitude of deforestation was particularly large in Brazil. As a result, the intensive occupation of new vital spaces by a large, growing number of susceptible individuals originally from nonmalarious areas is creating propitious conditions for the establishment of "economic frontier malaria" (Gusmão 1999). The predominant economic activities are based on small-scale, low-technology exploitation of lumber, gold, gems, and agricultural settlements. The epidemiological implication of this process has been a considerable increase in the prevalence of *Plasmodium falciparum* in the forested areas of the Andean subregion, mainly in the Amazon Basin (Gusmão 1999). Malaria transmission in this area is limited to the itinerant population because of two factors: difficult access to prompt diagnosis and immediate treatment, and risky behaviors (e.g., extraction of natural resources using low-technology means [subsistence agriculture, alluvial gold and gems mining, and timber exploitation]). Between 1994 and 1997, the population exposed to the highest risk of transmission increased from 9.8 million to 12.7 million, and the incidence of *P. falciparum* reached a high level for these areas: 1,988 cases per 100,000 exposed population (Gusmão 1999). Malaria-related implications of development and deforestation in the countries of Southeast Asia also are well documented (Sharma and Kondrashin 1991).

Occupational Migration and Malaria

Occupational migration has played a role in the epidemiology of malaria in many parts of the world. Development projects often involve the movement of workers from one location to another. In Swaziland, for instance, the combination of a development project (to provide irrigation for sugar cane production), an influx of agricultural workers (from Mozambique, where malaria was endemic), and the cancellation of malaria control measures led to a resurgence of malaria. The irrigation project provided favorable conditions for the growth of the anopheline vector, and the introduced workers were an infected population on which those vectors could feed.

Development projects are not the only reason for worker migration. In some locations, seasonal migrations are the norm because of animal husbandry or other agricultural activities. One such location is the Naya River valley in Colombia, which houses a growing population that migrates from the hills and terraces to its malarious delta. Approximately 60% of the population descend to the basin, where they cultivate and harvest their crops for four months of the year, then return to the hills the remaining eight months. Although malaria exists only in the basin, the large population density and large vector population maintain transmission (Sevilla-Casas 1993, cited in Martens and Hall 2000).

The highlands of western Kenya are another interesting example of how worker migration combined with other factors can change malaria epidemiology. They were the site of several malaria epidemics until the late 1950s. During the 1960s, the highlands were considered free of malaria, thanks to an extensive control program. Since the 1980s, however, malaria has been increasing in the region. Development and management of tea plantations required more workers than the highlands could supply. An influx of workers eventually resulted in a worker population of which approximately one-third came from the highlands, one-third came from areas where malaria was not endemic, and one-third came from areas where malaria was endemic.

Originally, all the cases of malaria were thought to have been imported, as a result of workers' annual visits to their malarious homelands. However, a recent epidemiological study of approximately 100,000 workers from the Kericho tea-growing area found that, although disease was imported, importation could not explain the increase that took place in the 1980s. Of the factors examined, changes in climate were ruled out, because weather data showed no obvious changes in average temperature or rainfall. An increase in the number of imported cases was ruled out, because the worker population had remained stable in terms of tribal and ethnic composition as well as number of employees (as indicated by the number of individuals with access to employer-provided health care) since the 1970s. Finally, changes in health care were ruled out, because the employer had maintained a high level of health care over the period.

Possible factors that could not be ruled out were increased vector habitat, brought about by the deforestation that accompanied expansion of the tea-growing area, and the development of pyrimethamine and chloroquine resistance in the malaria organism. In the latter case, it was hypothesized that incorrect use of various malaria medications had led to development of many semi-immune individuals who were symptom-free but also gametocyte carriers (Malakooti, Biomndo, and Shanks 1998).

Conclusion

The future consequences of population movement on malaria transmission and incidence will be very different depending on whether the receiving location is in the developed or the developing world.

Developing Nations

Population movement toward urban areas in Africa is likely to continue to play a dual role in the epidemiology of malaria. First, population pressure is likely to increase the rate of environmental changes that affect anopheline breeding through the preponderance of movement toward larger settlements. Second, urbanization might limit the increase of malaria in general (Bradely 1999).

On the whole, the malaria situation in African cities (and megacities in Asia and South America) will be determined by the balance achieved between two groups of factors. The first group consists of factors that might contribute to a decrease in the urban malaria problem. For example, many urban communities have better access to hospitals and doctors (in Africa, 75% of doctors and pharmacists are in the cities) than do rural communities. Malaria prevention and control programs are likely be more cost-effective in urban than in rural areas because of better information systems, higher educational and cultural levels, and easier access to international assistance.

The second group of factors are those that might contribute to an increase in the urban malaria problem. Because communal immunity is generally lower in urban communities, the malaria epidemic potential increases. International and domestic migrants carry new parasite strains with various degrees of virulence and drug resistance.

Developed Nations

The greatest concern for any developed nation vis-à-vis malaria is the reestablishment of malaria as an epidemic or endemic disease within its borders. International travel and immigration from areas where malaria is endemic ensure that cases of malaria will be imported into developed nations. Most if not all of the developed nations have competent vectors, but they are free of disease. The United States, for example, has been malaria-free since the 1950s but still has competent vectors in the 48 contiguous states. Nearly all of the U.S. cases diagnosed since the mid-1950s have been imported.

Since 1957, however, 76 reported cases do not appear to have been imported. Two of these cases were thought to be associated with recent blood transfusions, and the others appear to represent local mosquito-borne transmission. The vast majority of these cases (80%) were vivax malaria. Although cases have occasionally occurred in clusters, they never have resulted in a sufficiently large infected population to establish malaria in a continuous transmission mode (estimated to be 1,000 individuals [personal communication from D. Haile, 1989]). Most cases have been isolated or have occurred in small, well-identified groups (Zucker 1996). As such, these cases have been relatively easy to identify and manage.

Disclaimer

Opinions expressed in this chapter are the authors' only and do not necessarily reflect the policies and views of the World Health Organization.

References

APHA (American Public Health Association). 1995. *American Public Health Association Control of Communicable Diseases Manual,* edited by A.S. Benenson. Baltimore, MD: United Book Press.

Bradely, D.J. 1999. The last and the next hundred years of malariology. *Parassitologia* 41: 11–20.

CDC (Centers for Disease Control and Prevention). 1996. Summary of notifiable diseases: 1996. *Morbidity and Mortality Weekly Review* 45: 1–88.

Demissie, M., Y. Tekeste, S. Ayalew, R. Kouznetsov, and R. Somesawan Rao. 1977. Report of the External Malaria Review Team [unpublished document]. Addis Ababa, Ethiopia: Ministry of Health.

Esposito, F., S. Lombardi, D. Modiano, F. Zavala, J. Reeme, L. Lamizana, M. Coluzzi, and R.S. Nussenzweig. 1988. Prevalence and levels of antibodies to the circumsporozoite protein of *Plasmodium falciparum* in an endemic area and their relationship to resistance to malaria infection. *Transactions of the Royal Society of Tropical Medicine and Hygiene* 82: 827–832.

Frey, M., and U. Mammey. 1996. *Impact of Migration in the Receiving Countries: Germany.* Geneva, Switzerland: International Organization for Migration.

Gardiner, C., R.J. Biggar, W.E. Collins, and F.K. Nkrumah. 1984. Malaria in urban and rural areas of southern Ghana: A survey of parasitaemia, antibodies, and antimalaria practices. *Bulletin of the World Health Organization* 62: 607–613.

Gebre Mariam, N. 1988. Malaria. In *The Ecology of Health and Disease in Ethiopia,* edited by Z. Ahmed Zein and H. Kloss. Addis Ababa, Ethiopia: Ministry of Health, 136.

Gusmão, R.D. 1999. Overview of malaria control in the Americas. *Parassitologia* 41(1–3): 355–360.

Keyfitz, N. 1991. The growing human population. In *Managing Planet Earth.* New York: W.H. Freeman.

Kondrachine, A.V. 1998. Report on a Visit to Goa State of India [unpublished WHO document]. Geneva, Switzerland: World Health Organization.

Kondrashin, A.V. 1992. Malaria in WHO Southeast Region. *Indian Journal of Malariology* 29(3): 129–160.

Kondrashin, A.V., and V.S. Orlov. 1985. Malaria in Southern Asia: Migration of population in India and its role in epidemiology of malaria [in Russian]. *Meditzinskaya Parazitologia i Parazitarnie Bolezni* 2: 46.

Luxemburger, C., K.L. Thwai, N.J. White, H.K. Webster, D.E. Kyle, L. Maelankirri, T. Chong-suphajaisiddhi, and F. Nosten. 1996. The epidemiology of malaria in a Karen population on the western border of Thailand. *Transactions of the Royal Society of Tropical Medicine and Hygiene* 90: 105–111.

Malakooti, M.A., K. Biomndo, and G.D. Shanks. 1998. Reemergence of epidemic malaria in the highlands of West Kenya. *Emerging Infectious Diseases* 4(4) [online]. http://www.cdc.gov/ncidod/EID/eid.htm (accessed April 15, 2000).

Martens, P., and L. Hall. 2000. Malaria on the move: Human population movement and malaria transmission. *Emerging Infectious Diseases* 6(2): 103–109.

Martin, P., and J. Widgren. 1996. International migration: A global challenge. *Population Bulletin* 51 [online]. http://www.prb.org/bulletin.htm (accessed April 24, 2000).

Meskal, F.H., and H. Kloss 1989. Vector-borne diseases occurrence and spread as affected by labor migrations to irrigation schemes in Ethiopia. In *Demography and Vector-Borne Diseases*, edited by M.W. Service. Boca Raton, FL: CRC Press, 225–236.

Miller, L.H. 1995. Impact of malaria on genetic polymorphism and genetic diseases in Africans and African Americans. In *Infectious Diseases in an Age of Change: The Impact of Human Ecology and Behavior on Disease Transmission*, edited by B. Roizman. Washington, DC: National Academy Press.

Modiano, D., B.S. Sirima, A. Sawadogo, I. Sanou, and J. Paré. 1999. Severe malaria in Burkina Faso: Urban and rural environment. *Parassitologia* 41(1–3): 251–254.

NAS (National Academy of Sciences). 1992. *Emerging Infections: Microbial Threats to Health in the United States,* edited by J. Lederberg, R.E. Shope, and S.C. Oaks Jr. Washington, DC: National Academy Press.

Packard, R. 1986. Agricultural development, migrant labor, and the resurgence of malaria in Swaziland. *Social Science and Medicine* 22: 861.

Reuben, R. 1989. Obstacles to malaria control in India: The human factor. In *Service Book,* edited by M.W. Service. Boca Raton, FL: CRC Press, 143–154.

Rossi, P., A. Belli, L. Mancini, and G. Sabatinelli. 1986. A longitudinal entomologic survey on the transmission of malaria in Ouagadougou. *Parassitologia* 28: 1–15.

Roundy, R.W. 1985. Resettlement: A systematic overview of a diverse phenomenon and its impact on the environment and vector-borne disease transmission. Report PMO/PE/WP/85.1. Presented at the Fifth Annual Meeting Joint WHO/FAO/UNEP Panel Experts Environmental Management and Vector Control, Bangkok, Thailand.

Service, M.W. 1989. Urbanization: A hot-bed of vector-borne diseases. In *Demography and Vector-Borne Diseases,* edited by M.W. Service. Boca Raton, FL: CRC Press, 59–83.

Sevilla-Casas, E. 1993. Human mobility and malaria risk in the Naya River basin in Colombia. *Social Science and Medicine* 37: 1155–1167.

Sharma, V.P., and A.V. Kondrashin (eds.). 1991. *Forest Malaria in Southeast Asia.* New Delhi, India: Indian Council of Medical Research, Malaria Research Centre.

Trigg, P.I., and W.H. Wernsdorfer. 1999. Malaria control priorities and constraints. *Parassitologia* 41: 329–332.

Turner, M., D. Swezy, and J. Longstreth. 1992. *Potential Impacts of Global Climate Change in the U.S.: Importation/Exacerbation of Human Infectious Diseases.* Washington, DC: Office of Technology Assessment.

Zucker, J.R. 1996. Changing patterns of autochthonous malaria transmission in the United States: A review of recent outbreaks. *Emerging Infectious Diseases* 1(1) [online]. http://www.cdc.gov/ncidod/EID/eid.htm (accessed April 15, 2000).

Chapter 16

Human Population Movement
Recent Patterns

Ilya R. Fischhoff

In previous chapters, population movement has been identified as a key determinant of the spread of malaria. In this chapter, I discuss the categories and magnitude of population movement, emphasizing recent trends where possible. It is intended to be a quantitative footnote to Chapter 15.

Human mobility patterns have always been an integral component of infectious disease ecology. This factor has taken on greater importance as the magnitude, distances, and speed of human travel have greatly increased in recent centuries. People on the go bring novel parasites and vectors to their destinations, which in turn present disease agents unfamiliar to new arrivals. In addition to the interchange of people and pathogens, movement is linked with various other factors relevant to infectious disease: environmental change (e.g., deforestation, dam construction), political and economic patterns and processes (e.g., wage and employment discrepancies across borders, war), abiotic differences (e.g., temperature, precipitation), and disparities in health care and sanitation.

The effectiveness of humans as dispersal agents for infectious diseases depends partly on the mode of transmission. Pathogens spread by contact (e.g., influenza, HIV [human immunodeficiency virus]) may spread more efficiently via travelers than infectious diseases that have intermediate hosts, multistage life cycles, and restrictive environmental parameters (such as malaria). Spread of a disease via human movement is also mediated by access to health care and the immune status of potential hosts in the new location (Wilson 1995). Without discussing how travel affects malaria, I review the categories and scope of population movement, including recent trends where possible. Movements are broadly characterized by destination (domestic vs. international) and motivation (forced vs. voluntary).

Domestic Population Relocation

Internal Displacement

People forced to move within their country fall under the category of internally displaced persons (IDPs). Civil or international war, disease, famine, drought, flooding (due to weather or dam construction), and land expropriation are among the various causes of displacement. It usually is the result of conflict; less often, of natural disaster or longer-term environmental change. For example, among the 750,000 people uprooted in Colombia from 1996 to 1998, nongovernmental sources estimate that 54% were displaced due to paramilitary groups, 29% because of insurgents, and 6% because of the national military or police (Pettersson 1999). IDPs often are demographically different from the rest of their nation's population. In Africa, for example, children form the majority of many IDP populations, and women typically outnumber men (Deng 1998).

IDP populations are difficult to estimate for two reasons. First, no international agency is clearly responsible for these people. Situations that create refugees often cause even greater internal displacement. At least until recently, international recognition of IDPs associated with a refugee-creating situation has lagged one to three years behind that of refugees. The U.N. High Commissioner for Refugees (UNHCR) recently began accounting separately for IDPs but does so only if the IDPs are immediately connected to a refugee situation. The UNHCR currently considers itself responsible for 5 million IDPs. IDPs can be counted by their own government, but government inability or unwillingness may hamper the count. Many IDPs move into areas that are inaccessible to international aid organizations. Furthermore, inquiries about IDP populations may face sovereignty challenges at the national level.

Second, IDPs may move along routes similar to those they would use if moving by choice, and they may not seek help the way that refugees do. It may be unclear whether longstanding IDPs have decided to stay in their new location or intend to return to their original location when possible.

Based on data from UNHCR and the U.S. Commission for Refugees (USCR), regional IDP populations in 57 countries were estimated for 1964–1996 (Figure 16-1) (Schmeidl 1998). The numbers of IDPs have increased considerably but erratically over this period, from close to 0 in 1964 (when IDPs were essentially undocumented) to a

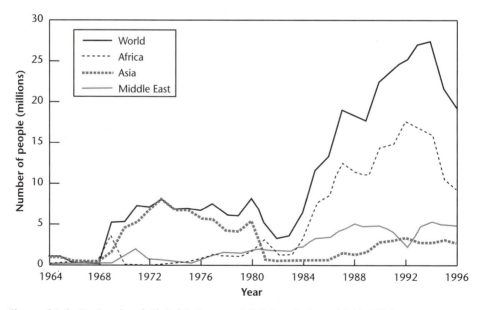

Figure 16–1. Regional and Global Estimates of IDP Populations, 1964–1996

Source: Schmeidl 1998.

Table 16-1. Change in IDP by Region, 1964–Present

	Change (%)					
Period	*Asia*	*Middle East*	*Eastern bloc*	*Latin America*	*Africa*	*Global*
1964–1970	NA	NA	NA	NA	NA	+400
1970–1980	+11	+50	NA	NA	NA	+60
1980–1990	−50	+200	NA	+1,300	+1,300	+188
1990–	−20[a]	0[a]	+67[a]	−14[a]	−24[b]	−9[b]

Note: NA = Data not available.
[a]Period: through 1996 (Schmeidl 1998).
[b]Period: through 1999 (USCR 2000).

peak of 27 million in 1994 and down to 19 million in 1996. By 1999, U.N. estimates ranged from 20 million to 25 million, and possibly as high as 30 million. The USCR (2000) has a more conservative current estimate of 21 million. Although the total number of IDPs declined in the 1990s, the number of countries with IDPs has increased to more than 50 (United Nations 1999).

As of 1996, about half of IDPs were in Africa, 20% were in the Middle East, and 10% were in Asia (Figure 16-1). Among affected nations, IDPs are distributed very unevenly: Afghanistan, Angola, and Sudan account for more than one-third of all IDPs (USCR 2000). IDP trends have been volatile, which is partly a reflection of reporting inconsistencies but also the result of real fluctuation. The percent increases in IDP populations by decade for each region and globally are listed in Table 16-1. Regional IDP ranges reflect the extent of fluctuation: 0–17 million in Africa; 0–7.5 million in Asia; 1 million to 5 million in Southwest Asia, North Africa, and the Middle East; 0–1.2 million in Latin America; and 1.5 million to 3 million in the former Eastern bloc. The former Eastern bloc nations have been the focus of growing numbers of IDPs in the past decade and now have more IDPs than Asia.

IDPs tend to remain displaced for longer periods than previously (Schmeidl 1998). The average length of displacement ranges from three years in the Eastern bloc to six years in Africa and Asia and seven years in Latin America.

Voluntary Relocation

To estimate the global volume of voluntary travel, it is necessary to piece together some fragments. Voluntary movements probably occur predominantly for "economic" reasons (e.g., education, employment, better living conditions, or access to land). In many countries, a large segment of the population moves seasonally for work (e.g., crop harvesting, herd grazing). For example, an estimated 40% of Azerbaijan's population moves annually for agricultural work (see Chapter 6).

Noneconomic motivations for travel include religious pilgrimage, family, and leisure. For example, an estimated 1.2 million Muslims currently make the Hajj to Mecca each year, supplemented by an additional 1 million pilgrims from within Saudi Arabia. Voluntary domestic military service also typically involves travel.

Domestic Air Traffic. One possible measure of voluntary travel is domestic air traffic. Domestic air traffic (including passengers, freight, and mail) increased by about 19% over the period 1990–1999 in the 185 countries reporting to the International Civil Aviation Organization (ICAO; 1999) (Figure 16-2). Domestic air traffic increased 40% in the

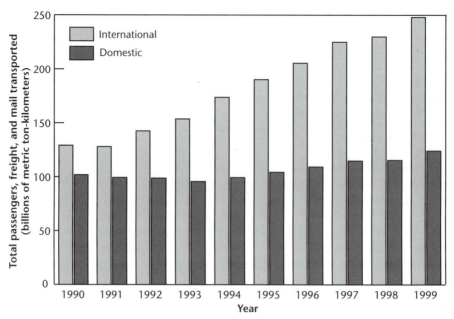

Figure 16–2. Total Passengers, Freight, and Mail Transported by Domestic and International Air Traffic (Billion Metric Ton-Kilometers), 1990–1999

Source: ICAO 1999.

United States from 1989 to 1999, according to the Air Transport Association, and travelers were projected to make 600 million domestic flights in 2000 (Leonhardt 2000; Wald 2000).

Domestic Ground Travel. Ground travel is not as well documented but at least as important as air travel, especially in less-developed countries (LDCs) and for short trips. Among nations of the U.N. Economic and Social Commission for Asia and the Pacific (ESCAP) with available data (22 of 56 nations reporting), rail travel increased 5% from 1980 to 1995 (from 679 billion to 713 billion passenger-kilometers). However, rail travel declined in 12 of the 22 countries, including all six reporting states of the former USSR (ESCAP 1998). (Some nations of the Middle East and Europe are included in ESCAP.)

Urbanization. Migration to cities is an important trend, especially in developing countries. The urban population is 75% of the total population in more-developed countries (MDCs), compared with 37% of the total population in LDCs. However, because of the absolutely greater populations of LDCs (where about 80% of all people live), 66% (1.7 billion) of the global urban population is located in LDCs and 34% (868 million) in MDCs. Among the projected 15 most populous cities in 2015, 14 are in Asia, Africa, or Latin America. Urbanization is comparatively stable in MDCs (Fornos 1997).

The global urban population has increased from 30% of the total in 1950 to 43% in 1990 and close to 50% in 2000. It increases at a rate of 2.5% per year, compared with 0.8% growth of the rural population (United Nations 1995). This difference is partly due to migration to cities, which includes both domestic and international movements. A city may include a significant population that migrates back and forth between the city and rural communities. The relative contributions of these sources to increasing urban population remain to be elucidated.

Agricultural Expansion. In some countries, especially in Southeast Asia and the Amazon Basin, people are moving to remote areas for new land and settlements. For example, the Indonesian government has sponsored the movement of an estimated 6.5 million to 8 million people to relatively sparsely populated areas (or those designated as vacant by the government). Whether such movements are wholly voluntary is unclear; displacement may be the impetus for some of these movements. In a few countries of the former Eastern bloc, people are moving out of cities and into rural areas in a process related to economic decline.

International

Involuntary

Distinguishing voluntary and involuntary international movements can be difficult. Refugees are accurately accounted for when they are concentrated and are being monitored by international agencies. People seeking asylum are counted when they seek residence in countries with tightly regulated immigration. But many people forced to leave their countries merge with those who leave by choice. Furthermore, people migrating of their own volition may have no practical alternatives (if, for example, there are no available jobs). Thus, the distinction between forced and voluntary cross-border movements is blurred. However, it is worth considering refugees as a separate category, because their living conditions and density put them at especially high risk for infectious diseases such as malaria.

Refugee populations, as recorded by UNHCR, increased globally from 6 million to 10 million, with a range of 2 million to 17 million, over the period 1964–1996 (Figure 16-3)

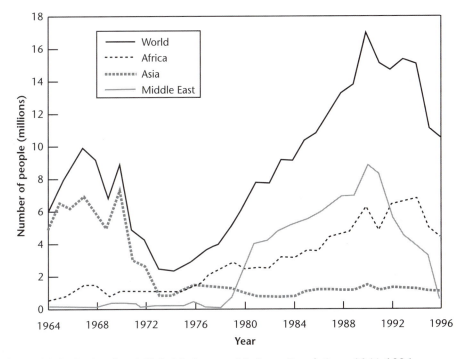

Figure 16–3. Regional and Global Estimates of Refugee Populations, 1964–1996
Source: Schmeidl 1998.

Table 16-2. Change in Refugee Populations by Region, 1964–Present

Period	Asia	Middle East	Eastern bloc	Latin America	Africa	Global
			Change (%)			
1964–1970	+40	+100	NA	+400	+100	+50
1970–1980	–86	+500	NA	–25	+100	–33
1980–1990	+50	+260	NA	+67	–50	+183
1990–	–33[a]	–61[a]	+100[a]	–80[a]	–50[b]	–18[b]

Note: NA = Data not available.

[a]Period: through 1996 (Schmeidl 1998).

[b]Period: through 1999 (USCR 2000).

(Schmeidl 1998). USCR (2000) estimated current global refugee populations at 14 million. In the first quarter of 2000, UNHCR recorded 4.8 million refugees taking asylum in 50 countries. Table 16-2 shows that, as with IDP populations, refugee numbers have fluctuated considerably over time, regionally and globally. An important recent trend has been the reduction in refugees in most regions, except for a marked increase in the former Eastern bloc. Refugees continue to be concentrated in Africa and the Middle East, each of which has about one-third the total refugee population.

When possible, refugees may seek residence in distant countries. Australia, the European Union, Japan, New Zealand, and North America received about 5 million asylum seekers between 1990 and 1996. Figure 16-4 shows the extensive variation in numbers of people seeking asylum in 10 major refugee destinations in North America and Europe over the 1990s.

In addition to people categorized as refugees, the USCR has documented 5.38 million people who are effectively but not officially refugees. These people are ignored or tolerated, are declared stateless or illegal aliens, or live in countries without "credible refugee determination procedures." Such refugee-like populations include 2 million Afghans in Pakistan and 140,000 stateless Kurds in Syria.

Voluntary

People choose to travel abroad for employment (temporary or permanent), military service, family, or leisure. Permanent emigration from MDCs to LDCs is much less common than the reverse. The relative importance of business and tourism travel from MDCs to LDCs is not well known. Globalization has increased business ties, and tropical countries have become popular vacation destinations.

One primary reason for migration from LDCs to MDCs is population pressure and underemployment in LDCs. Siem (1992) estimates that 70 million people, most from LDCs, work abroad annually.

Tourists and Visitors. Movement between Europe and LDCs has increased markedly, as reported by Sabatinelli (Chapter 6, Figures 6-8 and 6-9). Among 17 of 27 countries of the Organisation for Economic Co-operation and Development (OECD) reporting, 80% of 300.4 million visitors or tourists to OECD nations were from non-OECD nations (OECD 1997). These data indicate that the majority of travelers to the OECD were from LDCs.

Foreign tourists and visitor arrivals increased by 41% among 14 reporting OECD nations (Australia, Canada, France, Greece, Iceland, Ireland, Italy, Japan, New Zealand,

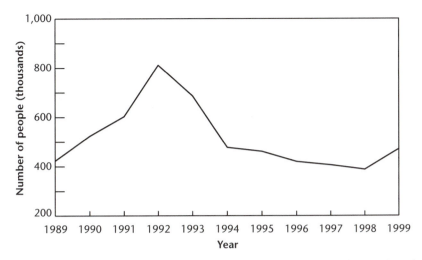

Figure 16–4. People Seeking Asylum in Select Destination Countries (Belgium, Canada, Denmark, France, Germany, the Netherlands, Sweden, Switzerland, United Kingdom, and the United States), 1989–1999

Source: USCR 2000.

Portugal, Switzerland, Turkey, United Kingdom, and the United States) from 1984 to 1995, from 286 million to 403 million people. In Asia, among 26 of 56 nations associated with the U.N. Economic and Social Commission for Asia and the Pacific, tourist and visitor arrivals increased 445% from 1980 to 1995, from 16.9 million to 91.8 million people (ESCAP 1998). Tourist and visitor arrivals to North America (excluding Mexico) increased 26% from 1984 to 1990, from 61.8 million to 77.6 million people; tourist arrivals in North America (including Mexico) increased 20% from 1990 to 1995, from 142 million to 170 million people (OECD 1997).

Migrants. International migrants, making longer or permanent moves, are about evenly split in their destinations between LDCs (54%) and MDCs (46%) but unevenly distributed within these two categories. Among LDCs, international migrants are concentrated in countries with labor-intensive natural resource extraction (e.g., diamonds in parts of Africa, oil in the Middle East) or manufacturing.

Among MDCs, seven wealthy nations—Canada, France, Germany, Italy, Japan, United Kingdom, and the United States—contain one-third of all migrants. In general, people making long-term moves are more likely to be going from LDCs to MDCs. From 1990 to 1995, Africa, Asia, and Latin America had net losses of migrants while Europe, North America, and Oceania (specifically Australia and New Zealand) had net gains (Table 16-3) (Martin and Widgren 1996).

International Air Traffic. Air traffic data show the scale and growth of international travel. The World Trade Organization estimated 657 million international air travelers in 1999, compared with about 460 million in 1990—a 40% increase for the decade. By another measure, international traffic increased 88% from 1990 to 1999, from 130 billion to 245 billion metric ton-kilometers (Figure 16-2).

In addition to travel on regularly scheduled commercial airlines, ICAO estimates an increase in unscheduled international air traffic from about 190 billion passenger-kilo-

Table 16-3. Average Annual International Migration by Region, 1990–1995

Region	Average annual net migration	
	Net no. of migrants (× 1,000)	Rate (per 1,000 people)
Sending regions		
Africa	−63	−0.1
Eastern	−128	−0.6
Central	+4	+0.1
Northern	+69	+0.5
Southern	+2	+0.04
Western	−10	−0.1
Asia	−1,366	−0.4
Eastern	−171	−0.1
South Central	−661	−0.5
Southwestern	−485	−1.1
Western	−46	−0.3
Latin America	−392	−0.9
Caribbean	−99	−2.9
Central America	−202	−1.7
South America	−91	−0.3
Receiving regions		
Europe	+739	+1.0
Eastern	−109	−0.4
Northern	+47	+0.5
Southern	−20	−0.1
Western	+821	+1.6
North America	+971	+3.4
Oceania	+111	+4.0
Australia and New Zealand	+122	+5.8
Other Oceania	−11	−1.7

Source: Martin and Widgren 1997.

meters in 1990 to 265 billion passenger-kilometers in 1999 (also a 40% increase). Certain regions serve as air traffic hubs. Of the 25 largest airports, through which 1,045 million passengers traveled in 1999, 17 are in North America, 5 in Europe, and 3 in Asia (ICAO 1999).

International Ground Travel. International ground travel is not well documented, but the available data suggest its importance. For example, data from China's Yunnan border with the Lao People's Democratic Republic and Myanmar indicate extensive travel back and forth. In 1996, 20 million people crossed official checkpoints in that region; about equal numbers of Chinese left and foreigners entered China (Kidson et al. 1999). Additional people moved across the border through unofficial channels.

It is unclear whether this situation represents an extreme case or whether proportional numbers cross at open borders in other regions. Even where borders are relatively closed, illegal and uncounted legal migration can be significant. For example, an estimated 300,000 people illegally cross into the United States annually, most through Mexico; however, these migrations constitute less than 10% of the 4 million illegal migrants in the United States, most of whom are on lapsed visas (Martin and Widgren 1997).

Human Movement and Malaria

Population movement—especially labor, development, and conflict-related migrations—has been associated with malaria epidemics and spread of disease resistance in developing countries. The acceleration of international travel between developed and developing countries generally has not led to the reestablishment of malaria in places from which it had been eradicated (see Chapter 15), despite sometimes heavy case loads from immigrants and returning soldiers. However, there are possible exceptions to this rule, including resurgent malaria associated with returning troops in Korea and Turkey. The E.U. countries currently treat more than 10,000 imported malaria cases annually. In the United States, more than 1,000 such cases are treated each year.

Population mobility is thus a risk factor for malaria predicated on the quality of the public health establishment of the receiving country. In the developing world, voluntary and involuntary population displacements represent increased public health challenges, the response to which is the dominant determinant of malaria risk.

Conclusion

Human movements within and across borders have increased greatly, with important implications for the incidence and range of malaria and other infectious diseases. Table 16-4 summarizes the trends in some of the major categories of moving populations: IDPs, domestic air traffic, refugees, and international visitors and tourists. The picture is fragmented but shows growth in almost all categories. Voluntary movements have consistently increased, both regionally and globally. Domestic and international air traffic rose 19% and 40%, respectively, from 1990 to 1999. Tourism increased to Asia, Europe,

Table 16-4. Change in Number of Travelers

	Change (%)							
Type of traveler	Asia	Middle East	Eastern bloc	Europe	North America	Latin America	Africa	Global
IDP[a]	+100	+433	+66	NA	NA	+1,100	+1,700	+1,800
Domestic air traffic[b]	NA	NA	NA	NA	+40	NA	NA	+19
Refugees[c]	−80	+1,300	+75	NA	NA	−33	+900	+66
International arrivals[d]	+445	NA	NA	+21	+39	NA	NA	NA

Note: NA = Data not available.

[a]Period: 1964–1996 for Asia, Middle East, Eastern bloc, and Latin America; 1964–1999 for Africa and Global (Schmeidl 1998; USCR 2000).

[b]Period: 1990–1999 for North America and Global (ICAO 1999; Leonhardt 2000).

[c]Period: 1964–1996 for Asia, 1970–1996 for Middle East, 1991–1996 for Eastern bloc, 1981–1996 for Latin America, 1976–1999 for Africa, 1964–1999 for Global.

[d]Period: 1980–1995 for Asia; 1984–1995 for Europe (nine countries of the Organisation for Economic Co-operation and Development) and North America (Canada and the United States) (OECD 1996; ESCAP 1998).

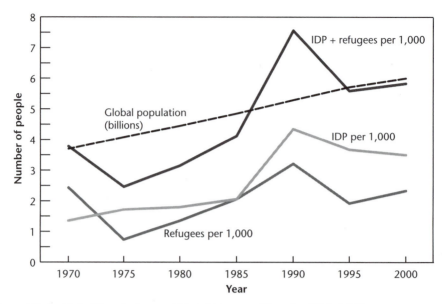

Figure 16–5. Global Population and Global Uprooted People, 1970–1999

Source: Schmeidl 1998; USCR 2000.

and North America. Permanent migration rates have, no doubt, also increased, but they are not as well documented.

The number of uprooted people (IDPs and refugees) increased fivefold from 1964 to the present, from 7 million to 35 million. Figure 16-5 shows that the rate of growth of populations of IDPs, refugees, and all uprooted people (IDPs and refugees) has increased at roughly the same rate as global population but with much greater variance. It indicates that the fraction of displaced people increases with global population. There are currently 14 million refugees and at least 21 million IDPs. During the past year, 7 million people were newly uprooted (USCR 2000). The problem of uprooted people is widespread; at last count, 96 countries have either produced or are host to uprooted people.

Population movements are variable and sensitive to world events, making it difficult to predict future trends from recent data. However, it is reasonable to expect that all types of population movement will continue to increase, as global population rises to a projected plateau in this century.

References

Deng, F. 1998. *Workshop on Internal Displacement in Africa.* http://www.brook.edu/fp/projects/idp/ conferences/contents.htm (accessed June 2000).

ESCAP (U.N. Economic and Social Commission for Asia and the Pacific). 1998. *Asia and the Pacific in Figures 1998.* UN ESCAP Statistics Division. http://www.unescap.org accessed June 2000).

Fornos, W. 1997 *World Population Overview.* http://www.populationinstitute.org (accessed June 2000).

ICAO (International Civil Aviation Organization). 1999. *Annual Report of the Council 1999.* http:// www.icao.int/cgi/goto.pl?icao/en/pub/rp99_c1.pdf (accessed June 2000).

Kidson, C., P. Singhasivanon, and S. Supavej (eds.). 1999. Mekong malaria: Malaria, multi-drug resistance, and economic development in the greater Mekong subregion of Southeast Asia (incorporating Geographical Information Systems databases). *Southeast Asian Journal of Tropical Medicine and Public Health* 30(Suppl. 4).

Leonhardt, D. 2000. Promises in the sky. *New York Times,* June 25, Travel 13.

Martin, P., and J. Widgren. 1996. International migration: A global challenge. *Population Bulletin* 51 [online]. http://www.prb.org (accessed June 2000).

OECD (Organisation for Economic Co-operation and Development). 1997. *Tourism Policy and International Tourism in OECD Countries, 1997 Edition.* http://www.oecd.org/ dsti/sti/transpor/ tourism/prod/e_97–173.htm (accessed June 2000).

Pettersson, B. 1999. *Internal Displacement in Colombia: Summary Report of the Workshop on Implementing the Guiding Principles on Internal Displacement.* Washington, DC: Brookings Institute. http://www.brook.edu/fp/projects/idp/conferences/contents.htm (accessed June 2000).

Schmeidl, S. 1998. Comparative trends in forced displacement: IDPs and refugees 1964–1996. *Internally Displaced People: A Global Survey.* London, U.K.: Earthscan. http://www.nrc.no/ global_idp_survey/internally_displaced_people/schmeidl.htm#schmeidl (accessed June 2000).

Siem, H. 1992. Migration and Health in 1990s. *International Migration* 30: 3–8.

United Nations. 1995. *World Urbanization Prospects.* New York: United Nations Publications.

———. 1999. *Internally Displaced Persons.* Note from the Secretary General. A/54/409. http:// www.brook.edu/fp/projects/idp/unreports.htm (accessed June 2000).

USCR (U.S. Commission for Refugees). 2000. *World Refugee Survey 2000.* http://www.refugees.org (accessed June 2000).

Wald, M. 2000. Getting there: A reality check. *New York Times,* June 25, Travel 12.

Wilson, M. 1995. Travel and the emergence of infectious diseases. *Emerging Infectious Diseases* 1: 39–46.

Chapter 17

Malaria Control and the Future of International Public Health

Socrates Litsios

Malaria control depends on the presence of certain essential public health functions. Health services systems in tropical malarious countries, following health models of the industrialized world, have not developed a public health capacity adequate for malaria control. To control malaria under current conditions requires an international response, one that builds national public health capacities capable of fully supporting local initiatives. In this chapter, my purpose is to explore the history of malaria control and public health in the twentieth century to bring to light certain critical features of the current situation that must be recognized and attended to before any agenda for the future can be placed on a solid foundation.

In a general sense, the fight against malaria has always been and will no doubt always be an instance of "public health." However, there has never been a consensus concerning just exactly what is meant by "control." In the early part of the twentieth century, control was generally taken to mean a reduction, if not elimination, of malaria transmission. This position helps explain why the League of Nations Conference in 1937, when it addressed malaria, pointed out that "the distribution of anti-malaria drugs ... is not so much malaria control as an alleviation of acute disease with reduction of mortality" (League of Nations 1937). Today, the reduction of mortality is seen as a legitimate goal for control programs to pursue. Nevertheless, the sentiment remains that control involves more than the diagnosis and treatment of malaria; in particular, it also should include the detection and containment of epidemics and the prevention of transmission where likelihood is strong that such action will reduce the incidence of disease and mortality (WHO 1993).

Where and when malaria was "king of the diseases," it was the most important public health problem present. Midway through the twentieth century, many looked to malaria control as an essential building block for the control of other diseases of public health importance. Instead, the eradication of malaria was attempted by an independent, vertical approach that kept malaria outside the mainstream of public health development. Once the great burden of malaria was dramatically reduced, it lost its priority. Today, it is seen by many as but one disease among others.

When malaria came back to the fold, so to speak, in the 1970s, most health systems where malaria was present were in a state of crisis that since has deepened. Instead of confronting the fact that public health infrastructures are lacking in most countries of the world where malaria is a major problem, malaria control has remained hostage to the idea that such infrastructures will be developed. Consequently, the reality today is that malaria control may be even less possible than it was 30 years ago. Confounding the problem even further is the fact the model health services system advocated by World Health Organization (WHO) initially grew out of the experiences of the industrialized countries and, later, from those of nontropical ones. These models largely ignored the special needs of malaria control under tropical conditions and consequently may be totally unsuitable for meeting such needs.

To justify these conclusions, I review the development of both malaria control and public health throughout the twentieth century. Because malaria control and public health have largely evolved along independent lines, I present the topics separately. Next, I review the past relationship between malaria control and public health. Most of this discussion is conceptual in nature, because little current practice exemplifies malaria control in the context of a national public health service. From this historical and functional review, several major deficiencies are identified, from which strategies for the future are suggested. A brief conclusion follows.

Malaria Control during the Twentieth Century

The global malaria eradication campaign was officially launched in 1955 and came to an unofficial end in 1969. Thus, the twentieth century can be seen as consisting of three periods: before, during, and after global eradication. None of these periods were homogenous in experience. Nevertheless, the global campaign was quite unlike what had preceded it, and the posteradication period, in which we still find ourselves, was radically altered by the earlier assumptions of the possibility of eradication.

Preeradication Era: 1900–1954

Prior to Ronald Ross' discoveries in 1898, the only sure method available to reduce the burden of malaria was the use of quinine, although the association of malaria with certain nefarious ground and wind conditions had led some towns and areas in Europe to attempt to control malaria by various environmental means, with occasional satisfactory results (Najera 1994). Ross' work opened up two new points of attack: reduction of mosquito numbers through larval and adult destruction, and reduction or elimination of contacts between man and the *Anopheles* mosquito (Bynum and Overy 1998). Although Ross was inclined toward a direct attack on the mosquito, Italian malariologists led by Giovanni Grassi and Angelo Celli explored all three possibilities during the early decades of the twentieth century, with varying degrees of success (Fantini 1998).

Ross was supremely confident that his work had opened the way for malaria to be controlled, if not fully eliminated. Before leaving India in February 1899, he wrote to Patrick Manson, "It is evident that the study of malaria has now entered on the third and last phase—prevention." He distinguished five classes of measures: public, isolated communities, medical men, travelers, and general private. He divided public measures into towns, rural areas, and general. With the exception of malaria cases that were to be "isolated in nets (with) treatment to be continued sufficiently long after the fever has ceased," all measures were directed against the mosquito. He also recognized that "little can be done in rural areas" (Bynum and Overy 1998).

Others soon joined Ross and the Italians in the battle against malaria, notably, William Gorgas, Sir Malcolm Watson, and Nicolaas Swellengrebel (Litsios 1996). Gorgas "conquered" malaria in the Panama Canal Zone; Watson achieved outstanding results in very specific plantation and mining conditions; Swellengrebel demonstrated the possibility of species sanitation, that is, altering the natural environment in such a way as to destroy the breeding of malaria-carrying anophelines (Takken et al. 1990; Bradley 1994). Nevertheless, whatever dream Ross and other early malariologists may have had that antivector work would eradicate malaria proved to be of very short duration, if it ever really existed at all. Even Gorgas and Watson, who achieved remarkable results in economically important areas and whose budgets were orders of magnitude greater than what could be expected to be available under "normal" circumstances, never eliminated malaria.

There was no escaping the fact that resources available for malaria control in typical rural areas of the tropics were totally insufficient. Furthermore, malaria was so intertwined with poverty that many malariologists concluded that its control depended on overall social and economic development (Litsios 1996). Paul Russell, commenting in 1936 on the situation in India, noted, "the ordinary rural community in India could not be expected to spend more than two and a half cents per capita per annum for malaria prophylaxis, yet malaria has never been controlled in such areas for less than twenty cents per capita per year and seldom for so little" (Russell 1936). What to do under such circumstances was one of the major questions discussed during a conference on rural hygiene organized by the League of Nations in Bandoeng, Indonesia, in 1937 (League of Nations 1937). Russell chaired the malaria technical working group.

To reduce costs for rural communities the conference recommended that "every effort be made (a) to extend the free distribution of *cinchona* products, (b) to enlist the aid of the people themselves in minor control methods, and (c) to explore cheaper methods of control which use time more than money." Of particular note is the conclusion that "persistence rather than perfection in control is required for rural areas." The so-called naturalistic methods were highlighted. Research was needed to obtain "a much more definite understanding of the relationship between malaria, malnutrition, famine, and poverty … as well as further elucidation of the factors concerned in malarial immunity." Also needed was "a good deal more investigation … to develop practical mosquito-nets for rural areas in the tropics" (League of Nations 1937).

Representative of this pre-DDT era were the conclusions reached by John Grant concerning malaria in rural India. A longtime (1917–1962) staff member of the International Health Division of the Rockefeller Foundation, Grant was "lent out" to be director of the All-India Institute of Hygiene and Public Health in Calcutta from 1939 to 1945. During that period, he played an important part in shaping the Bhore Committee recommendations concerning India's medical education and health-care systems. He judged in 1941 that malaria control could not be undertaken "solely through cash purchase," as it had been in Panama. But "considerable protection [could] be secured in Bengal provided there were education, organization, and methodology developed whereby citizens provided themselves with protection through local voluntary effort" (Grant 1963b).

With the arrival of DDT, as noted by the first WHO Expert Committee on Malaria in 1947, there was "at last a method of controlling malaria in many areas at costs within the economic means of the people" (WHO 1947). Expert committees are convened by WHO to give advice on technical and scientific matters. In the early years of the organization, the decision to convene a committee to address a particular subject reflected the priority being given to that subject by the WHO governing bodies.

In its first program statement concerning malaria, the WHO secretariat indicated that "the ultimate aim for WHO can, and should be, the eradication of malaria from the world" (WHO 1949a). Immediate aims, however, were confined to promotion, demonstration, and showing "the indirect benefits derived from malaria control, both with regard to public health in general and to increased agricultural or man-labour production." Methods to achieve these aims included, among others, "an attack on the problem of African malaria with a view to opening up the continent to large-scale development" and "the planning and carrying out, in collaboration with the U.N. Food and Agriculture Organization (FAO), of broad-scale programs of malaria control, of public-health improvements and of overall rural rehabilitation in large areas." These two points no doubt reflected the real sentiment, which stems from the conclusions of the Bandoeng conference, that the economic feasibility of malaria control was dependent on its socioeconomic importance.

The "economic importance of malaria in Africa" was one of the subjects discussed at the November 1950 Malaria Conference in Equatorial Africa (WHO 1951b). There, it was noted that "information relating to the economic importance of malaria in Africa is small and not always reliable." This was considered "the main cause of the lack of a unanimous consensus of opinion with regard to the appraisal of the effect of this most prevalent African disease on the distribution of population, on population movements, on demographic trends, on agriculture, industry, and transportation, education, and social welfare." The report highlighted in summary form the relationship seen to be present between malaria and these socioeconomic factors.

Although a joint effort on food production and malaria control had started between FAO and WHO in 1948, by 1953 it was no longer being pursued (Litsios 1997a). It collapsed for a combination of reasons. Suffice it to say, the cold war was probably enough to have killed it, although evidence suggests that the FAO secretariat would have dragged out the relationship long enough to have caused it to fail as well. Also, the fact that malaria control clearly stimulated rapid population growth placed in jeopardy the calculus of the malaria–economic development hypothesis. These factors contributed to the decision soon taken to drop intermediate objectives and to seek the aim of global eradication.

Eradication Era: 1955–1969

One aspect of the eradication era is worth noting for the purposes of this chapter. It relates to the generally accepted role of the health services to maintain eradication wherever it had been achieved. In 1960, WHO proposed the idea of preeradication projects, that is, building up the health services to the point where they could take over eradication in its final stages (Najera 1989). This proposal was driven in part by the large number of newly created African states that pressured WHO to extend the global eradication program to include the African continent.

Some eradicationists saw no role for the health services. Fred L. Soper—seen by many as almost single-handedly having forced WHO to undertake an eradication campaign—led this group (Litsios 2000). His position was rather simple: Eradication depended on steadily increasing the area where it was achieved until it covered the whole globe, or major regions of the globe. WHO, however, stressed the role of the health services in safeguarding whatever degree of eradication had been achieved, even if it were only confined to a national or subnational level. Soper argued that this approach doomed the campaign, because there were not enough resources to simultaneously pursue global eradication and develop health services capable of carrying out the epidemiological surveillance required to maintain eradication on a limited basis.

Soper's position was never expressed clearly in any public setting, as far as I am aware. Only in his diary notes did he express himself in unambiguous terms, as in this entry of May 4, 1964:

> I refuse to be pessimistic regarding the future ... the measures which are building up will eventually force the World Health Organization to abandon the Alvarado, Gonzales proposal for rural health infrastructures and will lead to the development of more highly specialized malaria eradication efforts with adequate technical and administrative support for efficient and honest services. (Soper 1964)

(Alvarado was director of WHO's Division of Malaria Eradication, having taken over that responsibility in November 1958 on Pampana's retirement, and Gonzales was the senior consultant who prepared the 1964 study group report concerning the integration of mass campaigns.)

Soper couched his public criticism in such vague terms as to make one doubt if even those sympathetic with his position were fully aware as to how strongly he was opposed to the manner in which WHO was engaging the eradication campaign. This possibly accounts for the fact that the debates that took place in the 1960s concerning the feasibility of eradication make no reference to his position.

Had such debates taken place, public health generalists would have learned not only that there was a major division in the eradication camp but also that the role of the health services in malaria control was a difficult, even controversial, subject of major importance. They would have learned, for example, that Arnoldo Gabaldón, who was responsible for the establishment of the first WHO Expert Committee on Malaria in 1946 and who had participated in almost all of its first 15 sessions, approached the question of malaria eradication in a manner that antagonized both Soper and WHO (Litsios 1998). He neither sought total eradication throughout all of Venezuela, nor did he rely at all on the general health services to maintain what the eradication program had achieved. Instead, he concentrated on controlling transmission using antivector methods. He went so far as to consider spraying as "natural" a public health measure as periodic vaccination.

Such a debate might have caused the eradication campaign to come to an end earlier. In any case, it would have led to discussions as to what role the health services, as such, had in malaria control. Lacking such a debate, the prevailing view well into the 1970s concerning the role of the health services was to see them solely in terms of protecting what had been obtained by the earlier eradication campaign. Those who favored the basic health services (BHS) were willing to accept this responsibility as the price that had to be paid to gain the upper hand over vertical campaigns. But the price paid was an unfortunate one, because the need to safeguard the gains of the eradication campaign placed the yet-to-exist services in a no-win situation. Instead of building services with the capacity to control disease outbreaks, attention was given to case detection by active and passive means, that is, the means advocated by the campaign for maintaining eradication gains. When malaria eradication campaigns were "integrated" with such services, outbreaks inevitably occurred that forced the return to specialized transmission control efforts.

Posteradication: 1969–Present

The transition from eradication to control did not occur quickly. Strictly speaking, the 1969 World Health Assembly (WHA) had not recommended the stoppage of eradication campaigns. On the contrary, it urged governments "to ensure the successful implementation of the [eradication] programmes" (WHO 1973b). Only in the 1975 and 1976 executive board and WHA resolutions can one clearly see the shift; for example, the 57th executive board meeting in January 1976 requested the director general "to assist countries to develop more realistic and flexible approaches in antimalaria programmes adapted to the different epidemiological and socioeconomic conditions" (WHO 1985a). Similarly, it was the last of the three Expert Committees that met in the 1970s—that is, the 17th Expert Committee in 1979—that was the first committee in which eradication, per se, was not discussed; control was its exclusive preoccupation (WHO 1979).

Around the time of the 1979 Expert Committee meeting, two of its participants, Mohyeddin Farid (an expert) and Leonard Bruce-Chwatt (a consultant), wrote revealing papers on the subject. Farid's (1980) was entitled "The malaria programme: From euphoria to anarchy," and Bruce-Chwatt's (1978) was entitled "The challenge of malaria: Crossroads or impasse?" Farid, a retired WHO malariologist who had worked with Soper in the 1940s, believed that the "goal of global malaria eradication—in its revised form—must be maintained" (a position that Russell totally agreed with in his comments on Farid's paper). Bruce-Chwatt, also a retired WHO malariologist, was less inclined to revert to the past. Nevertheless, he characterized the 1969 WHA decision as "the great leap sideways" and pointed out several critical issues associated with the newly accepted goal of control:

1. What degree of malaria, in terms of morbidity and mortality, is "acceptable"?
2. How can it be delineated where control should concentrate, especially in light of the fact that "beyond a certain degree of endemicity the adverse clinical and socioeconomic effects of malaria are directed not at the whole indigenous community but primarily at its youngest age-groups"?
3. How could a "great deal of steady devotion to a very distant goal" be obtained?
4. Should malaria control remain a "vertical target-oriented mass campaign," or should its responsibility be "transferred to the basic health services"?
5. How will the shortage of technically competent international and national staff be overcome?
6. Of greatest importance, would the technical and financial assistance that had so characterized the eradication era continue?

Much of WHO's activities in the years that followed can be seen as responding to these questions, particularly points 2 and 5. A major international training program was initiated in the early 1980s that has organized courses at national, regional, and international levels in all aspects of malaria control. With respect to point 2, considerable efforts have been undertaken to refine epidemiological information and evaluation systems that can be used to delineate where and what kind of malaria control should be undertaken. This has helped clarify issues related to point 1.

Point 6 has been addressed by the development of a global strategy for malaria control, which led to the adoption of the Amsterdam World Declaration on the Control of Malaria in 1992 (WHO 1993) and the more recent Roll Back Malaria initiative (Roll Back Malaria Partnership 1999). Point 4 has been addressed by all of the last five Expert Committees on Malaria that have convened since 1980. Point 3, however, has received far less attention. It is this point that has plagued many campaign efforts that are organized and carried out under the prevailing system of national health services. I will return to this important point later.

Public Health during the Twentieth Century

To facilitate an understanding of the parallel histories of malaria control and public health, this section covers the whole of the twentieth century, divided into approximately the same three time periods as above.

1900–1954

At the end of the nineteenth century, two different views existed concerning the control of epidemic disease, one old and one new (Litsios 2001a). The old view dated back to the Hippocratic ideas of "miasmas" and "epidemic constitution" in which disease was seen as intimately linked with the quality of the natural environment (i.e., air, water, and soil). The sanitary movement, which had taken place earlier in the century, largely was based on this view of disease causation. The new view grew out of the Pasteurian revolution, that all epidemic diseases were understood to have a microbial origin.

During the initial part of this period, the United States rapidly oriented its budding public health systems to incorporate the latest microbial developments, which were mostly emanating from European laboratories, particularly those in France and Germany. These same countries were slower than the United States to use antimicrobial methods, such as regular immunization against diphtheria (Newsholme 1932). Instead, Europe favored sanitary measures, improved diet, and the development of specialized hospitals for the different infectious diseases, such as fever hospitals.

Stimulated by the financing of private foundations, the United States took the lead in the development and promotion of public health during and immediately following World War I. This lead regressed as the private medical sector in the United States squelched further developments, particularly those related to developing a nationalized, compulsory health insurance system. Meanwhile, public health reestablished itself in Europe after the war and continued to develop along progressive lines. A common feature across the entire industrialized world was the rapidly growing importance given to the control of chronic illness and disability, a shift that relegated the infectious diseases to a much lower priority than they held earlier. In so doing, the center of gravity of public health efforts moved from community-based action toward individual care, especially preventive medical care. This brief, nutshell summary is expanded upon below.

Social reformers led the nineteenth-century sanitary movement in Europe. Differing somewhat from country to country, these reformers shared the desire to bring about broad economic and social change in order to break the link between poverty and disease. In England, for example, epidemic diseases were believed to be caused by environmental filth. Prevention was pursued by the provision of clean water supplies as well as effective sewerage and drainage; the removal of nuisances, such as refuse from all streets and roads; the control of industrial effluents; and the establishment of new standards of environmental and personal cleanliness (Fee and Porter 1991).

The United States was slow to take up the sanitary movement but quick to make practical use of the latest antimicrobial methods emerging from Europe's laboratories. William T. Sedgwick, a biologist with the Massachusetts State Board of Health, noted, "Before 1880 we knew nothing; after 1890, we knew it all; it was a glorious ten years" (Fee 1987). The period 1890 to 1910 marked "the start of an era that brought greater changes in medicine and medical practice than at any other time in (American) history" (Duffy 1990).

Stimulated by the promise and early accomplishments of the microbial revolution, Charles V. Chapin, chief medical officer for Providence, Rhode Island, argued in 1911 that health departments need no longer be responsible for social, economic, and environmental measures, because a clean environment "will make no demonstrable difference in a city's mortality." More important is to "learn the nature and mode of transmission of each infection [to] discover its most vulnerable point of attack" (Chapin 1934). Chapin used this philosophy to launch what became known then as "the new public health" (Rosenkrantz 1972). He brought together the new knowledge concerning infectious diseases in his book, *Sources and Modes of Infection*. In 1925, Carlos Chagas said that this book "still remains the most complete and most impartial documentary statement of our knowledge concerning the life and virulence of pathogenic microbes in the external world" (Winslow 1943).

The new knowledge concerning infectious diseases led the Rockefeller family to enter the field of medicine in 1901, when the Rockefeller Institute for Medical Research was established (Fosdick 1952). It was followed in 1907 with the creation of the Rockefeller Sanitary Commission, which launched a hookworm eradication campaign in the southern United States from 1909 to 1914 (Ettling 1981). This initiative brought to light the lack of suitably trained health workers to lead state and county health services. Public health schools were required to meet this need. The nucleus of such schools was seen to be an institute of hygiene, which should be autonomous but closely affiliated with a university and its medical school (Fosdick 1952). The first such school was the School of Hygiene and Public Health at Johns Hopkins University. It was built and endowed by the Rockefeller Foundation, and it opened in 1918.

The Rockefeller Foundation envisioned that the school would be used primarily for the training of low-level public health workers—those needed to fill positions in state health departments. William H. Welch thought otherwise. He successfully obtained the financial support of the foundation while establishing a school whose prime strength lay in research and the provision of "high-level education for an elite corps of public health professionals" (Fee 1987). Other medical schools that sought but did not receive support from the Rockefeller Foundation, including Columbia and Harvard, were more interested in the practical sides of public health, including social and economic reform. However, they were judged to have medical schools so oriented to private practice as to jeopardize the long-term survival of an independent school dedicated to the promotion of public health aims. So strong was the Harvard Medical School that it effectively blocked the creation of what would have been the first independent school of tropical medicine in the United States (Curran 1970). Johns Hopkins was different; there, the full-time medical professors were committed to research and teaching rather than to private practice. As a point of contrast, it is interesting to note that the London and Liverpool Schools of Tropical Medicine, which opened in 1898, had no formal affiliation with any medical school or university (Wiebe 1967).

With the establishment of new and largely independent institutions committed to the cause of public health, the vision of public health expanded much beyond its early sanitary orientation. Charles-E.A. Winslow defined public health in the following broad and sweeping manner:

Public health is the science and art of preventing disease, prolonging life, and promoting physical health and efficiency through organized community efforts for the sanitation of the environment, the control of communicable infections, the education of the individual in personal hygiene, the organization of medical and nursing services for the early diagnosis and preventive treatment of disease, and the development of social machinery to ensure to every individual a standard of living adequate for the maintenance of health, so organizing these benefits as to enable every citizen to realize his birthright of health and longevity. (Winslow 1923)

In practice, public health differed from county to county. Numerous projects were undertaken with the support of different foundations to help establish model county programs, especially in the rural areas. The Milbank Memorial Fund sponsored one such project in Cattaraugus County of New York State, with a population of around 75,000. This project, which met with Winslow's full approval, incorporated a county health unit, a school health service, a nursing program, tuberculosis control, a consultation service, a laboratory service, nutrition studies, the care of crippled children, and statistical studies. Whereas the unofficial national "standard" county health team had one nurse along with a full-time health officer, a sanitary inspector, and a clerk, that of Cattaraugus grew to have 27 nurses before the end of the project. The nursing service, which was responsible for home visits, bedside care, and school and sanitary inspections, cost more than 40% of the total budget. Winslow judged it to be a model that was "entirely sound and points the way along which other counties should seek to develop" (Winslow 1931).

Whatever vision that might have existed during the early decades of the twentieth century concerning a U.S. public health system along these lines had to give way to the prevailing political (and economic) reality. Most U.S. physicians favored sanitary measures, regulation of food and drugs, collection of vital statistics, and other public health measures. But by moving from the confines of sanitary engineering and taking on the battle against specific diseases, public health "entered the territory of medicine" (Fee 1987). By the 1920s, in fact, the American Medical Association's attitude toward preventive and public medicine was "actively hostile" (Cassedy 1991), as witnessed by the local County Medical Society's attack on the Rural Health Demonstration in Cattaraugus County (Winslow 1931). This negative attitude was fueled by increasing commercial prosperity (Hirshfield 1970) and by the social unrest following World War I, which led to a general distrust of any ideas that smacked of socialism (Wiebe 1967).

Preventive and public medicine fared far better in parts of Europe, where different models were explored in different countries. Under the leadership of Ludwig W. Rajchman, the League of Nations Health Organization (LNHO) blended the Rockefeller Foundation with Yugoslavian, German, and Soviet initiatives into a new program for rural health (Weindling 1995). Although the United States did not join the LNHO and Rajchman was considered too radical by many, the Rockefeller Foundation contributed importantly to these developments (Dubin 1995). The foundation not only financed much of the work of LNHO, it also invested $25 million in the renovation and building of public health institutions and developed a system of fellowships for graduate training along with refresher courses for those already trained as public health officers and teachers (Fosdick 1952). Through this system, an informal international network of public health institutions grew that in time provided the international public health leaders for the post–World War II period. This network brought together public health schools in the United States with those in Ankara, Athens, Belgrade, Bucharest, Budapest, Calcutta, Cluj, Copenhagen, London, Madrid, Manila, Oslo, Prague, Rome, São Paulo, Sofia, Stockholm, Tokyo, Toronto, Warsaw, and Zagreb.

The hope that creating independent public health schools would suffice to establish a cadre of public health workers who would lead the way to develop national public health systems around the world proved overly optimistic. Grant, for example, who became a faculty member of the Peking Union Medical College in 1921, came to realize that the college was totally irrelevant to the real needs of China (Farley 1980). Modeled after Johns Hopkins, it did not address the diseases, poverty, and problems of "the sick man of Asia." Nevertheless, the network of schools contributed to the spread of innovative ideas, many of which did lead to important developments in the field of public health.

One important development was the emergence of a model for regionalized health services, one that was largely based on the work of Andrija Stampar, inspector general for health in Yugoslavia (Grmek 1966). The Central Institute of Hygiene in Belgrade served as the technical and methodological center for a network of hygiene institutes. Each regional institute technically and administratively supervised health centers that were responsible for hygienic and epidemiological services in one or more districts. Services included environmental sanitation, drinking water supply, public health education, as well as the administration of antimalaria stations, venereal dispensaries, antitrachoma centers, and other specific disease services where conditions required them. The 1931 congress on rural hygiene recommended that such health centers should be the basis of all new health-care systems (Dubin 1995).

This model was closely linked with *social medicine*, a way of conceptualizing health that had its roots in nineteenth-century social reforms (Rosen 1948). Stampar fought for the introduction of social medicine into the regular curriculum of medical schools (Grmek 1966). A special Institute of Social Medicine was founded at the Zagreb Medical School under his influence. As formulated earlier in the century by the German physician Alfred Grotjahn, social medicine recognized that the etiology of disease is biological and social. Social conditions may create or favor a predisposition for a disease, cause disease directly, transmit the causes of disease, or influence the course of a disease (Rosen 1948).

Social medicine "places the emphasis on man" (Ryle 1948). When confronted by an ailing individual, the physician would move beyond attempting to determine "what's he got and what's good for it" and seek to determine "the overall performance of the individual according to his position in life; that is, in the light of his age, educational, vocational, social, and other prerogatives and obligations" (Galdston 1954). According to John A. Ryle, who in the 1940s was professor of social medicine at Oxford University, social medicine derives its experience from the field of clinical experience and thus finds its place in hospital practice in the form of "social diagnosis and social therapeutics— the investigation of conditions, the organization of after-care, and the readjustment of the lives of individuals and families disturbed or broken by illness" (Ryle 1948).

The growing (theoretical) importance given to social medicine was largely due to the dramatic reduction of certain infectious diseases and the parallel growth in importance of many chronic conditions. As early as 1919, Sir George Newman, chief medical officer of the Ministry of Health of the United Kingdom, declared, "there is a relatively light burden of epidemic and infectious disease, which, with certain exceptions, is steadily decreasing in incidence and mortality" (Newman 1919). In 1926, Winslow noted that "communicable diseases and environmental diseases have been so substantially reduced that the problems of the future are heart disease, the acute respiratory diseases and cancer" (Winslow 1926).

Social medicine probably peaked in importance just when WHO was being founded. Its biases and assumptions were commonly accepted by many of the founders of WHO, particularly Stampar (known as the "father of WHO"). It provided the key ideological base on which WHO's early conception of a national health system was built. This conception took the form of a hierarchical set of health units, which dealt with both preventive and clinical work. Such a system looked to the practice of preventive medicine, per se, to control infectious diseases. Traditionally, this "involves some action which in many instances can be compelled by law, and in which the individual is acted on by some one authorized to perform the action" (Galdston 1954).

Strongly conditioning the above history was the industrial world's limited experience with the tropical diseases particularly related to environmental factors, such as malaria, plague, and yellow fever. Yellow fever and plague were much too short-lived and too marginal in the U.S. twentieth-century experience to allow the natural environment to remain as important in disease etiology as microbes. The "environment" that social medicine explored was a social and economic one; there was little, if any, place for a consideration of vector biology and ecology, human-made malaria, and a host of other issues of importance in the control of malaria and other diseases mostly found in the tropics.

Also of importance in this history is the fact that tropical medicine, as such, developed along lines that "diverged from contemporary European public health policies." This divergence was most pronounced in England, where Ross' discoveries served to help stake out new "professional territory." Malaria control took central place in the "new" profession of tropical medicine, a profession that focused on the parasite, the vector, and transmission, "at the expense of immunity, educational programmes and self-help" (Worboys 1996).

One unfortunate consequence of these earlier developments was the neglect of an independent consideration of the health needs of the tropics at the time of WHO's establishment. The tropical medicine model for malaria control was a vertical one, which was out of tune with the horizontal tendencies of public health in the temperate countries. Leading public health voices were from the north; tropical medicine was relatively "marginal ... in world medicine" (Worboys 1996).

Further undermining the development of an independent approach to public health in the tropics was the earlier shift in the field of infectious disease epidemiology, from operational field investigations to laboratory research studies. When the Rockefeller Foundation carried out its hookworm program earlier in the century, the purpose was not to control hookworm, per se, but "to make demonstrations which will lead ultimately to the enlistment of local agencies in the work" (Ettling 1981). In effect, each demonstration was an applied research project where innovative solutions to the different scientific and operational problems encountered were developed in the field. There was no separating out of any work that might on its own qualify as scientific. Particularly important was the supporting role of public health laboratories, which were used for education and training as well as public health investigations initiated in response to the appearance of "serious gaps in the knowledge essential to successful control" (Farley 1995).

This policy remained in force until Frederick Russell, appointed director of the International Health Division (IHD) of the Rockefeller Foundation in 1928, pushed for the creation of a central laboratory in New York that could carry out more fundamental research, especially in the field of yellow fever. Most reaction from IHD staff was negative. Winslow and Victor Heiser were adamantly opposed, the latter arguing "there is still a tremendous amount of needless suffering and death because existing scientific knowledge has not found its way into the lives of the people." Heiser was an international public health specialist who began his career with the U.S. Public Health Service before joining the Rockefeller Foundation in the Far East. Wade Hampton Frost, professor of epidemiology at Johns Hopkins University School of Hygiene and Public Health, warned that a central laboratory would be acceptable if it were directly geared to the problems in the field, but workers in such laboratories have a tendency to initiate studies from "the standpoint of their attractiveness as intramural laboratory investigations" (Farley 1995).

As greater attention was given to laboratory research, central or otherwise, some began to worry that the whole nature of public health was being undermined. Louis W. Hackett, one of the leading malariologists at the time, interpreted Russell's "field research" as "lab research in the field rather than … public health and statistical investigation" (Farley 1995). More foreboding was his observation that the IHD began to offer more support to the "advanced, cultured, and prosperous nations" of the north than to the "poorer, ignorant, and backward countries" of the south. When the IHD closed down its experimental malaria stations in Italy, Hackett pointed out that the absence seemed to have changed the entire character of malaria work in Italy. Field stations, he believed, were "the life of a malaria laboratory." Without them, laboratories would study bird and monkey malaria to the exclusion of the practical and applied.

All these trends were present when WHO was established in 1948. However, the WHO constitution, adopted in 1946, did not attempt to conceptualize a model health system according to the thinking of advocates of social medicine or other variants that were current then. Instead, it listed various functions related to the health system, such as health services; administrative and technical services, including epidemiological and statistical services; work to eradicate epidemic, endemic, and other diseases; improvement of nutrition, housing, sanitation, recreation, economic or working conditions, and other aspects of environmental hygiene; maternal and child health and welfare; mental health; research in the field of health; and an informed public opinion among all peoples on matters of health.

The WHO Expert Committee on Environmental Sanitation was the first WHO-affiliated body to present a systems view of public health, one based on the premise that the "sanitation of the environment is literally the foundation on which a sound public-health structure must be built" (WHO 1950a). This committee held three sessions, in 1949, 1951, and 1953 (WHO 1950a, 1951a, 1953). The first report was judged by the executive board to have placed "undue emphasis on the engineering aspect of the problem rather than on the sanitation viewpoint" (WHO 1950b). While approving the publication of this report, the executive board requested that the director general, when developing proposals for the future, bear in mind "the advantages of activities in the nature of self-help, education, and stimulation of local interest in favor of general improvement of environmental conditions." The third report confined its attention to rural sanitation and, in doing so, avoided the question as to what kind of organization is needed to administer rural sanitation programs.

The Expert Committee on Environmental Sanitation did not meet again to consider the totality of environmental health services until 1969 (Litsios 1998). Instead, environmental health services were incorporated in what came to be known as the BHS model, developed by the Expert Committee on Public-Health Administration during its second session in 1953 (WHO 1954). This committee continued in the direction established by the first (WHO 1952), which had met in 1951 and had adopted Winslow's 1920 definition of public health (amended to include mental as well as physical health). It defined the BHS model in terms of maternal and child health, control of communicable diseases, environmental sanitation, maintenance of records for statistical purposes, health education of the public, public-health nursing, and medical care (to an extent varying with the needs of the area and the accessibility of larger hospital centers). Although the functions of a public health service remained more or less the same as those identified earlier by the first committee, staff requirements were greatly enlarged by the second committee. A team consisting of only a physician, a nurse, a sanitarian, and auxiliary workers was judged to be "uneconomical." Rural health units, to provide the greatest efficiency, should have, in addition to a physician in charge, "some five to ten nurses, several sanitarians, and a substantial number of auxiliary workers (including clerical staff)."

This is more or less where matters stood, conceptually, concerning the international view of public health, when the global malaria eradication campaign was launched in 1955.

1955–1974

This period is difficult to characterize. The Expert Committee on Public-Health Administration had defined a model for the health services system that, with hindsight, appears totally unrealistic. The world was caught up in a cold war that made rational discussion of the pros and cons of alternative approaches to social and economic development, including health, almost impossible. It certainly did not help that the U.S. system of health had moved even farther away from providing a model that was in line with the more progressive social health developments of Europe. Not only was the U.S. health system largely dominated by curative medicine, its public health officers were reluctant to take any initiative with respect to public health research or new health problems (Duffy 1990).

In light of the evidence that basic health services were not evolving as it had been hoped they would, it became apparent that studies were needed in individual countries to determine what specific mix of programs and services best suited each situation. The third report of the Expert Committee on Public-Health Administration, in 1959, called for the execution of pilot studies on local health services (WHO 1960). The report outlined how such studies might be carried out and encouraged all countries to make such studies "a routine procedure in health administration." Grant pointed out how important it was that such studies (demonstration projects) conform to "an already existing political unit of the administration of the country in question" under the responsibility of an authority "in the central government for the technical services in question" (Grant 1963c). He viewed such studies as a form of "operations research aimed at developing methods and procedures to secure a greater return on the health care dollar"; particularly important for "developing areas" was the "development of a research arm to facilitate innovation and experimentation with alternative ways of meeting the people's health and social needs" (Grant 1963d).

As the malaria eradication campaign began to falter in the early 1960s, calls for the integration of such campaigns into the general health services intensified. A study group was convened by WHO in 1964 to address this subject (WHO 1965). Study groups differ from expert committees in that they address problems of a highly uncertain character, such as one where expert consensus may not be possible. The 1964 study group reviewed the role of mass campaigns in the evolution and development of health services, assessed the comparative advantages of the two approaches, and reviewed the factors influencing the process of integration. Aware that there was inadequate experience to demonstrate the series of steps involved in developing the general health services in a manner acceptable to the continuing execution of mass campaigns, the study group concluded that "this is a challenging opportunity for WHO to stimulate and sponsor useful operational research." The subjects for study identified were "the acquisition and analysis of data on the staffing needs of mass campaigns and general health services in terms of both general and specialized personnel, the financing and organization of campaigns, the methodology of training, and the evaluation of results in terms of economics and of benefits to the health of the people" (WHO 1965).

WHO's Division of Research in Epidemiology and Communications Sciences (RECS), established in 1967, undertook several operational research studies related to the organization of health services. Most were attached to public health schools supported by the Rockefeller Foundation, particularly those in Cali, Colombia, and Teheran, Iran, where strong professional and personal links existed between Kenneth Newell, the director of the division, and leading faculty members of each school. The idea behind these studies was to demonstrate the utility of population-based epidemiology to the planning of local and regional health services. Also foreseen was the involvement of several North American schools of public health.

Although this effort led to an important health services project in Iran (King 1982), it did not lead to the creation of a network of public health schools as Newell had hoped. None of the North American public health schools that were approached accepted the condition of being involved in a study where someone else would choose their study subject. Nor did most staff in RECS, many of whom were already involved in unrelated studies in Colombia. Instead, these and other public health schools became part of an international clinical epidemiology network established around 1970 by the Rockefeller Foundation. Although in theory the network was designed to sensitize clinicians to community health, the program "focused entirely on hospitals and medical schools" to such a degree that it fueled "perceptions that the Rockefeller Foundation had 'abandoned' public health altogether" (Chen 1997). A more critical interpretation of this movement is that it was trying "to stop the development of prevention and public health" as part of a "retrogressive movement ... [where] the medical profession is trying to recoup its fortunes" (Milton Terris, quoted in PAHO 1988). This history provides further evidence of the failure of developing countries to escape the dominating trends of the industrialized world.

RECS, which was disestablished in 1972, did cooperate with the WHO malaria program in the development and carrying out of the Garki Project (Molineaux and Gramiccia 1980). However, whereas RECS staff members were working from the premise that malaria could not be eradicated, the participating staff members from the malaria program were hoping that Garki would demonstrate that eradication was feasible even in the savanna of West Africa (personal communication from L. Molineaux, Sept. 10, 1982). How far apart RECS views were from those of the eradicationists can be judged by contrasting the views of René Dubos (whose works were essential reading for RECS staff) and those of Soper (Litsios 1997b). Soper used his successful attack on *Anopheles gambiae* in Brazil in the 1930s and Egypt in the 1940s to argue in favor of attempting the global eradication of malaria, whereas Dubos argued that what worked in one area might not work in another, owing to the fact that malaria is "a huge congeries of disease, occupying a large number of ecological provinces each with its particular conditions ... (where) the climate, the topography, the plant and animal populations are different, to say nothing of the habits of the human populations" (Dubos 1965).

Although WHO efforts in the field of operational research had faltered, the WHO secretariat continued to promote the idea that each country had to work out its own approach to the development of health systems. In a major report presented to the executive board in January 1973, it was found "improbable" that any international model for health services would be developed. Each country "will have to possess the national ability to consider its own position (problems and resources), assess the alternatives available to it, decide on its resource allocation and priorities, and implement its own decisions" (WHO 1973a). This same report announced the failure of the BHS approach, a failure that Halfdan Mahler, WHO director general from 1973 to 1988, characterized as "the most signal failure of WHO as well as the Member States ..." (Mahler 1974).

The resolution adopted by WHA in May 1973 (WHO 1985b) in response to a paper presented to the executive board recommended, among other things, that the organization

- concentrate on specific programs that would assist countries in developing their health-care systems for their entire populations, with special emphasis on meeting the needs of those populations that have clearly insufficient health services;
- improve its capability for assisting national administrations to analyze their health delivery systems through organized research projects, with the goal of increasing their efficiency and effectiveness;
- design its programs so as to encourage member states to develop a strong national will to undertake intensive action to deal with their long-term health-care problems as well as their immediate requirements in a form designed for the orderly development of health services; and
- further develop management methods suited to health service needs and assist countries in developing a national capability of applying these methods.

The executive board also requested that the director general report "on a comprehensive long-term research programme with systems of health care organization on local and country-wide levels ...." Such a program was never presented to the board. Instead, in January 1975, the secretariat presented a paper on a conceptual approach called *primary health care* (PHC), its principles and assumptions, and a list of ongoing activities that could be considered part of the proposed program, such as technical material for the training of PHC workers and the preparation of technical packages that detail the functioning of select types of PHC services (WHO 1975). Concerning research, the report indicated that "the objectives of each country's programme should be the prime determinant of the research (health service, epidemiological, operations research, managerial) to be sponsored and conducted." WHO could be expected to contribute to the evaluation of such research, an activity that it considered should be pursued both nationally and internationally.

From 1967 to 1975, the socialist bloc countries, led by the Soviet Union, pushed for WHO to recognize their centrally planned and administered health services system as a model suitable for other countries to follow. WHO countered, at first, with the call for greater self-reliance on the part of individual countries to develop their own health services system model, and then with a conceptual approach (PHC) that opposed the Soviet model. Whereas the Soviet model was heavily oriented to centrally determined norms and standards, PHC was to evolve from and to be shaped "around the life patterns of the community" (WHO 1975). Furthermore, instead of consisting of a hierarchical series on independent health units, PHC was to be "fully integrated with the services of the other sectors involved in community development." Although the Soviets failed to have their model officially sanctioned by WHO, they did succeed in forcing the organization to hold an international conference in 1978, in Alma-Ata, then-capital of the Kazakh Soviet Socialist Republic (Litsios 2002).

Marcolino Candau, WHO director general from 1953 to 1973, in his 1972 review of WHO's first 25 years, commented that "much of the developing world has had imposed upon it a manpower pattern that is foreign to it and that is unlikely to function properly in the conditions obtaining there" (Candau 1972). Surprisingly, this observation did not seem to attract any attention at the time. Possibly, those who agreed with him believed that the ongoing review of the BHS would make more explicit his concern, which it did not. My guess is that Candau, who started out his career as a malariologist in Brazil, came to this conclusion under the influence of Gabaldón and Soper, both very close to him.

Gabaldón was of the opinion that "the health risks in tropical countries are not only quantitatively different from those of temperate countries, but also qualitatively different." Despite these differences, however, "Latin America continues to imitate the temperate zone health schemes as intensely as possible" (Gabaldón 1969). Soper, who is rumored to have been responsible for Candau being elected WHO director general in 1953, believed that disease campaigns were a necessary prelude to the building of general health service. Lack of enthusiasm (for mass campaigns), he believed, could be attributed "in great part to the previous predominance of schools of public health in the United States as international centers for the training of public health administrators" (Soper 1963). From his review of the past, Soper concluded that the first generation of international health workers—that is, Americans and those trained in the United States involved in the earlier hookworm campaigns—had "moved too fast in [their] attempts to transform the campaigns for the prevention of a specific disease into a general health service." He particularly criticized the attention given to maternal and child health, noting that such services depended on public health nurses who, although available in the industrialized countries, particularly America, were "nonexistent or scarce" in undeveloped countries. Furthermore, they were not needed for any mass campaign.

How far apart the industrialized world was from the developing world during this immediate postwar period can be judged by Grant's observation concerning public health nurses. Whereas Soper noted that none existed in the developing countries, Grant, when examining trends in health care in social welfare in the United Kingdom in 1949, noted that "an outstanding administrative problem with respect to the practice of social medicine in the community ... is the relationship of the public health nurse and the social worker" (Grant 1963a). In other words, even as early as 1949, industrialized countries were facing the problem of redundancy and conflict involving different categories of health workers, a luxury that the developing countries were not yet in a position to afford.

A look at the names of the leading public health specialists who took part in the meetings that led to the creation of WHO and the establishment of its public health program shows that almost all were from nontropical countries. Gabaldón was an exception, but he confined his attention, in Geneva at least, only to malaria, although as I note below, his interests were far broader. Those concerned with the development of the BHS were from temperate countries. They had no practical experience concerning the development of such services or the control of common diseases under tropical conditions.

1975–2000

Mahler (1976) called for a "social revolution in public health." Noting that "social evolutions and revolutions have taken place because the social structures were crumbling," he saw signs that the "scientific and technical structures of public health are also crumbling, because they cannot cope with social needs at a price that most societies can afford to pay." Conditions "appear to be ripe for a truly critical reevaluation in social terms of the means for attaining health." Mahler believed that four key factors were necessary to bring about the "adoption of an approach to the solution of community health problems that is completely new." It is necessary for any society

- to determine what social health goals it wishes to attain;
- to identify the health technologies that serve those social health goals;
- to select those health technologies that are not merely sound but that it can afford; and
- to manifest the political will to determine health policies and to create the necessary mechanisms for formulating health programs and developing appropriate health-care systems to implement them.

Social health goals should be shaped by a social justice whereby individual care would be provided beyond what can be afforded for the population as a whole "only when the total population has been provided with a level of care that society considers essential and is able and ready to pay for, even to the extent of making sacrifices in other areas" (Mahler 1976).

As noted earlier, it was during this period that the PHC concept emerged. Another important development was the decision in 1977 that the principal social target in health of member states and WHO was "the attainment by all the citizens of the world by the year 2000 of a level of health that will permit them to lead socially and economically productive lives." In 1978, the Alma-Ata Declaration identified PHC as the key for achieving "health for all by the year 2000," known as HFA 2000. The clearest distinction between BHS and PHC was the latter's call for the use of "appropriate technology" and "community health workers," the latter to include "traditional medical practitioners and birth attendants."

Even before the ink was dry at Alma-Ata, the conservative medical community in many industrial countries attacked PHC. They believed that WHO had been overly influenced by the example of the Chinese barefoot doctor and that attention to appropriate technology, as exemplified by the concept of "essential drugs," would lead to second-rate care. Within WHO, both PHC and HFA 2000 were derided. Those leading the development of PHC did not appreciate that although a "far cry from the definition of the WHO constitution, (but) at least [HFA] is nearer to reality" (Howard-Jones 1981). Instead of exploring how a society might define the contribution of health to social and economic productivity, the impossibility of achieving anything so grandiose by a fixed date was ridiculed.

Even the friends of PHC were undermining its development. Development agencies, in their rush to help countries implement PHC, imposed their particular versions of appropriate technology, setting out timetables for implementation that were totally unrealistic. It was not unusual to find countries where regions were being assisted by different aid agencies and where no single national health system pattern was being followed. Thus, community health workers in different regions were trained differently and for different tasks and responsibilities. Governments were hard pressed to use assistance, and assisting agencies judged their success not by any real progress but by the mere spending of money.

All of these developments led Mahler to denounce the "development crisis," which he characterized as "too many countries, too many bilateral and multilateral agencies, too many influential individuals [having] become too disillusioned with the prospects for genuine human development to be ready to continue the struggle for it" (Mahler 1985).

The replacement of a universal model such as BHS with a set of principles and general objectives proved particularly unsatisfactory for those who wished specificity concerning exactly what the peripheral health services would be delivering. A counterrevolution set in, which Newell claims already had started at Alma-Ata, where PHC was identified in terms of a list of health problems—adequate food supplies, maternal and child health care, immunization, and so forth—that needed to be dealt with (Newell 1988). The counterrevolution took a sharper form in the notion of "selective primary health care" (Walsh and Warren 1979). Selective PHC purported to place the choice of what to do in terms of the cost and effectiveness of available interventions (Warren 1988). Selective PHC and any other form of priority listing deprive people of their ultimate responsibility to decide what problems their health system should address. The responsibility of the health sciences should be "to describe possible interventions and their implications and costs, but not to choose"; no "collective or world list of health service actions should exist" (Newell 1988).

The counterrevolution gained further ground with the development of indicators such as the disability-adjusted life year (DALY) and the quality-adjusted life year (QALY). These indicators have been and are being used to estimate the total global burden of disease from which alternative interventions in terms of DALY/QALY gained per dollar invested are ranked and national and international health research priorities are established. The use of DALYs suit those in the international community who lobby for the achievement of specific global targets through well-defined interventions, as witness their importance in guiding "efforts in prioritization at all levels of government" and "the direction of investment in international health programs" (NAS 1995). But such prioritization undermines any long-term investment in the improvement of public health systems that meet the criteria called for by Newell and Mahler, that is, building a system that promotes human dignity through an informed and active public role in decisionmaking, a decreasing gap between the haves and the have-nots, preferential allocations to the social periphery, and achievement of a level of health that contributes to socially and economically productive lives. That DALYs divert attention from these goals can be seen most simply by the fact that the total disability attributed to a local disease outbreak that affects the working population is the same whether that population group happens to be employees in secure jobs covered by health insurance or poor farmers who lose their crops and are pushed into a state of destitution.

Concerning malaria, the use of DALYs would not have captured any of the economic benefits achieved during past control and eradication campaigns, such as increased agricultural productivity and the opening up of new lands. DALYs might even not be useful in portraying the importance of epidemic detection and containment. This is reflected in the latest WHO publication concerning health systems, where only "case management (early assessment and prompt treatment) and selected preventive measures (e.g., impregnated bed nets)" are rated as "interventions with a large potential impact on health outcomes" (WHO 2000). Consciously or unconsciously, the use of DALYs and DALY-related indicators favors a magic bullet approach to preventive medicine.

Even if DALYs were accepted as a proper basis for portraying disease burden, the fact that estimates are based on an entire population, national and global, means that the nature of the disease burden among the poor is not properly appreciated. Thus, for example, communicable diseases, which account for 63.8% of DALY loss among the global poor, account for only 10.9% of DALY loss among the global rich (Gwatkin and Guillot 1999). The shift from estimating the impact of disease on the poor in developing countries to estimating global burden has led to a lowering of the priority given to communicable as opposed to noncommunicable diseases.

These criticisms aside, the use of DALYs provided the World Bank with a quantitative justification for a new agenda for action, one that called for increased investment in "basic public health services and essential clinical care" (World Bank 1993). Health reform is required that eliminates spending on "discretionary clinical services" so that governments can concentrate on ensuring cost-effective clinical care for the poor. An "essential public health package" would be expected to include immunization and micronutrient supplementation; school health programs to treat worm infections and micronutrient deficiencies and to provide health education; programs to increase public knowledge about family planning and nutrition, self-cure or indications for seeking care, and vector control and disease surveillance activities; programs to reduce consumption of tobacco, alcohol, and other drugs; and AIDS [acquired immune deficiency syndrome] prevention programs with a strong component for sexually transmitted diseases. However, it should be noted that this public health package is largely if not uniquely dominated by interventions whose success depends on their acceptance by individuals, as opposed to the earlier nineteenth-century approach to public health, which called for governments to do "for the health of the individual [that] which the individual cannot do for himself" (Galdston 1954).

The weak state of public health was the subject of several global meetings in the first half of the 1990s. For a while, WHO flirted with the idea of a "new public health" to focus attention on the crisis situation that was seen to exist almost worldwide (WHO 1995). Instead, "new challenges" were recognized, and the call for reforms and change was incorporated in the policy introduced as Health for All in the 21st Century (WHO 1997). The new challenges include globalization, ecology and environment, public–private interaction, governance, social change, community action, and political advocacy. More relevant for this discussion is the introduction of "essential public health functions" that include, among other things, preventing and controlling disease and protecting health; developing health information systems and ensuring active surveillance; and securing adequate and sustainable financing. These functions are discussed next as they apply to malaria control.

Malaria Control and Essential Public Health Functions

In the posteradication period, a situation has emerged in which malaria control has made and continues to make increasing demands on public health systems whose capacity, for all intents and purposes, does not exist. It is precisely the lack of such a capacity that led to the resurrection of the notion of "essential public health functions." Furthermore, malaria has received very little attention in the general public health literature over the past 30 years or so. Even the fact that malaria is one of the major obstacles to socioeconomic development has only recently returned to the central stage of global thinking. This neglect seems to have been a sort of punishment aimed at those responsible for malaria control for having attempted eradication. Not appreciated by diehard proponents of PHC and HFA was the fact that the shift from infection control to disease control, which was led by the Expert Committees on Malaria in the 1980s, represented a major policy shift for the malaria community. Instead, disease control has been derided because it "does not inevitably lead to health or to what people necessarily want" (Newell 1988). By indicating that health is "not merely the absence of disease," the WHO constitution had possibly set the tone for later criticism of efforts that "merely" sought to control or eradicate disease.

Also, from the counterrevolution point of view, the control of a specific disease still has connotations of having been selected by a committee meeting in Geneva; this extreme view condemns disease control programs for being "ideologically similar to the malaria eradication disaster and ... a regression to the very qualities of imposed systems" (Newell 1988). However, instead of imposing a model to be followed by all countries, the global malaria control strategy, which has evolved over the past 20 years, emphasizes the integration of malaria into the national health services system. The idea of integration is not new, but it did get sidetracked during the eradication era.

What follows is a review of certain aspects of malaria control that relate to three essential public health functions. In this review, the function of preventing and controlling disease and of protecting health is considered from an infrastructure point of view—in other words, the kind of organizational arrangements envisioned that include malaria control. Most of this section reflects conceptual positions that have been taken at one time or another by the international community concerned with the malaria problem.

Malaria Control as Part of a Wider Public Health Infrastructure

Most of the early twentieth-century efforts to control malaria were undertaken independently of any other public health problem; they were carried out either as demonstration projects or where control was deemed economically necessary. No doubt there are instances where other public health problems were addressed at the same time (for example, Gorgas' control of yellow fever at the Panama Canal), but they were exceptions and did not follow any preconceived model.

Only in the 1920s and 1930s, when malaria control in rural areas of tropical countries was under study, was malaria's relationship with the rest of the health system addressed. The Bandoeng report, for example, indicated that where "malaria is an outstanding social and health problem, the resources of the health administration, specially augmented where necessary, should be directed chiefly towards malaria control, even if this should entail the restriction of other public health activities, until malaria is no longer of major importance." The responsibility for malaria control "should rest squarely on the minister or other officer in charge of the public health policy of a country and not on the technical expert." Furthermore, "since malaria is a focal disease ... absent in some rural areas, lightly prevalent in others, and moderately or heavily endemic elsewhere, the structure of, and programme for, rural health organization, including health units and health centers, should not be stereotyped, but flexible" (League of Nations 1937).

This model applied to rural tropical countries. Nontropical industrialized countries were able to control malaria (more or less) using independent means. For example, in the United States, the Malaria Control in War Areas program was established in 1942 to control malaria in the southern United States, where malaria threatened the health of soldiers stationed at the many military facilities located there (Mullan 1989). In 1946, this program evolved into the Communicable Disease Center, which had the responsibility of controlling all communicable diseases. This is a rare if not unique example of a malaria control effort, admittedly relatively short-lived but intense and costly, evolving into a specialized national communicable disease control program. However, malaria was already on the way out; its eradication may not even have required any application of DDT. Had malaria been more extensive and more difficult to control, the separation of disease control from other related public health concerns in the United States, particularly environmental sanitation and housing, might have been less acceptable.

Those who outlined the concept of BHS in the early 1950s, although allowing that malaria campaigns might precede the development of more general health services, preferred to approach campaigns with the belief that the local health services would be intimately involved with campaign implementation. Thus, health services staff "will lay the groundwork for these major campaigns, by education of the people and in other ways" (WHO 1954). They would obtain special training so that they could "undertake contact-tracing, follow-up of cases, and 'mopping-up' operations when the intensive campaign is over, as well as participate in the evaluation of results." Contrary to the conclusion reached by the Bandoeng meeting, specially trained teams of experts would direct the campaign itself. Why this difference existed needs additional historical exploration.

Although PHC replaced BHS in the mid-1970s, the relationship between malaria control and the health services has been described in terms similar to those above. Where a strong health infrastructure exists guided by "strong leadership oriented toward primary health care and preventive services," most routine antimalaria activities, including some vector control ones, "could be undertaken as an integral part of primary health care" (WHO 1986). Where the infrastructure is less developed, "a specialized unit" may be required for some "vector control operations," but where malaria "is a high priority problem" and where PHC is weakly developed, "a special project may be the only effective means of implementing antimalaria action."

Although most attention has been given to placing malaria control in a well-structured and hierarchical health services system, other structural contexts have been suggested that are worth examining, even if only briefly. Mention has already been made of the link between malaria control and agricultural development. Historically, that link goes back many centuries to early efforts to drain swamps and adopt irrigation methods to control mosquito breeding (Najera 1994). Just before the arrival of DDT, the so-called naturalistic measures to control breeding were investigated and their use promoted, "especially such methods as primarily will improve agricultural yields of the land" (Russell 1936). With DDT, a more proactive malaria–agriculture policy engaged the international community for a while.

Malaria control has also been linked with the control of other vector-borne diseases. In 1949, for example, the Italian delegate to WHA proposed that the Expert Committee on Malaria be transformed into one that dealt with malaria and other vector-borne diseases. He described how house disinfection was a common response to several diseases, concluding that it would be "highly desirable that personnel should be trained in the whole field of insect control as a measure of public health" (WHO 1949b). The issue was referred to the executive board, where it was voted down, eight votes to three.

Instead, the control of other insect-borne diseases was addressed in the context of environmental sanitation. The first session of the Expert Committee on Environmental Sanitation took place in 1949. The committee singled out the projected FAO/WHO scheme for combined agricultural development and malaria control to be of particular importance for the development of environmental services. In later sessions (1951 and 1953), the committee strengthened the link between environmental sanitation and general community development, particularly with agricultural progress. This line of thinking ceased rather quickly when eradication became the leitmotif of the program. Still, some malariologists, including George Macdonald, who chaired the third Expert Committee on Environmental Sanitation, foresaw that the malaria effort would form the backbone of an epidemiological service and a system of environmental sanitation (Macdonald 1956). At the least, when eradication was achieved, malaria epidemiologists were expected to serve as public health epidemiologists. However, this did not happen even in Taiwan, where eradication was achieved and a substantial project with that aim had been put in place (Manning 1968).

Venezuela, under the leadership of Gabaldón, chose a strategy that was close to the model promoted by the Expert Committee on Environmental Sanitation (Litsios 1998). Having become minister of health of Venezuela in 1959, in 1960 Gabaldón transformed the Division of Malariology into the Ministry of Malariology and Environmental Health, incorporating the Divisions of Sanitary Engineering, Rural Water Supply and Rural Housing, and Ankylostomiasis and other Helminthic Diseases. How drastically different this program was can be seen from the fact that it was able to develop a credit plan for rural families that led to more than 89,000 housing units being built by 1970.

Not only was Gabaldón's association of malaria with environmental programs in line with what the early Expert Committee on Environmental Sanitation foresaw as a natural development, it also anticipated the direction that environmental health would take in the 1970s as additional environmental problems emerged. For example, the Panel of Experts on Environmental Management for Vector Control, created jointly in 1981 by WHO, FAO, and the United Nations Environmental Program, has stressed the importance of preventing diseases such as malaria from becoming major public health problems in the wake of water resources development, among other issues. For large national projects, such as large-scale irrigation schemes, two institutional arrangements have been useful for ensuring the collaboration needed to "reduce adverse effects of development through early detection of potential problems and resource sharing for their prevention and mitigation": the establishment of interministerial linkages through memoranda of understanding, and the establishment of a special body with elevated executive powers that can operate in a fully integrated manner either alone or through existing structures (WHO 1999). These concepts have led to a broader understanding of the health impact assessment of development projects, which embraces all health issues related to all kinds of development (Birley 1995).

Many of the major and successful early twentieth-century malaria control projects were conducted under similar intersectoral arrangements. For situations where smaller schemes are being undertaken, the problem of protecting health is more difficult to organize as a result of lacking the necessary expertise and means of enforcing agreed-upon standards. This problem is analogous to controlling malaria in remote situations where no formal public health system is present and, thus, is a critical part of the challenge for public health and malaria in the twenty-first century.

Information and Surveillance for Malaria

Information is needed about each malaria situation to decide on specific program targets and objectives, measures to be undertaken, and resources required as well as to measure progress and to evaluate the effectiveness and efficiency of control strategies and measures implemented. What makes malaria information particularly hard to define is the large number of factors involved in determining the distribution of malaria and the epidemiological uncertainty that still surrounds the importance of each factor. Obviously, the simplest situations are those in which malaria is homogenous and relatively straightforward control tools are used, but such situations are few, and their number will decrease even more as different types of malaria spread around the world.

The nineteenth Expert Committee on Malaria specifically addressed the question of "development of epidemiological skills in the health services" and arrived at this position:

> The areas where malaria is most prevalent are also those where personnel trained epidemiologically to evaluate the information obtained by community health workers are in shortest supply. These epidemiological workers are usually stationed at the district health facility (the second referral level), and should have a qualification in biology equivalent to the B.Sc. They require in-service training in stratification, in planning and implementing the programme as it applies to their assigned area, in consolidating and analyzing epidemiological data, and in evaluating the progress of the campaign. They should be trained to identify vectors and changes in vector habits and patterns, ecological changes, vector resistance to insecticides and parasite resistance to drugs, human migration both into and out of their districts, and (to the extent possible, using previous seasonal records and current climatic and parasitological data) to forecast epidemics. These epidemiologists may have to undertake a range of duties, and deal with other vector-borne and communicable diseases which may have epidemiological characteristics in common with malaria. It is particularly important to appreciate that existing personnel already trained only in malaria, or those trained only for other diseases, will require reorientation. (WHO 1992)

Some concerns identified, such as drug resistance, human migration, and climate changes, go far beyond concerns of the district level. For example, the lack of a regional perspective on the spread of multiple-drug-resistant falciparum malaria, the epicenter if which is in southeast Asia, impedes the development of a system of information that would form the backbone of any resistance-containment policy (Kidson, Indaratna, and Looareesuwan 2000). The challenge is more than a simple harmonization of information; the countries involved have conflicting, largely vertical strategies regarding malaria. And the relationship between these vertical programs and PHC is so weak that it "needs to be urgently addressed. There is a great deal of ferment about health sector reform: malaria control is on the sideline in that great debate, it must be brought into the main game" (Kidson, Indaratna, and Looareesuwan 2000).

Molecular-level factors need to be added to this list as well:

> The most pressing intellectual challenge, requiring collaboration between researchers and operational workers … will be to take the rapidly growing body of detailed epidemiological understanding at the micro level and the unfolding work on molecular mechanisms of pathogenesis and so of risk, and to incorporate them, together with socioeconomic considerations, into a macro-epidemiological understanding that can be the basis of operational control programmes. (Bradley 1991)

A personal anecdote shows the size of the gap between malaria specialists and public health generalists concerning how information might be processed at the periphery of PHC. As a faculty member in an international malaria training course, it was my task (as the generalist) to lead a discussion on the relationship between malaria control and PHC. Having just joined the Malaria Action Programme in 1981 after having been chief of Primary Health Care and Rural Development in the Strengthening of Health Services Division of WHO, I had a deep professional interest in developing the issue to the maximum extent possible. In one exercise, I distributed a detailed map of a cluster of villages in Turkey and asked the students to develop a control strategy appropriate to each village situation. They did so, but during the discussion one student, who in fact was head of a major national (vertical) malaria control program, rejected the whole exercise. In his mind, it was impossible for any health service system to be so knowledgeable and sensitive to each local situation.

At the time, I took his position to reflect the thinking of a nonrepentant eradicationist and hoped that others with a more open mind would think differently. Now I realize that I had presumed a certain epidemiological capacity on the part of the general health services that normally might not be present. In fact, nowhere in the report to Alma-Ata on PHC can the role of epidemiology be found! Reference is made to multidisciplinary planning teams that include only the disciplines of economics, political science, and other social sciences. In addition, the brief discussion on information is technically nondescriptive. Mention is made of the importance of identifying relevant information, the need for two-way exchange between levels, and the need for information gathering and analysis to be an integral part of PHC activities.

Others had noted that PHC was not incorporating epidemiology in the logic of its functioning, or as one editorial put it, PHC "seems to be bypassing the epidemiological intelligence on which it should be based" (*International Journal of Epidemiology* 1976). But in reality, according to a follow-up editorial, the problem lay in the rank-and-file epidemiologists who questioned their own utility in "health policy" work (*International Journal of Epidemiology* 1977). "Real" epidemiology was a research activity; epidemiology within the health services had been reduced to a routine one that was preoccupied with the analysis of data to develop norms. Furthermore, the editorial continues, epidemiologists were "deliberately relieved of responsibility for program operations and field activities." PHC programs were being implemented in the Americas "without the essential components of epidemiological surveillance and disease prevention and control" (*International Journal of Epidemiology* 1978). Ironically, the past existence of vertical programs such as malaria eradication was cited as one reason for epidemiology being isolated from program operations.

PHC has not led to the resurgence of interest in surveillance and monitoring over the past quarter-century. Instead, the combined threat of a deteriorating global environment and the emergence of new infectious diseases has mobilized countless new initiatives, many of which offer the potential of radically altering the availability of information at the grassroots level, that is, at the individual malaria foci in the world.

Although it is beyond the scope of this chapter to summarize the current status of developments in this field, some indication of how information for decisionmaking is being approached is relevant for the future direction outlined below. This subject was explicitly addressed at the U.N. Conference on Environment and Development held in Rio de Janeiro, Brazil, in 1992. Chapter 40 of Agenda 21 outlines the commitment taken at that time. One of the major objectives identified is to "strengthen local, provincial, national, and international capacity to collect and use multisectoral information in decision-making processes and to enhance capacities to collect and analyze data and information for decision-making, particularly in developing countries" (United Nations 1992). Indicators for sustainable development are required. Governments are expected to establish "comprehensive information frameworks," and the international organizations are expected to help create such frameworks along with "supporting mechanisms to provide local communities and resource users with the information and know-how they need to manage their environment and resources sustainably."

Various global information networks that address different aspects of Agenda 21 are being established. Similar developments are beginning to occur in the field of emerging diseases. For example, the U.S. Centers for Disease Control and Prevention (CDC) has developed a strategy for preventing emerging infectious diseases in the twenty-first century in which four interdependent goals are identified: surveillance and response, applied research, infrastructure and training, and prevention and control (CDC 1999). The program of WHO, "the CDC for the world," calls for global monitoring, global information access, strong national surveillance and control, and international preparedness. WHO's Division of Emerging and Other Communicable Diseases was created following the international turmoil caused by plague in India and the Ebola outbreak in Zaire. The division brought together expertise in disease surveillance and viral, bacterial, and zoonotic diseases (diseases of animals potentially transmissible to humans) to address the problem of emerging and reemerging communicable diseases that could become international threats to public health.

Financing Malaria Control

Malaria control, like any other organized affair, requires secure financing if it is to thrive and perform well. Watson was able to find the funds to control malaria in Malaya's rubber plantations and Zaire's copper mines because the relationship between a healthy work force and profits was understood and was immediate (Watson 1953). Gorgas, on the other hand, only managed to obtain a free hand to control yellow fever and malaria while the Panama Canal was being constructed because he had the full backing of the president of the United States (Gorgas and Hendrick 1924; Litsios 2001b). Without that backing, the engineers in charge of the project would never have agreed to allocate the funds needed for his efforts.

When Winslow spoke to the 1952 WHA, he urged that careful records be kept of the cost of health programs and of the actual results attained, including economic ones, so a "sum equal to one half such economic gains be appropriated for the further expansion of the public-health programme" (Winslow 1952). Myrdal, who spoke on the same occasion, argued that the demographic explosion that no doubt would follow any major investment in health would overwhelm resulting economic gains (Myrdal 1952). Myrdal's view cast a deep shadow across the whole rationale for malaria control; as Russell put it, "the satisfaction of malariologists has thus been disturbed" (Russell 1955).

In any case, even if economic productivity could be assured, there was no obvious method for ensuring that a reasonable percentage of health-driven economic gains would be invested in public health. Early efforts in the twentieth century offer no useful example. All major malaria control programs associated with economic projects, for example, never contributed to the building of a public health infrastructure.

When the malaria eradication program was being pressured by WHA in the late 1960s to revise its strategy, it attempted to argue that the economic gains that had been achieved where malaria had been significantly reduced justified maintaining a high priority for malaria eradication and control. Most of that argument fell on deaf ears. Malaria had had its turn; international funding shifted to other global priorities, particularly that of family planning (Gramiccia and Beales 1988).

The threat of epidemics has always been used to mobilize political and economic support for some form of preventive action. Soper did not hesitate in 1938 to superimpose a map of the region in Brazil where *An. gambiae* had invaded on a map of the state of New York to suggest that the whole of the United States was threatened by this invasion. Some "millions of dollars and many years of constant effort" might be needed, but "the problem is such a serious one that such an expenditure might well be justified" (Packard and Gagdelha 1994). Similarly, when the funding of state mosquito control boards is threatened, a mass propaganda campaign is launched to remind the public of past epidemics and the need to remain vigilant. Even better is the appearance of a new mosquito-borne disease, as witness the emergence of the West Nile virus in the United States, which has led many states to reinvest in their antimosquito programs, which had been severely cut back over the past few decades.

The use of threats can go only so far; it is certainly no way to build a permanent public health capacity anywhere. Stable financing is required. Today, the financing of public health work is threatened more than ever by the increasing privatization of the health services. It is not obvious what economic arguments can be used to reverse these trends. Even when improved health can be demonstrated to have positive economic benefits, of the kind Winslow identified 50 years ago, the means for investing some part of those benefits into building and strengthening essential public health functions are still lacking.

Where malaria and poverty contribute significantly to environmental degradation, there is the possibility of justifying malaria control and the alleviation of poverty to preserve ecological wealth. In the past decade or so, a new economics has arisen that attempts to develop realistic arguments that, once accepted, would dramatically alter the way prices are determined and investments are valued. Such an economics, for example, would "impose worldwide prices that reflect approximate real costs (including environmental externalities, worker health, and livable wages)" (Meadows 2000). Where environmental externalities involve saving malarious tropical forests, worker health and livable wages would apply to the whole population living in such areas. (For an example of current thinking on the subject, see the South African New Economic Foundation website at http://www.sane.org.za/).

It is important to remember at this point that many of the malaria control programs attempted in the immediate pre-DDT era were built on the premise that malaria could be controlled only if the measures undertaken were intimately related to rural development. Equally important was how the mere presence of DDT led to a dramatic cutback in funds available for such control and development efforts. For example, John McArthur, who proposed experimental villages in Borneo where agricultural practices would suppress mosquito breeding, was denied such funding (McArthur 1947). Today, there is as much risk as then that malaria control will follow the path of the magic bullet, when the long-awaited vaccines for malaria are finally developed and that history will repeat itself.

Malaria and Public Health in the Twenty-First Century

This chapter's highly selective review of the twentieth-century history of public health and malaria control has brought to light several trends that continue and that greatly undermine the future prospects for health development in malarious countries.

- The policies of western industrialized countries have dominated international public health concepts and priorities. These policies have favored the control of infectious and noninfectious diseases by means of medical treatment. Consequently, the control of vector-borne infectious diseases, especially those that strike in epidemic form, has been increasingly problematic, especially in tropical countries, where resources are very scarce but still largely consumed by the provision of curative services.

- Public health is in a state of crisis. As Berlinguer (1999) put it, "The model of primary health care as fundamental to the prevention and treatment of diseases has almost been abandoned. The trend is now toward dismantling the machinery of public health. Even in countries with minimal resources, priority is given to costly technologies, to the exclusive benefit of the happy few. Community services are increasingly replaced by private insurance …. This is, in brief, a step back to nineteenth-century Europe."

- Largely opposed to curative services, the discipline of public health exists today in a heavily fragmented manner, where it exists at all, a far cry from its comprehensive, early twentieth-century roots. Dominant decisionmaking methodologies in public health, as evidenced in the use of DALYs, further favor fragmentation.

- Epidemiology, instead of becoming the scientific arm of public health, has become a sophisticated research-oriented practice, more and more remote from the needs of communities. Furthermore, epidemiological research is no longer oriented to the solution of problems encountered in the field, such as those met in the course of efforts to control diseases.

- Malaria control over the past 20 years or so has been pursued under the false assumption that essential public health functions either are present or in the process of being developed. As I demonstrate above, these developments are not taking place. Many malariologists have concluded that the control of malaria in the future must be pursued as an independent, vertical approach, as exemplified by the eradication campaigns of the 1950s and 1960s. Yet it is doubtful, under prevailing political realities, that an independent effort would be allowed to materialize.

Currently, malaria is receiving priority attention on many fronts, with WHO's Roll Back Malaria initiative—calling to halve the malaria burden by 2010—leading the way. A group of senior health economists has restudied the economic costs of malaria in Africa and concluded that they are many times higher than previously thought. Presented at a malaria summit held in Abuja, Nigeria, in April 2000, this evidence suggests that malaria has impeded development in Africa and that its control is essential if Africa's poor economic performance is to be reversed. After the call for funding, several multilateral and bilateral donor agencies came forward in Abuja with pledges totaling about $750 million for malaria. How this funding will be managed remains to be worked out.

One must hope that these initiatives will be successful and reduce the burden of malaria in such a way that what is achieved can be sustained for periods well beyond the initial target date of 2010. Yet many disturbing signs suggest the contrary. What seems to be emerging is an initiative driven by a vertical mentality, so that interventions will not be a consequence of a strengthened local health infrastructure but rather special efforts largely driven by external assistance, technically and financially. History suggests that such initiatives may achieve short-term gains (at high cost) but will not survive far beyond the day external inputs are no longer present. Donors want quick results for their investments, and few malarious countries are in a position to absorb such inputs effectively or efficiently. In other words, many millions of dollars may be spent, but the results will not be as hoped.

If the current push against malaria fails to achieve significant results, the international community could very well abandon the pursuit of malaria control and await newer technologies, particularly vaccines, before reengaging the battle against malaria.

This risk could be greatly reduced if, instead of combating malaria head-on, so to speak, malaria control became part of a much longer-term commitment to build local public health capacities to the level necessary to control all major infectious diseases. Something different is needed, something analogous to the early twentieth-century efforts of the Rockefeller Foundation to strengthen local health units in the southern United States. That program envisaged, but never achieved, the creation of a network of supporting services, including laboratories, that would be on call to serve the needs of the local level.

Each local project needs to demonstrate a local capacity to control malaria. It clearly involves bringing to bear the most up-to-date technical understanding of malaria. It also involves demonstrating the socioeconomic feasibility of maintaining whatever results are achieved. In this regard, one of the key questions to be addressed is to what degree malaria control contributes to economic gains that can justify increased investment in the strengthening of related public health functions. But perhaps the greatest problem facing such a program is the question raised by Bruce-Chwatt, namely, how to obtain a great deal of steady devotion to a very distant goal. It is perhaps here where one can hope to achieve results that have not been possible to date, owing to the growth in recent decades of extraordinarily powerful means of communication. These means allow individuals and communities to be in constant communication with others. Properly organized, such communication should provide a continuous source of encouragement, both psychologically as well as technically. This is a power that opens up new possibilities for developing public health capacities from the ground level up with the active involvement of communities and the active support from all higher levels. Although still largely confined to the industrialized world, modern communication is rapidly coming to the fore in many developing countries, as well. The Chennai-based M.S. Swaminathan Foundation (http://www.mssrf.org), for example, provides villages with free technology and information in exchange for the villages' promise to house the computers and staff of their operation. Although primarily oriented to sustainable agriculture and rural development, many of the project specifics concern community health issues as well.

How such grassroots efforts will materialize is for national and international public health leaders to determine. Nevertheless, some elements can be gleaned from history, in addition to points already made above, that should be taken into account in such a development. They are addressed below.

Strengthening Local Managerial Capacities

Community development projects have probably been the most successful in their approach to strengthening local managerial capacities. These projects have used various methods; for example, the Montana Study, funded by the Rockefeller Foundation in the 1940s, used a group study guide as a form of community self-analysis with the aim of discussing "in an objective way the economic, social, and cultural problems" present, to find "ways of stabilizing and improving the local economy, and to help people make life in their own town more enjoyable and more secure" (Posten 1950). Another approach, which stems from late nineteenth-century Scandinavian tradition, is the use of adult education to stimulate communities to address major problems they were facing (Adams 1975).

From these studies and empowerment efforts, a wide range of methods have arisen to help local leaders organize their efforts to help the community better address their priority concerns. Today, these methods can readily be found on the Internet; see, for example, http://nrm.massey.ac.nz/changelinks/, which is dedicated to "improving community participation in the environment and development."

Where malaria is a concern, local studies might take several, nonmutually exclusive, forms, for example,

- historical accounting of past malaria outbreaks and control efforts,
- understanding the impact of malaria,
- building an epidemiological model of malaria, or
- developing an adaptive management approach to malaria control.

Adaptive management has its roots in more analytic and quantitative efforts from the 1960s to address specific environmental problems (Holling 1978). Whereas the traditional community involvement efforts are largely qualitative in form, adaptive management seeks to develop quantitative models of the problem being addressed. Such models invariably involve extensive field investigations to gather data, interspersed with highly structured workshops that focus on the key question "what would I do with the information if I had it?" This area, too, has extensively grown over the past few decades. A website entitled The Adaptive Management Forum (http://www.mnr.gov.on.ca/MNR/arm98/amfinfo5.html) provides URLs of "the various groups, agencies, and universities which are currently at the forefront of the development of adaptive management approaches and their links."

The local development of quantitative models is clearly benefiting from the increased ability to obtain needed information concerning malaria and other public health problems from external sources, when needed (Fraser and McGrath 2000). Particularly important in this connection is the development and use of geographic information systems (Omumbo et al. 1998).

Active Involvement of Communities, Especially Schoolchildren, in Public Health Projects

Community involvement has been seen primarily as a means of getting local communities to adopt approaches developed at higher levels of government. However, efforts have been made, admittedly on a much more limited scale, to approach involvement as a means of empowering the local level. Although found mostly in community development projects of one kind or another, it was proposed by health development specialists as part of the 1970s PHC movement (Banerji 1978).

The involvement of communities in public health work is nothing new. The special role of schoolchildren has been demonstrated over and over again, but rarely has the power of children been developed and sustained over any length of time. For example, when head of the U.S. Public Health Service in the Philippines in the early 1900s, Heiser (1936) made a point of involving children in educational campaigns undertaken to improve personal hygiene of adults. These campaigns were developed with the Bureau of Education and the active cooperation of churches. One subject was taken at a time—beriberi, cholera, tuberculosis, or "whatever was important at the time." Similarly, the Rockefeller Foundation hookworm campaigns underscored the community education role that children could play. They were the ones who attended lectures concerning health in full force and who carried "the message home to the older ones" (Ettling 1981).

Malaria history also offers some outstanding instances of children's involvement. In 1916, when Wilhelm Schüffner attempted to control malaria by destroying adult anophelines, he taught schoolchildren to identify *Anopheles sundaicus, Anopheles hyrca-*

nus, Anopheles annularis, Anopheles aconitus, and *Anopheles vagus*. When he visited villages, as the first ceremony, the schoolmaster, with some of his senior students, would carry bamboo tubes containing freshly caught specimens of each species. They were able to reduce "a pile of hundreds of mosquitoes to five or six smaller heaps of one species each, even without the use of a hand lens—and they never made a mistake" (Swellengrebel 1950).

Education played an important role in the control of the 1930s malaria epidemic in Natal and Zululand (Park Ross 1936). Native schoolmasters were taught how to treat the disease and complications, take blood slides, conduct spleen examinations, and search for *Anopheles* larvae and adults. They addressed meetings and led village discussions to promote the methods being used to control the epidemic. A weekly nature study on mosquitoes was made compulsory for all children from Standard IV upwards.

In one district in India, a health assistant, on his own, developed a system whereby the schoolchildren of one particular year became responsible for educating their parents concerning malaria as well as the students of the lower grade who would take over that responsibility from them the following year (personal communication from D. Clyde, Jan. 20, 1976).

Use of Graduate Students to Support Local Efforts

College-level students are traditionally involved in community activities, as exemplified by the Montana Study. In that study, students from the University of Montana were actively involved to "find ways to enrich the quality of living in Montana" (Posten 1950). This approach also has been used for health development; for example, the Narangwal Studies in India included a rural internship to prepare doctors for rural service and to develop a rural orientation as part of their medical training (Taylor et al. 1967). Many countries have made compulsory service in rural areas part of the program for obtaining a medical degree, but under the prevailing conditions of isolation, lack of immediate support, and total lack of preparedness for the task, this approach has filled a resource need but little more.

With modern communication methods, it is tempting to suggest that attractive and productive ways of making community service for health development compulsory exist. Medical and public health students could be trained to lead certain school health activities, such as field investigations, microscopic analyses, computer simulations of local epidemic possibilities, and video preparation.

Local schools also should be involved, with their curriculum redesigned to incorporate malaria-related topics. Courses in geography, mathematics, computers, history, and so forth have relevance to disease control efforts and, with the use of modern multimedia approaches, courses often thought dull and a waste of time could be made interesting and—why not?—even exciting while meeting vital needs in the community.

Additional problem-solving programs organized at the community level could also benefit from the input of graduate students who have been fully trained in the use of one or more of the methods indicated above. In countries where participatory management disciplines are taught at colleges and graduate schools, student involvement in local public health projects could be sought.

Making Local Information Available to the Community

Much knowledge concerning malaria and all of its determinants has been accumulated over the past century. But almost all of it rests in institutions far removed from where that knowledge has been obtained. Even within countries, certain facts gathered in the course of major campaign efforts have not been made public. For example, many countries did not make publicly available maps that were being used by the eradication campaign, fearing that the maps could be used for military purposes by unfriendly nations.

The communication and information revolution that is in the process of taking place, in theory, should increase the free and easy access to information. It is encouraging many institutions to code their information into electronically readable forms and to provide easier access to these sources. Individuals with strong personal interests (professional or otherwise) are taking the time to create websites concerning very specific subjects.

All needed information is not to be found on the Internet, however, despite claims to the contrary. Malaria history, for example, is still largely an archival affair, with historians delving into diaries, books, and records, mostly covered with dust and not easily found. Bringing local but old historical information back to the communities may require the active involvement of malaria historians. One could imagine a network of historians willing to be involved in historical work in local communities engaging the malaria problem, where, of course, there was sufficient indication that such delving into the past would resurrect points of view as well as actual results of direct relevance to the current situation.

International Role

The international health community has a major role to play in ensuring that the skills needed for the strengthening of local and national public health systems, including nongovernmental initiatives, form part of the information revolution. Malaria should be one of the leading priorities in the future, because 60% of malaria deaths occur among the poorest 20% of the total global population (Gwatkin and Guillot 1999). This percentage is higher than any other disease condition, including respiratory infections, diarrheal diseases, and tuberculosis. Clearly, the percentage would be near 100% if, instead of including all countries of the world, only malaria-endemic countries were included.

Health economists are also looking at malaria more carefully to better understand how costly this disease is in direct as well as indirect economic terms. Preliminary conclusions indicate that "despite important local differences ... the burden of malaria is great" (Hamoudi forthcoming). These results support the call for a sustained and integrated global effort against malaria. The recognition that the goals of malaria interventions should be place-specific and should be adapted to particular local ecological, epidemiological, economic, and social conditions suggests that such a global effort must adopt strategies that are designed to build capacities to control malaria is each specific place, that is, in each malarious community.

The strategic elements outlined above suggest the following tasks for international organizations:

- Carry out demonstration projects aimed at enhancing local capacity to control malaria.
- Develop prototype approaches for local capacity building using adaptive management workshop protocols.
- Integrate such projects within wider efforts to strengthen national public health functions.
- Extrapolate the information needed concerning malaria to other situations of the world and make that information readily and easily available on the Internet.

- Encourage national governments to adopt information policies that are supportive of local public health initiatives.
- Encourage and support, technically and financially, national governments in their efforts to reform their educational systems to provide needed support to local public health initiatives.
- Invite the global applied research community, including historians, to be on-call when specific skills are in short supply, locally and nationally.
- Ensure that a representative sample of local initiatives are well evaluated.

Such an agenda is not a quick fix to the problem of malaria. The history of the twentieth century suggests, however, that no such quick fix exists. If the twenty-first century is not to follow the same mistakes that have been made during the past 60 years, then the problem of malaria must be taken seriously; it can only come about when site-specific efforts to control malaria become the common approach, as it was during the pre-DDT period of the twentieth century.

Conclusion

Malaria remains special. Its specialness lies less in the absolute burden of illness and death that malaria imposes than in the fact that its control demands a response from public health systems that few, if any, are in a strong enough position to provide. Malaria exemplifies a problem worthy of a different approach to public health than has been used thus far. It calls for an educated response; no brute force, top-down method will solve it. If active community collaboration is not obtained, available control methods will fail. Malaria is technically as complex as any problem that humankind has had to face until now and thus should attract the attention of the entire scientific community.

Acknowledgements

Thanks to Andrew A. Arata, Robert Bos, Randall M. Packard, V.P. Sharma, and Burton Singer for constructive comments. Remaining faults and omissions are those of the author, and no one else.

Disclaimer

Opinions expressed in this chapter are the author's only and do not necessarily reflect the policies and views of the World Health Organization.

References

Adams, F. 1975. *Unearthing Seeds of Fire: The Idea of Highlander.* Winston-Salem, NC: John F. Blair.

Banerji, D. 1978. Health as a lever for another development. *Development Dialogue* 1: 19–25.

Berlinguer, G. 1999. Globalization and global health. *International Journal of Health Services* 29(3): 579–595.

Birley, H. 1995. *The Health Impact Assessment of Development Projects.* Norwich, U.K.: Her Majesty's Stationery Office.

Bradley, D.J. 1991. Malaria—whence and whither? In *Malaria: Waiting for the Vaccine,* edited by G.A.T. Targett. Chichester, U.K.: John Wiley & Sons.

———. 1994. Watson, Swellengrebel and species sanitation: Environmental and ecological aspects. *Parasitologia* 36(1–2): 137–147.

Bruce-Chwatt, L.J. 1978. The challenge of malaria: Crossroads or impasse? In *Tropical Medicine: From Romance to Reality,* edited by Clive Wood. London, U.K.: Academic Press.

Bynum, W.F., and C. Overy. 1998. *The Beast in the Mosquito: The Correspondence of Ronald Ross and Patrick Manson.* Amsterdam: Rodopi.

Candau, M.G. 1972. International public health: Some reflections after 25 years. *WHO Chronicle* 35: 225–235.

Cassedy, J.H. 1991. *Medicine in America: A Short History.* Baltimore, MD: The Johns Hopkins University Press.

CDC (Centers for Disease Control and Prevention). 1999. *Preventing Emerging Infectious Diseases: A Strategy for the 21st Century.* Atlanta, GA: CDC.

Chapin, C.V. 1934. *Papers of Charles V. Chapin, M.D.* New York: Commonwealth Fund.

Chen, L. 1997. World Health and the Rockefeller Foundation: Can History Inform the Future? [unpublished paper]. March 9.

Curran, J.A. 1970. *Founders of the Harvard School of Public Health with Biographical Notes 1909–1946.* New York: Josiah Macy Jr. Foundation.

Dubin, M.D. 1995. The League of Nations Health Organisation. In *International Health Organisations and Movements 1918–1939,* edited by Paul Weindling. Cambridge History of Medicine. Cambridge, U.K.: Cambridge University Press.

Dubos, R. 1965. *Man Adapting.* New Haven, CT: Yale University Press.

Duffy, J. 1990. *The Sanitarians: A History of American Public Health.* Chicago, IL: University of Illinois Press.

Ettling, J. 1981. *The Germ of Laziness: Rockefeller Philanthropy and Public Health in the New South.* Cambridge, MA: Harvard University Press.

Fantini, B. 1998. Unum facere et alterum non omittere: Antimalarial strategies in Italy 1880–1930. *Parassitologia* 40(1–2): 91–101.

Farid, M.A. 1980. The malaria programme: from euphoria to anarchy. *World Health Forum* 1: 8–33.

Farley, J. 1980. John Black Grant '12: The Rockefeller Bolshevik. *Acadia University Alumni Bulletin* 74: 10–12.

———. 1995. The Rockefeller Foundation: The Russell years 1920–1934. In *International Health Organisations and Movements 1918–1939,* edited by Paul Weindling. Cambridge History of Medicine. Cambridge, U.K.: Cambridge University Press.

Fee, E. 1987. Cited in *Disease and Discovery: A History of the Johns Hopkins School of Hygiene and Public Health 1916–1939.* Baltimore, MD: The Johns Hopkins University Press, 19.

Fee, E., and D. Porter. 1991. Public health, preventive medicine, and professionalization: Britain and the United States in the nineteenth century. In *A History of Education in Public Health,* edited by E. Fee and R.M. Acheson. Oxford, U.K.: Oxford University Press.

Fosdick, R.B. 1952. *The Story of the Rockefeller Foundation.* New York: Harper and Brothers.

Fraser, H.S.F., and S.J.D. McGrath. 2000. Information technology and telemedicine in sub-Saharan Africa. *British Medical Journal* 321: 465–466.

Gabaldón, A. 1969. Health services and socioeconomic development in Latin America. *Lancet* 7598: 739–744.

Galdston, I. 1954. *The Meaning of Social Medicine.* Cambridge, MA: Harvard University Press.

Gorgas, M.D., and B.J. Hendrick. 1924. *William Crawford Gorgas: His Life and Work.* New York: Doubleday, Page and Co.

Gramiccia, G., and P.F. Beales. 1988. The recent history of malaria control and eradication. In *Malaria: Principles and Practice of Malariology,* edited by W.H. Wernsdorfer and Sir I. McGregor. Edinburgh, U.K.: Livingstone.

Grant, J.B. 1963a. Mutatis mutandis. In *Health Care for the Community: Selected Papers of Dr. John B. Grant,* edited by Conrad Seipp. American Journal of Hygiene Monograph Series, no. 21. Baltimore, MD: The Johns Hopkins University Press, 169–184.

———. 1963b. Public health as a social service. In *Health Care for the Community: Selected Papers of Dr. John B. Grant,* edited by Conrad Seipp. American Journal of Hygiene Monograph Series, no. 21. Baltimore, MD: The Johns Hopkins University Press, 11–20.

———. 1963c. The health program of the International Cooperation Administration. In *Health Care for the Community: Selected Papers of Dr. John B. Grant,* edited by Conrad Seipp. American Journal of Hygiene Monograph Series, no. 21. Baltimore, MD: The Johns Hopkins University Press, 64–73.

———. 1963d. Trends of health care in social welfare. In *Health Care for the Community: Selected Papers of Dr. John B. Grant,* edited by Conrad Seipp. American Journal of Hygiene Monograph Series, no. 21. Baltimore, MD: The Johns Hopkins University Press, 35–41.

Grmek, M.D (ed.). 1966. *Serving the Cause of Public Health: Selected Papers of Andija Stampar.* Monograph Series, no. 3. Zagreb, Yugoslavia: University of Zagreb.

Gwatkin, D.R., and M. Guillot. 1999. *The Burden of Disease among the Global Poor: Current Situation, Future Trends and Implications for Strategy.* Washington, DC: World Bank.

Hamoudi, A. (ed.). Forthcoming. *Economics of Malaria.* Cambridge, MA: Harvard University Press.

Heiser, V. 1936. *An American Doctor's Odyssey.* New York: W.W. Norton.

Hirshfield, D.S. 1970. *The Lost Reform: The Campaign for Compulsory Health Insurance in the United States from 1932 to 1943.* Cambridge, MA: Harvard University Press.

Holling, C. 1978. *Adaptive Environmental Assessment and Management.* New York: Wiley Interscience.

Howard-Jones, N. 1981. The World Health Organization in historical perspective. *Perspectives in Biology and Medicine* 16(3): 467–482.

International Journal of Epidemiology. 1976. Epidemiology for primary health care [Editorial]. *International Journal of Epidemiology* 5(2): 224–225.

———. 1977. Epidemiology and health policy [Editorial]. *International Journal of Epidemiology* 6(2): 99–100.

———. 1978. Editorial. *International Journal of Epidemiology* 7(1): 3–5.

Kidson, C., K. Indaratna, and S. Looareesuwan. 2000. The malaria cauldron of Southeast Asia: Conflicting strategies of contiguous nation states. *Parassitologia* 42(1–2): 111–115.

King, M. 1982. *Primary Health Care in Iran.* Oxford, U.K.: Oxford University Press.

League of Nations. 1937. *Report of the Intergovernmental Conference on Far-Eastern Countries on Rural Hygiene.* Geneva, Switzerland: League of Nations.

Litsios, S. 1996. *The Tomorrow of Malaria.* Wellington, New Zealand: Pacific Press.

———. 1997a. Malaria control, the Cold War, and the postwar reorganization of international assistance. *Medical Anthropology* 17: 255–278.

———. 1997b. René J. Dubos and Fred L. Soper: Their contrasting views on vector and disease eradication. *Perspectives in Biology and Medicine* 41(1): 138–149.

———. 1998. Arnoldo Gabaldón's independent path for malaria control and public health in the tropics: A lost "paradigm for WHO. *Parassitologia* 40: 231–238.

———. 2000. Criticism of WHO's revised malaria eradication strategy. *Parassitologia* 42(1-2): 167–172.

———. 2001a. *Plague Legends: From the Miasmas of Hippocrates to the Microbes of Pasteur.* Chesterfield, MO: Science and Humanities Press.

———. 2001b. William Crawford Gorgas (1854–1920). *Perspectives in Biology and Medicine* 44(3): 368–378.

———. 2002. The Long and Difficult Road to Alma-Ata: A Personal Reflection. *International Journal of Health Services* 32(4): 709–732.

Macdonald, G. 1956. *Public Health Policy in Relation to Malaria Eradication Programmes.* WHO/MAL/165. Geneva, Switzerland: World Health Organization.

Mahler, H. 1974. An international health conscience. *WHO Chronicle* 28: 207–211.

———. 1976. A social revolution in public health. *WHO Chronicle* 30: 475–480.

———. 1985. *Faith in Development, Address to 38th World Health Assembly.* WHA38/Div/4. Geneva, Switzerland: World Health Organization.

Manning, R.L. 1968. Assignment Report China (Taiwan) [unpublished WHO report]. September. Geneva, Switzerland: World Health Organization.

McArthur, J. 1947. The Transmission of Malaria in Borneo. *Transactions of the Royal Society of Tropical Medicine and Hygiene* 40(5): 537–558.

Meadows, D. 2000. A kind WTO. *Whole Earth* Spring: 44.

Molineaux, L., and G. Gramiccia. 1980. *The Garki Project.* Geneva, Switzerland: World Health Organization.

Mullan, F. 1989. *Plagues and Politics: The Story of the United States Public Health Service.* New York: Basic Books.

Myrdal, G. 1952. Economic aspects of health. *WHO Chronicle* 6: 203–218.

Najera, J.A. 1989. Malaria and the work of WHO. *Bulletin of the World Health Organization* 67(3): 229–243.

———. 1994. The control of tropical diseases and socioeconomic development (with special reference to malaria and its control). *Parassitologia* 36(1–2): 17–34.

NAS (National Academy of Sciences). 1995. *Metrics for Health, Proposed Project for Institute of Medicine.* Washington, DC: NAS.

Newell, K. 1988. Selective primary health care: The counter revolution. *Social Science and Medicine* 26(9): 903–906.

Newman, G. 1919. *An Outline of the Practice of Preventive Medicine.* London, U.K.: Ministry of Health.

Newsholme, A. 1932. *Medicine and the State.* London, U.K.: George Allen and Unwin.

Omumbo, J., J. Ouma, B. Rapuoda, M.H. Craig, D. Le Sueur, and R.W. Snow. 1998. Mapping malaria transmission intensity using geographical information systems (GIS): An example from Kenya. *Annals of Tropical Medicine and Parasitology* 92(1): 7–21.

Packard, R.M., and P. Gagdelha. 1994. A land filled with mosquitoes: Fred L. Soper, the Rockefeller Foundation, and the *Anopheles gambiae* invasion of Brazil. *Parassitologia* 36(1–2): 197–213.

PAHO (Pan American Health Organization). 1988. *The Challenge of Epidemiology: Issues and Selected Readings.* Discussed and compiled by Carol Buck, Alvaro Llopis, Enrique Njera, and Milton Terris. Washington, DC: PAHO.

Park Ross, G.A. 1936. Insecticide as a major measure in control of malaria. *League of Nations Quarterly* 5(4): 114–133.

Posten, R.W. 1950. *Small Town Renaissance.* New York: Harper and Brothers.

Roll Back Malaria Partnership. 1999. *Halving the Malaria Burden by 2010.* Geneva., Switzerland: WHO, World Bank, UNDP, and UNICEF.

Rosen, G. 1948. Approaches to a concept of social medicine: A historical survey. *Milbank Memorial Fund Quarterly* 26(1): 7–21.

Rosenkrantz, B.G. 1972. *Public Health and the State: Changing Views in Massachusetts 1842–1936.* Cambridge, MA: Harvard University Press.

Russell, P.F. 1936. Malaria in India: Impressions from a tour. *American Journal of Tropical Medicine* 16(6): 653–664.

———. 1955. *Man's Mastery over Malaria.* London, U.K.: Oxford University Press.

Ryle, J.A. 1948. "Social medicine" and "public health." In *Changing Disciplines,* edited by J.A. Ryle. London, U.K.: Oxford University Press.

Soper, F.L. 1963. The Relation of the Mass Campaign for the Prevention of a Specific Disease to the General Health Services. PHA/Mass Campaign/5 [unpublished document].

———. 1964. Diary entry. May 4. From the Manuscript Collection of the National Library of Medicine, Division of History of Medicine, Bethesda, MD.

Swellengrebel, N.H. 1950. How the malaria service in Indonesia came into being 1898–1948. *Journal of Hygiene* 48: 146–157.

Takken, W., W.B. Snellen, J.P. Verhave, B.G.J. Knols, and S. Atmosoedjono. 1990. *Environmental Measures for Malaria Control in Indonesia: An Historical Review on Species Sanitation.* Wageningen Agricultural University Papers 90.7. Wageningen, The Netherlands: Wageningen Agricultural University.

Taylor, C.E., et al. 1967. *Doctor for the Villages: Study of Rural Internships in Seven Indian Medical Colleges.* Bombay, India: Asia Publishing House.

United Nations. 1992. *Earth Summit '92, The United Nations Conference on Environment and Development.* New York: United Nations.

Walsh, J.A., and K.S. Warren. 1979. Selective primary health care: An interim strategy for disease control in developing countries. *New England Journal of Medicine* 301(18): 964–967.

Warren, K. 1988. The evolution of selective primary health care. *Social Science and Medicine* 26(9): 891–898.

Watson, M. 1953. *African Highway.* London, U.K.: John Murray.

Weindling, P. 1995. Social medicine at the League of Nations Health Organisation and the International Labour Office compared. In *International Health Organisations and Movements 1918–1939,* edited by Paul Weindling. Cambridge History of Medicine. Cambridge, U.K.: Cambridge University Press.

WHO (World Health Organization). 1947. *Expert Committee on Malaria, First Session.* WHO.IC/Mal./6. April 22–25. Geneva, Switzerland: WHO.

———. 1949a. *Operating Programme and Estimates, Annex 2.* Geneva, Switzerland: WHO.

———. 1949b. Proceedings of the World Health Assembly. *WHO Official Records* No. 21: WHO, 192.

———. 1950a. *Expert Committee on Environmental Sanitation, Report of the First Session.* WHO Technical Report Series No. 10. Geneva, Switzerland: WHO.

———. 1950b. *Fifth Session of the Executive Board.* EB5/Min/4. Geneva, Switzerland: WHO.

———. 1951a. *Expert Committee on Environmental Sanitation, Second Report.* WHO Technical Report Series No. 47. Geneva, Switzerland: WHO.

———. 1951b. *Report of the Malaria Conference in Equatorial Africa.* WHO Technical Report Series No. 38. Geneva, Switzerland: WHO.

———. 1952. *Expert Committee on Public-Health Administration, First Report.* WHO Technical Report Series No. 55. Geneva, Switzerland: WHO.

———. 1953. *Expert Committee on Environmental Sanitation, Third Report.* WHO Technical Report Series No. 77. Geneva, Switzerland: WHO.

———. 1954. *Methodology of Planning an Integrated Health Programme for Rural Areas. Second Report of the Expert Committee on Public-Health Administration.* WHO Technical Report Series No. 83. Geneva, Switzerland: WHO.

———. 1960. *Local Health Service, Third Report of the Expert Committee on Public Health Administration.* WHO Technical Report Series No. 194. Geneva, Switzerland: WHO.

———. 1965. *Integration of Mass Campaigns Against Specific Diseases into General Health Services.* WHO Technical Report Series No. 294. Geneva, Switzerland: WHO.

———. 1973a. Organizational study on methods of promoting the development of basic health services. *WHO Official Records* No. 206, Annex 11: 103–115.

———. 1973b. WHA resolution WHA22.39. In *WHO Handbook of Resolutions and Decisions of the World Health Assembly and Executive Board, Volume I: 1948–1972.* Geneva, Switzerland: WHO.

———. 1975. The promotion of National Health Services: Report of the director-general to the 55th session of the executive board. *WHO Official Records* No. 226, Annex 15: 112–119. Geneva, Switzerland: WHO.

———. 1979. *Seventeenth Report of the Malaria Expert Committee.* WHO Technical Report Series No. 640. Geneva, Switzerland: WHO.

———. 1985a. Executive Board resolution EB57.R26. In *WHO Handbook of Resolutions and Decisions of the World Health Assembly and Executive Board, Volume II: 1973–1984.* Geneva, Switzerland: WHO.

———. 1985b. WHA Resolution WHA26.35. In *WHO Handbook of Resolutions and Decisions of the World Health Assembly and Executive Board, Volume II: 1973–1984.* Geneva, Switzerland: WHO.

———. 1986. *Expert Committee on Malaria: Eighteenth Report.* WHO Technical Report Series No. 735. Geneva, Switzerland: WHO.

———. 1992. *WHO Expert Committee on Malaria, Nineteenth Report.* WHO/CTD/92.1. Geneva, Switzerland: WHO.

———. 1993. *A Global Strategy for Malaria Control.* Geneva, Switzerland: WHO.

———. 1995. *New Challenges for Public Health, Report of an Interregional Meeting.* Geneva, Switzerland: WHO.

———. 1997. *Health for All in the 21st Century.* Geneva, Switzerland: WHO.

———. 1999. *Water Resources Development and Vector-Borne Diseases in Malawi.* WHO/SDE/PHE/99.2. Geneva, Switzerland: WHO.

———. 2000. *The World Health Report. Health Systems: Improving Performance.* Geneva, Switzerland: WHO.

Wiebe, R.H. 1967. *The Search for Order.* New York: Hill and Wang.

Winslow, C.-E.A. 1923. *The Evolution and Significance of the Modern Public Health Campaign.* New Haven, CT: Yale University Press.

———. 1926. Public health at the crossroads. *American Journal of Public Health* 16(11): 1075–1085.

———. 1931. *Health on the Farm and in the Village.* New York: Macmillan.

———. 1943. *The Conquest of Epidemic Disease.* Princeton, NJ: Princeton University.

———. 1952. The economic value of preventive medicine. *WHO Chronicle* 6: 191–202.

Worboys, M. 1996. Germs, malaria and the invention of Mansonian tropical medicine: From "diseases in the tropics" to "tropical diseases." In *Warm Climates and Western Medicine,* edited by D. Arnold. Amsterdam, The Netherlands: Rodopi.

World Bank. 1993. *World Development Report: Investing in Health.* Washington, DC: World Bank.

PART 4

Synthesis

Chapter 18

Integrated Assessment of Malaria Risk

Baruch Fischhoff, Ilya R. Fischhoff, Elizabeth A. Casman, and Hadi Dowlatabadi

Malaria risk is enormously complex. Dealing with such a complex issue requires assembling all the relevant pieces and then arranging them in proper relationship to one another. If pieces are missing, then interventions may not have the intended effects. Or, they may work as planned but still be inferior to overlooked alternatives. Without a common, comprehensive perspective, it is difficult to interpret historical experiences or to pool them to reveal recurrent problems. Without a shared overall understanding, it is difficult to coordinate the parties that play the many roles needed for a successful intervention. Without a big picture of malaria, it is easier for a fashionable research issue or intervention to capture undue attention and resources.

One possible strategy for addressing such challenges to create an integrated assessment of malaria risk (Dowlatabadi and Morgan forthcoming; Fischhoff 2000). Developed in the context of other complex problems (e.g., acid rain, climate change, and infectious disease), integrated assessments attempt to capture the critical relationships among the factors that determine a risk (or other focal outcome, such as morbidity or mortality rate, temperature, precipitation, or accident probability). If successful, an integrated assessment allows experts to communicate across areas by focusing on those expressions of their knowledge that are most relevant to the overall problem. Doing so draws together current research while focusing future research on relevant issues. Integrated assessments also can help to structure communications with nonspecialist audiences, helping them to create coherent mental models of the problem by identifying the set of facts most worth knowing (Fischhoff 1999; Fischhoff and Downs 1997).

Ideally, an integrated assessment model allows computing either the overall risk associated with a given situation or the change in risk subsequent to some change (planned or unplanned). However, a model misses the point if it achieves computability at the price of ignoring difficult issues because they are difficult to estimate or integrate with other factors. As a result, the process of creating an integrated assessment begins by qualitatively assembling the set of potentially relevant factors and identifying the relationships among them. In successive stages, these factors and relationships are developed into a computable model. That means specifying variables and functional relationships in terms that can be estimated, if sufficient data (or acceptable expert judgment) are available. Even if that goal proves impossible (for the model as a whole, or for some subcomponent), the process encourages clarity of thought while identifying the research needed to complete the work. It also shows just how much of the overall problem the computable part of the model covers.

Mature fields may provide models that cover some sections of an integrated assessment (e.g., the sensitivity of vector reproduction to temperature mean and diurnal variation). However, the developers of those models still need to integrate them with other knowledge, which may require new bridging research. With malaria, some relationships are well understood, and parameters have been estimated with considerable precision (for at least some circumstances). However, these models provide an incomplete picture until they are integrated with contextual determinants of how those pieces of the risk picture play out.

In this chapter, we present the first step toward developing an integrated assessment for malaria risk, addressing the suite of issues raised in this volume. Although the model might eventually be given in computational form, our purpose here is to provide a shared framework for discussing the issue. First, we explain the logic of the model, at two levels of detail (Figures 18-1 and 18-2). Then, we apply the model to the conditions of malaria in each region of the World Health Organization (WHO) and neighboring regions described in other chapters of this book, modestly supplemented by additional citations. Such mapping is the next step toward elaborating the model and testing its applicability.

We begin the mapping with a case study of Sri Lanka, described in terms of each component of the general model. We then survey the issues from each chapter, choosing examples that illustrate the various processes associated with malaria, particularly those addressed by the cross-cutting chapters on climate, population growth, and population movement (Chapters 11, 13, and 15). To conclude, we consider the work needed to take the approach further.

A General Model of Malaria Risk

Top-Level Model

The goal of an integrated assessment is to predict some important variable(s). In this case, it is *Malaria Risk*. (*Note*: Terms in text that are boldface italics on first mention correspond to the "nodes" in the figures.) In a computational model, that risk could be expressed simply as the expected annual mortality rate for the focal region. More complexly, it could be the morbidity or mortality rate, as a function of time (during and over years). More complexly still, the vector of risk outcomes could differentiate among population groups (e.g., by age). And so on.

As indicated in Figure 18-1, Malaria Risk is a function of the extent to which the region's *Conditions for Malaria* are conducive to the disease and its *Host Population* is capable of serving as hosts (and victims). Whether the disease potential of this combination is realized depends on the region's *Public & Private Health Capability* for preventing cases from occurring and limiting their health effects. *Climate* is, obviously, an essential factor in determining how favorable the conditions are for malaria. It has more indirect effects on malaria risk through its impacts on public and private health capability. These impacts might arise through such routes as a region's agricultural productivity (hence economic strength, hence ability to afford public health services) or its road system (hence ability to deliver health services to outlying regions during the rainy season). Different aspects of climate may be relevant to these direct and indirect pathways,

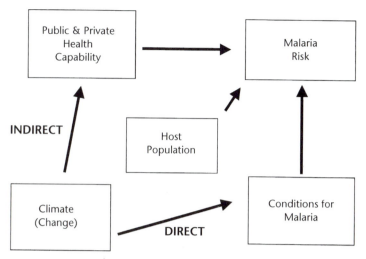

Figure 18-1. General Model: Conceptual Overview of the Factors That Affect Malaria Risk and Their Linkages

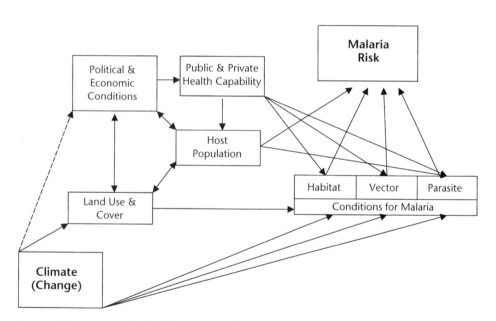

Figure 18-2. Specific Model: Elaboration of the General Model Presented in Figure 18-1

expressed as variables in the vector (in the mathematical sense) that characterizes climate. Any climate changes would be expressed through changes in these variables. The overall impact on malaria risk, of course, depends on other factors in the system. The factors might have a large effect in a region already on the brink of economic collapse but a negligible one in a region that has the resources needed for flexible adaptation.

The special role assigned to climate in Figure 18-1 could be assigned to other contextual drivers of malaria risk, both those that are stable and those that are susceptible to change. For example, an equivalent figure could be drawn for global economic development. Current malaria risk reflects the state (and practices) of the global economy (e.g., how logging and mining practices affect vector habitat and the exposure levels of vulnerable populations, or how the distribution of profits affects investments in public health). A change such as increased international commerce could affect the conditions for malaria directly, if it affected the distributions of vector, parasite, and vulnerable human populations. Indirect effects could come through impacts (good or bad) on the attention that health services pay to poor and marginalized populations. The increased flow of information that accompanies globalization might improve the distribution of scientific research on malaria and the dissemination of advice to citizens. It also could concentrate attention on fashionable strategies whose advocates are particularly effective communicators.

Second-Level Model

Figure 18-2 provides the next level of elaboration in the model. Conditions for Malaria is expanded into **Habitat**, **Vector**, and **Parasite** nodes. Each is characterized in terms of the variables relevant to predicting malaria risk (e.g., the distribution of each mosquito species over space and time). This is a portion of the overall model in which knowledge is often both deep and expressed in the quantitative, functional terms needed by a computational model (for predicting malaria risk). For some regions, other models link these factors with weather and climate (and, by inference, to changed climate). These predictions are necessarily weaker unless they also incorporate other contextual factors. For example, the implications of rainfall patterns on malaria risk will depend on such **Land Use & Cover** variables as the prevalence of pits from gem mining and of salinated soils from intensive irrigation.

A qualitative expression of the link between Land Use & Cover and Habitat would be a scenario that involves that connection. A quantitative expression would specify land use and cover in terms that predict vector-related habitat. For example, the intensity of logging practices might predict a reduction in breeding habitat for shade-loving species such as *Anopheles dirus*; the acreage in rice or aquaculture might predict the habitat available to other vectors, as might the prevalence of different cropping practices. The extent of peri-urban slums without in-home running water can predict concentrations of some mosquito species.

Land Use & Cover can affect and be affected by **Political & Economic Conditions**. For example, agriculture can provide prosperity that strengthens social institutions; exploitative gold mining can do the opposite, especially when profits go outside the region or to a privileged elite within it. Internal corruption or external coercion can affect Land Use & Cover, with myriad consequences—often negative. Poverty alone can encourage unsustainable practices, such as agriculture on sensitive lands, deforestation, and unplanned urbanization.

Climate might affect these "upstream" variables in many ways that could, eventually, cascade into changed Malaria Risk. One general route is by affecting the rate of other environmental changes, although the specifics of these scenarios may be quite varied. For example, increased ocean temperatures may lead to coral bleaching, reducing offshore fisheries and increasing migration to urban or inland areas. Decreased precipitation may reduce forest regeneration, whereas increased precipitation may enhance it. Changed precipitation timing may affect the viability of traditional agriculture, for which substitutes may or may not be feasible (depending on what will grow under the new conditions and whether forecasts and institutional support for making the transition are adequate).

Both Land Use & Cover and Political & Economic Conditions can affect the human population available as hosts (Host Population), thereby affecting Malaria Risk. For example, opening an area to agriculture or mining may encourage the in-migration of populations that lack previous exposure to malaria. It also may force the migration of populations with prior exposure, who then bring parasites to regions without previous exposure. Those migrant populations may pose significant burdens on a region's Land Use & Cover and Political & Economic Conditions.

Anything that affects Political & Economic Conditions can affect the Public & Private Health Capability to manage malaria risk. Also, any other large-scale driver, such as global development or war (each of which has many faces), could become dominant.

The next section is a worked example of Figure 18-2 for one focal area, Sri Lanka, then applies the framework broadly to the six world regions, thereby highlighting key factors that belong in assessments of their malaria risk (taken from Chapters 4–10).

Focal Area: Sri Lanka

Parasite. In Sri Lanka, as elsewhere in the WHO Southeast Asia region, vivax malaria causes high morbidity but few deaths; falciparum malaria is more frequently fatal, and drug-resistant strains have reached Sri Lanka. The *Plasmodium falciparum* parasite is more prevalent than *Plasmodium vivax* in Sri Lanka (Amerasinghe et al. 1999).

Vector. *Anopheles culicifacies* is the primary human vector. However, malaria parasites have been found in six other mosquito species, several of which may be secondary vectors (Amerasinghe et al. 1999). For example, *Anopheles subpictus* is found, but it rarely feeds on humans. *An. culicifacies* feeds relatively early in the evening, making it likely to feed on humans before they go indoors for the night. These mosquitoes can move up to 3 kilometers at night to bite and lay their eggs.

An. culicifacies exhibits a high degree of resistance to DDT; many mosquitoes are resistant to malathion and about 25% to permethrin (Karunaratne 1999). The species is highly heterogeneous among populations in pesticide resistance and ecotype (arid, semi-arid, and dry deciduous zones).

Habitat. *An. culicifacies* breeds primarily in streams but also is found in village water tanks, irrigation works, and gem pits. Although it prefers clear, sunlit water, it also has been found breeding in turbid, shaded water (van der Hoek et al. 1998).

Land Use & Cover. Rice fields have long provided breeding grounds for this species. Since the late 1960s, gem pits have become important *An. culicifacies* breeding sites. Irrigation and dam creation also have expanded mosquito habitat.

Host Population. Many people live close to streams and associated breeding sites as well as in poor housing, both factors that increase exposure to mosquitoes (Gunawardena et al. 1998). Gem pits have increased human exposure to infected mosquitoes by bringing nonimmune people, from other areas, to work at the sites.

Displacement due to civil war is an important factor in population movement and density. The population of internally displaced persons (IDPs) has grown from an estimated 560,000 people in 1993 to more than 800,000 in 2000. More than half of the malaria cases and 80% of deaths occurred in districts containing most of the country's IDPs (Global IDP Project 2000).

Public & Private Health Capability. Sri Lanka's malaria eradication program, begun in 1958, reduced malaria to 17 cases by 1968. The indoor DDT spraying program was declared a needless expense and discontinued. Almost immediately, large epidemics ensued, and malaria incidence quickly reached preeradication levels. Spraying resumed, using DDT, malathion, and later, synthetic pyrethroids (as resistance evolved to successive pesticides). Pesticide shortage has limited indoor residual spraying at times. In 1998, as part of the civil war, the government began to limit the distribution of "war-related medical items" (including those related to malaria) and food, further compromising public health.

Political & Economic Conditions. Since 1983, the Liberation Tigers of Tamil Elam have been fighting the government for control of the northern part of the country, with violent acts throughout. During this period of political chaos, economic disruption and internal displacement have been extensive.

Climate. In areas of Sri Lanka that receive more than 2,500 millimeters of rain per year (wet zone), constant precipitation maintains stream flows, preventing stagnant water from forming and limiting mosquito breeding areas and malaria. Major epidemics have occurred in this zone when the southwest monsoon failed (i.e., did not bring as much precipitation as usual) and *An. culicifacies* populations increased. (The effect of climate on malaria is discussed in detail in Chapter 11.)

In areas that receive less than 2,000 millimeters of rain per year (dry zone), stagnant pools are common, and malaria is endemic. The malaria case rate is correlated with rainfall, with a two-month lag. Northeast monsoon rainfall may increase malaria by expanding breeding sites. However, unusually high rainfall is not followed by periods of unusually high malaria incidence (van der Hoek et al. 1997). Although *An. culicifacies* females feed more frequently at night at high ambient temperatures, the biting rate is unrelated to humidity (Amerasinghe and Amerasinghe 1999).

WHO South East Asia Region

Parasite. *P. vivax* is more prevalent in Asia than *P. falciparum*, but the latter is spreading quickly, including multiple-drug-resistant strains. Of the estimated 20 million drug-resistant cases that occur globally, 30% are present in this region.

Vector. *An. culicifacies* is, overall, the most important and widespread vector in Asia. But at least eight other significant vectors are present in the region, some of which are primary in other areas, including *Anopheles stephensi, Anopheles fluviatilis, An. dirus, Anopheles minimus, Anopheles balabacensis, Anopheles maculatus, Anopheles umbrosus,* and *Anopheles sundaicus.*

Habitat. The habitats, breeding and feeding habits, and pesticide resistance of the nine major vectors vary. In addition, secondary vectors are found in a wide range of habitats (forest, urban, desert, and rural). For example, *An. stephensi* is prevalent in urban and industrial areas. *An. culicifacies* and some other vectors can breed opportunistically in anthropogenic water sources. Malaria has been on the rise in forest and hill areas.

Land Use & Cover. In addition to gem mining, other risk factors arise from such diverse actions as deforestation for agriculture, irrigation and dams, rice fields, roads, urban construction, fish ponds in Java (if salinity is low), and cattle grazing.

Host Population. Blood polymorphisms throughout Asia (e.g., Duffy group antigens, sickle hemoglobin, thalassemia) appear to affect susceptibility to *Plasmodia*. Having survived previous malaria infections also imparts some level of protection to individuals. Various kinds of population movement bring nonimmune individuals into endemic areas and individuals who carry the parasite (or a resistant strain) to susceptible populations at their destinations. Refugees, IDPs, and purposeful migrants typically experience high exposure to mosquitoes due to working conditions (e.g., mining gems, constructing dams, or collecting firewood in forests) or poor housing. Peri-urban populations also are at high risk of malaria.

Public & Private Health Capability. Many areas have knowledgeable health officials, but few have resources for sustained, coordinated programs. Services are particularly lacking in border areas occupied by marginalized populations. In various places, spraying and medical care have been disrupted by unrest or the recent economic downturn. Larvicides have been effective in controlling *An. stephensi* and *An. maculatus* in urban areas (Litsios 1996).

Political & Economic Conditions. Recent financial crises and poverty, warfare, border disputes, internal conflicts, poverty, and unplanned urbanization are among the factors that people and governments must confront.

Climate. Malaria epidemics in India are associated with heavy rainfall. Flooding in Rajasthan associated with the El Niño–Southern Oscillation (ENSO; see details in Chapter 11), for example, was linked with epidemic malaria when it extended the rainy season into September (Akhtar and McMichael 1996; Gupta 1996). Similarly, high temperatures in ENSO years correlate with high malaria incidence in Pakistan.

WHO Oceania and East Asia Region

Parasite. In the Mekong River region (through Cambodia, southern China, Lao People's Democratic Republic [Lao PDR], Myanmar, Thailand, and Vietnam), both *P. vivax* and *P. falciparum* are prevalent. Why one predominates in a particular locale is unclear. Falciparum malaria is dominant where incidence is high (Kidson, Singhasivanon, and Supavej 1999). The Mekong River region has been a global epicenter of multiple-drug-resistant falciparum malaria.

Vector. Numerous significant vectors (at least 15) are present. At least five vectors (*An. sundaicus, An. maculatus, An. minimus, An. subpictus,* and *An. dirus* complex species) are important vectors in several countries.

Habitat. Some of the many vectors range over coastal areas (*Anopheles farauti*), brackish rice fields and aquaculture and other delta areas (*An. sundaicus* and *An. subpictus*), forests (*An. dirus*), and hilly areas and forest fringe (*An. minimus* and *An. maculatus*).

Land Use & Cover. Malaria is more prevalent in densely forested areas than in cultivated or otherwise cleared areas (Kidson, Singhasivanon, and Supavej 1999). Deforestation, proceeding at a rapid pace across most of the region, may eventually reduce malaria transmission by removing exophilic forest vectors, especially *An. dirus*. Dam construction creates new habitat while displacing people. Rapidly expanding aquaculture, especially in Cambodia, Thailand, and Vietnam, increases vector breeding areas. Brackish rice agriculture offers similar vector habitat. Conversely, soil desalination for agriculture has eliminated the vectors that need brackish water from parts of Vietnam. Water pollution also has limited some vectors. Breeding silkworms in and near homes precludes insecticide use in parts of Cambodia, Lao PDR, and Vietnam.

In Cambodia, Myanmar, Papua New Guinea, Thailand, and Vietnam, mining increases both vector habitat and exposure of nonimmune hosts, who then take malaria back to their places of origin. Dam projects often displace people, who relocate in the forest (as in Lao PDR and Vietnam), increasing their exposure to malaria vectors.

Host Population. Ethnic minorities, highland peoples, border populations, and mobile populations (refugees, soldiers, migrants, tourists, and resettled people) are at high risk for malaria. Multiple-drug-resistant strains are spread by migrating forest workers returning to their homes.

Deforestation puts some people at high risk for malaria, but after an area is cleared and settled, malaria often declines. Slash-and-burn and other forms of subsistence forest agriculture require people to settle the forest continually, because soil fertility may rapidly decline in newly deforested areas.

Public & Private Health Capability. Most affected areas have insecticide-treated net (ITN) programs, the impact of which varies depending on the scope of coverage and public understanding. Among the countries of the Mekong River region, malaria prevention, surveillance, and treatment activities are generally better in China, Thailand, and Vietnam than in Cambodia, Lao PDR, and Myanmar. Thailand has a policy of providing free treatment to all, regardless of nationality. Low-density populations, especially minorities, tend to receive the least attention. Among Pacific countries with endemic malaria, public health efforts are effective in Vanuatu but poor in Papua New Guinea and the Solomon Islands. Lack of public understanding of malaria transmission is a barrier in some countries (e.g., the Philippines and Vietnam). The traditional use of bed nets in some areas (e.g., China) facilitates ITN programs.

Political & Economic Conditions. Civil unrest and international wars have created refugees and IDPs in many countries: Cambodia, the Thailand–Myanmar border, Papua New Guinea, the Solomon Islands, and China's borders with Myanmar, Lao PDR, and Democratic People's Republic of Korea (North Korea). Border areas are often porous and occupied by marginalized populations.

Climate. One outbreak in Vietnam may have resulted when El Niño–associated drought drove people into the forest. Malaria occurs seasonally in some areas, and weather effects on particular vectors have been observed.

WHO European Region (Including Western Asia)

Malaria was nearly eradicated by the campaign begun in the 1950s but has reemerged over the past decade. Epidemics are ongoing in Armenia, Azerbaijan, Tajikistan, and Turkey. International travel, war, political and economic crises, and changes in land use are the important factors in this resurgence.

The number of cases in western Europe, imported by immigrants and tourists, is increasing. However, because of the low densities of potential vectors and infected people as well as the effective public health care in most western European countries, malaria is unlikely to become endemic in Europe or the Balkans. Even so, infrequent local transmission is possible. In central Asia and the Caucasus, countries struck by warfare and economic collapse have become foci. From these nations, the disease has spread to neighboring states, whose own capacity for control has been reduced by these destabilizing events.

Parasite. Although *P. falciparum* cases have been imported from tropical countries to Europe, the endemic parasite is almost solely *P. vivax*. *P. falciparum* caused 3% and *Plasmodium malariae* 1% of cases in Kazakhstan, for example. *P. falciparum* cases have been on the rise in Tajikistan. *P. falciparum* infection also has increased to 70% of imported cases in the European Union. In areas without local transmission, such as the European Union, it is unclear whether native potential vectors are susceptible to infection by exotic imported *Plasmodia*.

Vector. Vectors that are present in multiple countries include *Anopheles sacharovi*, *Anopheles maculipennis*, *Anopheles claviger*, *Anopheles messeae*, *Anopheles hyrcanus*, *Anopheles superpictus*, and *Anopheles pulcherrimus*. Anopheles vectors generally are more common in rural areas than in cities. *An. superpictus* is especially effective as a vector because it is endophilic and anthropophilic. *An. sacharovi* is frequently resistant to pesticides. At least in Turkey, mosquito resistance to pesticides is the inadvertent result of the quantity and variety of agricultural pesticides used.

Habitat. Malaria control efforts generally have been directed toward killing vectors. This approach has left breeding areas intact and allowed vectors to return after control was abated, increasing the receptivity of regions where malaria had been interrupted to reintroduction of the disease.

Land Use & Cover. Subsistence rice fields located near houses provide vector breeding grounds in Kyrgyzstan, Tajikistan, and Uzbekistan. Extensive wetlands and irrigation systems, especially those that have fallen in disrepair, also serve as breeding places in some newly independent states and in Turkey.

Host Population. In central Asia and the Caucasus, the migration of infected people and the living conditions of people on the move have been major factors in the reemergence of malaria. The disease has spread via human hosts from countries in upheaval (especially Azerbaijan, Tajikistan, and Kyrgyzstan) to surrounding states, in which local transmission may begin. For example, malaria has moved from Afghanistan to Kyrgyzstan, Tajikistan (directly and via Kyrgyzstan), and Turkmenistan. Other countries affected by these sources include Armenia, Georgia, Kazakhstan, the Russian Federation, and Uzbekistan. Throughout the region, most imported cases are recorded in cities.

Population movement includes voluntary migration among the newly independent states for employment; the return home of troops, including peacekeepers, from Afghanistan, Azerbaijan, and Tajikistan; and refugees from these states. Internal migrations are also significant. About 40% of Azerbaijan's population migrates annually; Turkey has 560,000 such seasonal workers. An estimated 3 million IDPs live in Armenia, Afghanistan, Azerbaijan, Georgia, and the Russian Federation; Tajikistan also has significant IDP populations (Global IDP Project 2000). These people are often on the move and are routinely exposed to malaria vectors. As elsewhere in the world, the distinction between forced and voluntary migration is often blurred.

Cases of malaria imported to western Europe have increased dramatically. The number of imported cases peaked at 12,860 in 1997, with the largest numbers occurring in France, Germany, and the United Kingdom. This increase reflects both increasing numbers of European tourists traveling to Africa, Asia, and South America (from 2 million in 1978 to 12 million in 1996) and the increase in legal and illegal immigration from malarious countries to the European Union.

Public & Private Health Capability. Diagnosis and treatment help prevent imported cases from leading to local transmission in the European Union. In contrast, poor public health responses in central Asia and the Caucasus have allowed imported cases to initiate local epidemics (e.g., in the Russian Federation). Economic difficulties and the near absence of malaria for decades have resulted in an insufficient supply of malaria experts and technicians in central Asia. A shortage of public health personnel is one reason for the low level of public understanding of malaria and control options (e.g., how to protect oneself). Spraying and ITN programs are not widespread.

Warfare has interrupted control efforts in several countries and contributed to epidemics. However, it need not be an insurmountable obstacle, as seen near Tajikistan's border with Afghanistan, where a recent malaria control campaign achieved a 70% reduction in cases. International assistance is a major factor in the effectiveness of malaria campaigns.

Political & Economic Conditions. Economic problems throughout the former USSR and wars in Afghanistan, Armenia, Azerbaijan, and Tajikistan have contributed to malaria in the region. Armenia, Azerbaijan, Georgia, and Kyrgyzstan have been especially hard hit economically. Poverty levels exceed 50% in some of the newly independent states. Conversely, malaria epidemics have locally hindered economic growth (e.g., in Turkey).

Climate. Winter temperatures seasonally interrupt transmission in this region. Historically, malaria was endemic over much of this region, so that its (current and recent) climate per se is not a barrier to the disease.

WHO Eastern Mediterranean Region

The Middle East is generally considered to include the countries along the southern and eastern Mediterranean Sea, the Arabian Peninsula, and some countries of western Asia. The 23-nation WHO Eastern Mediterranean Region includes the Islamic Middle East (excluding Israel), Somalia, and Sudan. This area encompasses three ecogeographic regions, each of which has different disease ecology: Afrotropical, Oriental, and Palearctic (see region descriptions and detailed discussion in Chapter 9). Malaria has been largely eradicated from the Palearctic areas. Malaria in Oriental areas has been successfully interrupted with greater difficulty. Afrotropical malaria appears impossible to eradicate.

Parasite. With the exception of the rare transmission of *P. malariae*, *P. falciparum* and *P. vivax* are the dominant parasites in the WHO Eastern Mediterranean Region. *P. falciparum* predominates in Africa south of the Sahara, where it is well adapted to the vectors. Both are present about equally in the Oriental region. *P. vivax* remains in the Palearctic region, whereas *P. falciparum* has been almost eliminated.

Vector. In the Afrotropical region, mosquitoes of the *Anopheles gambiae* complex transmit malaria efficiently due to their biomics, preference for feeding on human blood, and susceptibility to *Plasmodia*. Secondary but also effective Afrotropical vectors include *Anopheles funestus, Anopheles moucheti,* and *Anopheles nili*. Palearctic vectors are of the *An. maculipennis* complex. Two Oriental vectors, *An. stephensi* and *An. fluviatilis*, extend west into the Palearctic Gulf states, but *An. culicifacies* occurs only in the Oriental region.

Habitat. Generally speaking, *An. gambiae* is heliophilic. *An. funestus* favors permanent waters with vegetation, shade, streams, and seepages. *An. moucheti* is found in riverine forests, *An. nili* in streams, and *An. maculipennis* in fresh and brackish marshes and lagoons.

Host Population. Historically, malaria has significantly affected settlement patterns. For example, transmission in fertile African lowlands has motivated people to live in highlands (e.g., in Ethiopia). The region has nomadic and refugee populations as well as excluded minorities.

Land Use & Cover. Reclamation projects were important in earlier malaria declines. Irrigation and excavation projects and expansion of poorly drained peri-urban areas increased malaria risk. *An. gambiae* is favored by forest clearing and the replacement of papyrus marshes with cultivated fields as well as the proliferation of sunlit temporary freshwater pools, dams, irrigation channels, rice fields, and hoof prints. *An. funestus* multiplies in fallow rice fields and grassy edges of rice impoundments, and *An. maculipennis* by rice fields.

Public & Private Health Capability. Economic difficulties and the near absence of malaria for decades has severely reduced the pool of malaria experts in the region. Several countries (e.g., Morocco) have experienced cycles in which control efforts succeed in nearly interrupting malaria, leading to lower concern and relaxation of spraying campaigns and surveillance. Epidemics then recur, initiating renewed antimalaria campaigns.

Political & Economic Conditions. The conditions in this area vary widely, ranging from wealthy countries to poor nations strained by war and refugees.

Climate. Periods of high temperatures were linked to epidemics in the 1990s. Epidemics have been associated with heavy rains that follow long droughts. Malaria risk in highland and desert fringe areas is expected to be most sensitive to climate change.

WHO Americas Region

Malaria eradication campaigns begun in the 1940s and 1950s sharply reduced the range and incidence of the disease in North America and South America, eliminating it from some countries (e.g., the United States) and restricting it to rural areas in other countries. Disease burden was high before this effort, although not as severe as in Africa south of the Sahara. DDT spraying was a major component of control efforts, which were sharply relaxed in the 1970s. Since then, the disease has resurged and is currently endemic in Brazil, Paraguay, and Bolivia and north through Mexico and Haiti.

Parasite. There is a general cline, first defined in 1949, of *P. falciparum* increasing relative to *P. vivax* from south to north. *P. falciparum* is predominant in the West Indies and

Guiana shield countries, but *P. vivax* is more prevalent in Central America. *P. malariae* also occurs but is of minor importance.

Vector. *Anopheles darlingi* is the most important inland vector in South America, breeding in flowing water by major waterways, where people also congregate. It is endophilic and can travel up to 7 kilometers to feed. *Anopheles pseudopunctipennis* is found from Mexico to Argentina and is prevalent in the foothills of the Andes Mountains, breeding in sunlit drying pools. Endophilic and anthropophilic, this species is the predominant vector in highland valleys.

Anopheles albimanus* and *Anopheles aquasalis* are important coastal vectors. *An. albimanus* is found on both coasts in Central America and on the Pacific Coast of South America. Its effectiveness as a vector is increased by its biting early in the evening, while people are outdoors. *An. aquasalis* is limited to coastal areas from Brazil to Ecuador and does not stray far inland. The coastal vectors are zoophilic and more endophagic than the other species, making them less effective as human vectors except at high density and in the absence of plentiful domestic animals.

Insecticide resistance is prevalent in Central America (Litsios 1996).

Habitat. Malaria control has focused on killing vectors through indoor spraying, which leaves vector habitat intact and allows vectors to rebound after spraying is discontinued. Limiting vector reproduction by removing their egg-laying habitat seems intractable, except perhaps in cities. *An. albimanus* is found in mixed forest and agricultural areas. *An. pseudopunctipennis* is found in this vegetation zone as well as in more arid and barren areas. *An. darlingi* is found in the interior lowland forests of the Amazon Basin as well as in the agricultural and secondary growth vegetation in this region.

Land Use & Cover. *An. darlingi* has benefited from an expansion of breeding habitat provided by aquaculture ponds. Irrigation systems provide breeding grounds for *An. albimanus*. Deforestation, slash-and-burn agriculture, cattle grazing, and mining in forests all affect mosquito habitat in ways that increase malaria risk. Agricultural developments in Latin America have expanded breeding habitat. Peri-urban areas have expanded.

Host Population. Fewer people are displaced in Latin America than in some other WHO regions. There are currently an estimated 100,000 refugees and 1.2 million IDPs, with longstanding displacement in Colombia, El Salvador, Guatemala, and Peru. Extensive human movements in the Amazon Basin have been associated with changes in land use. Many people have come from outside the region to live and work in the forest, and indigenous people have become increasingly concentrated.

Although malaria has been a characteristically rural disease in Latin America, it has become an increasingly urban problem in the Amazon Basin. This change has coincided with increasing urbanization throughout much of Latin America and the influx of infected ex-farmers back to villages and cities.

Public & Private Health Capability. This region has been adapting to the decentralization of the international malaria eradication campaign for three decades. Faced with rapidly changing settlement patterns, the various national and international programs to control malaria have struggled with resource constraints and evolving malaria challenges (see Chapters 4 and 5).

Political & Economic Conditions. Civil unrest is a persistent problem in some parts of the Americas. Poverty and economic disparity are problematic in Latin America; economic development occurs without proportional social development.

Climate. A large zone of South America is characterized by relatively warm and moist conditions that allow year-round transmission (see Chapter 4). A smaller zone farther south is cooler and drier and has greater seasonality in malaria because winter conditions are not conducive to *Plasmodium* or vectors. A third, cooler zone of the Andes is even less favorable to malaria, which nonetheless occurs, transmitted by *An. pseudopunctipennis* in some valleys.

Africa South of the Sahara

Most of Africa south of the Sahara is characterized by stable holoendemic malaria, with control possible but eradication currently not. About 90% of global malaria cases and mortality occur in this region.

Parasite. *P. falciparum* resistance to chloroquine is widespread, especially in cities, with resistance to amodiaquine and sulfadoxine–pyrimethamine becoming more prevalent. In West Africa, *Plasmodium ovale* is prevalent and *P. vivax* rare.

Vector. *An. funestus, An. gambiae,* and *Anopheles arabiensis* account for an estimated 95% of transmissions. The *An. gambiae* and *An. funestus* complexes are highly anthropophilic. *An. gambiae* is long-lived and very susceptible to falciparum infection. Secondary vectors, of primary importance in some localities, include *Anopheles melas* and *Anopheles merus,* both of which breed in saltwater, and the freshwater species, *An. nili* and *An. moucheti.*

Habitat. *An. gambiae* breeds in small turbid water sources, such as puddles in hoof prints. *An. funestus* prefers more lasting water sources. Highlands are inhospitable to vectors because of the scarcity of water sources and the low temperatures.

Land Use & Cover. Papyrus swamp drainage for agriculture in highland Uganda resulted in a higher density of indoor-resting *An. gambiae* (a correlate for malaria risk) (Lindblade et al. 2000). Swamp clearing for agriculture also has been linked to higher malaria rates in Rwanda and Burundi.

Rice agriculture has had varied effects on malaria. In the savannas of West Africa, it has had little effect. However, rice cultivation has led to local epidemics at higher elevations, apparently as a result of increased vector populations. Peri-urban rice agriculture has led to high malaria incidence in Madagascar.

Dams and deforestation have had a more consistent effect of increasing malaria. Deforestation for agriculture is linked with the arrival and increase of vectors (*An. gambiae sensu stricto* and *An. funestus*) and an increase in *P. falciparum* infection.

Urbanization has a complex effect on malaria transmission. Peri-urban areas and urbanization in forest landscapes tends to result in high transmission rates because of ample breeding grounds and poor living conditions. However, some towns have lower transmission than nearby rural areas. After cities are built up, open water sources are reduced.

Host Population. Human genetic variation is an important factor in malaria susceptibility. The Duffy blood group (relatively common in West Africa) affects *P. vivax* susceptibility. Sickle-cell trait also is an important factor. Survival of repeated bouts of malaria imparts a specific but partial and transient immunity; children and nonimmune individuals are most vulnerable.

Africa has more IDPs (estimated 10 million) and refugees (5 million) than any other continent. These problems affect many if not most countries in the continent: five countries in the WHO Eastern Mediterranean Region (Djibouti, Eritrea, Ethiopia, Somalia, Sudan) plus Angola, Burundi, Democratic Republic of the Congo, Kenya, Liberia, Mali, Nigeria, Rwanda, Sierra Leone, Togo, and Uganda (Schmeidl 1998).

Public & Private Health Capability. Insecticide-treated curtain and bed net programs have the potential to reduce childhood mortality. For example, one such program in rural Burkina Faso markedly reduced vectors and transmission, contributing to a 15% overall decline in childhood mortality (Diallo et al. 1999). One goal of the Roll Back Malaria initiative (a program of intensified support to control malaria started in 1998 with special WHO and external funds) is to bring nets treated with pyrethroid insecticide to 60 million families in Africa. The slogan of the program is "One bed net for every African child."

Inadequate funding, personnel and medicine shortages, and urban bias in health access are among the problems that affect malaria control. Control efforts have been more effective in southern Africa, where transmission is less intense and funds more readily available.

Political & Economic Conditions. Many countries are affected by war or border disputes. Poverty is widespread. Road building and economic development programs have increased population mobility and the mixing of immune with nonimmune populations.

Climate. Monthly mean temperatures below 15 °C seasonally interrupt malaria transmission. Such conditions are found in southern Africa and in the highlands of eastern and central Africa and Madagascar. Frost, in South Africa and Zimbabwe, appears independently to exclude *An. gambiae sensu lato*.

Above-normal rainfall in 1997 was associated with increased *An. gambiae* populations and may have contributed to an epidemic in Uganda (Lindblade et al. 1999). In Senegal, declining rainfall and increasing temperatures have been associated with decreasing malaria rates over the past 40 years. Dry conditions in some other areas (e.g., southern Africa) probably limit vector abundance. However, the relationship between precipitation and malaria transmission is difficult to generalize. High rainfall in equatorial areas may not make much difference, given the baseline of extensive breeding areas and stable endemicity.

Elaborating the Integrated Assessment

Transitional Strategies

Though synoptic, the preceding exposition attempted to show how the various contextual factors associated with malaria risk could be accommodated within a common conceptual framework. If it made that case, then the analysis can be pursued in terms of both comprehensive case studies and individual predictive factors.

Mapping a case study of malaria risk (past or predicted) into an integrated assessment framework provides a quick way to determine which contextual factors have been considered and which ignored. Somewhat more work can show how clearly the included factors have been specified and, then, how well the presented evidence matches the research literature. These are, of course, the issues considered in any critical review. The practical question is whether that review is more effective when reports are mapped into an integrated assessment—or even submitted in that format.

Were such mapping standard, it would be easier to pool results from studies dealing with a particular factor or relationship (e.g., everything known about deforestation, travel malaria, or the effect of climate change on land use). It would facilitate both accessing and summarizing such information. It might help specialists to find the place for their work in ongoing analyses and to understand the connections that need to be made before that potential relevance is realized. It might increase the chances that factor specialists will be sought out by case specialists to complete the picture of a case study. Such a graphic depiction can facilitate discussion and communication of the issues, both among experts and between experts and laypeople, including policymakers (Fischhoff 1999; Morgan et al. 2001) .

In these ways, implementing the qualitative version of an integrated assessment can reduce the risk of fundamental mis-specification, when creating models to explain or predict malaria risk. However, it does not provide quantitative estimates—for absolute risk levels or for the relative risk associated with different conditions (e.g., two possible climate regimes or three alternative medical interventions). Conceptualizing the model in terms of potentially measurable variables ensures that the qualitative version is upwardly compatible with more quantitative ones.

In the next section, we explain how that elaboration might proceed, looking at work in progress on one segment of the overall model.

Next Steps for Some Factors

One set of issues, critical to determining malaria risk, is captured in the basic reproduction rate (R_0) (Macdonald 1957). A derivative index, epidemic potential (or transmission potential), is the central component of the MIASMA model (Martens 1998; see also Chapter 4), which has been used to predict the effects of climate change on malaria distribution. Figure 3-1 shows the formula for R_0, embedded in an integrated assessment for predicting its value, as a function of average temperature, vector and parasite species, and public health interventions. This particular representation is an influence diagram (Morgan and Henrion 1990). In such diagrams, an arrow between two nodes means that the value of the variable at its head depends on (i.e., is influenced by, or can be better predicted by knowing) the value of the variable at its tail. As noted in the discussion of Figures 18-1 and 18-2, these "variables" may actually be multivariate vectors, each of which captures a feature of the concept represented by that node. To one extent or another, all these variables and relationships are context-dependent.

In some cases, existing research provides an estimate that can be incorporated directly in the model. In other cases, estimates must be derived from an understanding of related conditions. The overall uncertainty in the estimate reflects the uncertainty in the component variables as well as the relationships among them.

Other estimates are more complex. For example, Figure 18-3 shows the submodel for the node **Reduction of Human–Mosquito Contact** illustrated in Figure 3-1. Any of several procedures can achieve this public health objective. The success of a given intervention is some fraction of its maximum possible effectiveness (e.g., what percentage of a particular vector's attempts will be thwarted by perfectly used bed nets) multiplied by

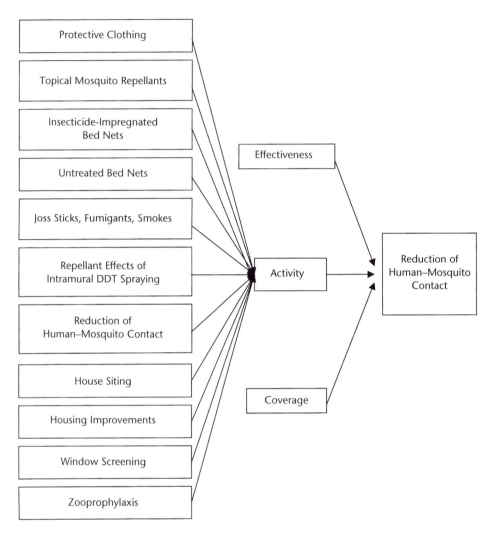

Figure 18-3. Contents of the "Reduction of Human–Mosquito Contact" Node Illustrated in Figure 3-1

an average actual effectiveness multiplied by the fraction of the population served. These values are determined by the resources available for the program, the fraction of the population applying the intervention, and participants' skill and motivation. These factors depend, in turn, on the quality of the associated health education and outreach. Thus, the reduction in contact from a given measure is a multiplicative function of these factors. This variable is scaled from 0 to 1, with 0 indicating that the intervention has not been applied. The relationships among the interventions vary. Some substitute for one another (e.g., completely effective home screening could eliminate the need for bed nets); some provide defense in depth, also captured by a multiplicative function (e.g., the percentage of mosquitoes that get through home screening that are then stopped by bed nets—the use of which is realistically estimated); and some are complementary (e.g., bed nets at night and protective clothing during the day).

Completing such a module is a difficult task. It requires the collaborative efforts of individuals from many disciplines. Its complexity reflects that of the interplay among this subset of contextual determinants of malaria. As a result, in order to have any meaning, this module must be applied at the local scale. Some of the parameters and functions will have to be specified separately for each locale, human population sub-group, and vector. Estimating the parameters for this submodel is a daunting task. However, as with any complex model, there is likely to be much cumulative learning from application to application.

Conclusion

Given the essential role of these contextual factors in determining malaria risk, even judgmentally derived estimates may be preferable to completely ignoring the factors that are hard to quantify—even if all that those judgments do is assess the incompleteness of an analysis and the uncertainty surrounding its outputs. Systematic analysis of contextual factors within a common conceptual framework offers some chance of more accurate and efficient analyses of malaria risk as well as how that risk evolves in response to deliberate and inadvertent human interventions.

In this chapter, we emphasize the special role that climate might play as a cross-cutting driver of malaria risk. Climate can have direct effects on the life cycles of the malaria vectors and parasites as well as on the physical habitats that they require. However, it also can have potentially powerful indirect effects on malaria risk. Unpredictable or unmanageable changes in climate can precipitate the collapse of already tottering economies and ecosystems. They can set populations in motion and undermine public and private health capabilities.

Moreover, climate is not the only large-scale driver in determining malaria risk. For example, in Figure 18-2, "globalization of the world economy" could be added as an external driver, having connections to many other variables. In complex ways, climate affects political and social conditions as well as land-use patterns of countries around the world. It can set populations in motion, in search of opportunities or safe havens. It might strengthen some public health capabilities and undermine others.

Global economic trends are a subtext of many chapters in this book, especially those that deal with the impacts of deforestation, agricultural development projects, and mining on malaria risk. However, they deserve a full treatment, assembling the relevant research and translating its implications on malaria risk under different specific circumstances. That knowledge, too, could be incorporated into an integrated assessment model, augmenting the one begun here.

References

Akhtar, R., and A.J. McMichael. 1996. Rainfall and malaria outbreaks in western Rajasthan. *Lancet* 348(9039): 1457–1458.

Amerasinghe, P.H., and F.P. Amerasinghe. 1999. Multiple host feeding in field populations of *Anopheles culicifacies* and *An. subpictus* in Sri Lanka. *Medical and Veterinary Entomololgy* 13: 124–131.

Amerasinghe, P.H., F.P. Amerasinghe, F. Konradsen, K.T. Fonseka, and R.A. Wirtz. 1999. Malaria vectors in a traditional dry zone village in Sri Lanka. *American Journal of Tropical Medicine and Hygiene* 60: 421–429.

Diallo, D.A., A. Habluetzel, N. Cuzin-Ouattara, I. Nebié, E. Sanogo, S.N. Cousens, and F. Esposito. 1999. Widespread distribution of insecticide-impregnated curtains reduces child mortality, prevalence and intensity of malaria infection, and malaria transmission in rural Burkina Faso. *Parassitologia* 41: 377–381.

Dowlatabadi, H., and M.G. Morgan. Forthcoming. *Integrated Assessment*. New York: Cambridge University Press.

Fischhoff, B. 1999. Why (cancer) risk communication can be hard. *Journal of the National Cancer Institute Monographs* 25: 7–13.

———. 2000. Scientific management of science? *Policy Sciences* 33: 73–87.

Fischhoff, B., and J. Downs. 1997. Overt and covert communication about emerging foodborne pathogens. *Emerging Infectious Diseases* 3: 489–495.

Global IDP Project. Global IDP Project Database. http://www.idpproject.org (accessed June 2000).

Gunawardena, D.M., A.R. Wickremasinghe, L. Muthuwatta, S. Weerasingha, J. Rajakaruna, T. Senanayaka, P.K. Kotta, N. Attanayake, R. Carter, and K.N. Mendis. 1998. Malaria risk factors in an endemic region of Sri Lanka, and the impact and cost implications of risk factor-based interventions. *American Journal of Tropical Medicine and Hygiene* 58: 533–542.

Gupta, R. 1996. Correlation of rainfall with upsurge of malaria in Rajasthan. *Journal of the Association of Physicians of India* 44(6): 385–389.

Karunaratne, S.H. 1999. Insecticide cross-resistance spectra and underlying resistance mechanisms of Sri Lankan anopheline vectors of malaria. *Southeast Asian Journal of Tropical Medicine and Public Health* 30: 460–469.

Kidson, C., P. Singhasivanon, and S. Supavej. 1999. Mekong Malaria. *Southeast Asian Journal of Tropical Medicine and Public Health* 30(Suppl. 4).

Lindblade, K.A., E.D. Walker, A.W. Onapa, J. Katungu, and M.L. Wilson. 1999. Highland malaria in Uganda: Prospective analysis of an epidemic associated with El Nino. *Transactions of the Royal Society of Tropical Medicine and Hygiene* 93: 480–487.

———. 2000. Land use change alters malaria transmission parameters by modifying temperature in a highland area of Uganda. *Tropical Medicine and International Health* 5: 263–274.

Litsios, S. 1996. *The Tomorrow of Malaria*. Wellington, New Zealand: Pacific Press.

Macdonald, G. 1957. *The Epidemiology and Control of Malaria*. London, U.K.: Oxford University Press.

Martens, P. 1998. *Health and Climate Change: Modelling the Impacts of Global Warming and Ozone Depletion*. London, U.K.: Earthscan.

Morgan, M.G., and M. Henrion. 1990. *Uncertainty*. New York: Cambridge University Press.

Morgan, M.G., B. Fischhoff, A. Bostrom, and C. Atman. 2001. *Risk Communication: The Mental Models Approach*. New York: Cambridge University Press.

Schmeidl, S. 1998. Comparative trends in forced displacement: IDPs and refugees 1964–1996. In *Displaced People: A Global Survey*. London, U.K.: Earthscan.

van der Hoek, W., F. Konradsen, D. Perera, P.H. Amerasinghe, and F.D. Amerasinghe. 1997. Correlation between rainfall and malaria in the dry zone of Sri Lanka. *Annals of Tropical Medicine and Parasitology* 91: 945–949.

van der Hoek, W., F.D. Amerasinghe, F. Konradsen, and P.H. Amerasinghe. 1998. Characteristics of malaria vector breeding habitats in Sri Lanka: Relevance for environmental management. *Southeast Asian Journal of Tropical Medicine and Public Health* 29: 168–172.

Chapter 19

Importance of Context in Defining Malaria Risk
Summary and Discussion

Elizabeth A. Casman, Reid E. Basher, Andrei E. Beljaev, Martin Birley, Robert Bos, Jonathan St. H. Cox, Robert S. Desowitz, Hadi Dowlatabadi, Baruch Fischhoff, Dana A. Focks, Duane J. Gubler, Renato d'A. Gusmão, Chev Kidson, Anatole Kondrachine, R. Sari Kovats, Lester B. Lave, Socrates Litsios, Janice Longstreth, Wolfgang Lutz, Anthony J. McMichael, M. Granger Morgan, Jean Mouchet, Paul Reiter, Donald R. Roberts, Guido Sabatinelli, Allan Schapira, Michael E. Schlesinger, Vinod Prakash Sharma, Kenneth M. Strzepek, Tang Lin-hua, and Mark L. Wilson

Recent analyses have focused attention on the effects of climate change on malaria, suggesting the possible spread of malaria into areas currently free of the disease. The goal of this book is to present the contextual determinants of malaria, including climate and climate change, and to attempt to understand their relative importance to malaria risk. In this chapter, we summarize our findings, focusing on the factors that influence the present and future geographic distribution of malaria.

Contextual Determinants of Malaria

In this volume, a diverse set of contextual determinants has been described, often with complex linkages. In case after case, the authors highlight disease risks associated with poverty, limited access to health services, population movement, inadequately funded (or negligent) public health systems, and water management methods that increase vector habitat near human habitation. Climate plays a central role in determining a region's underlying ecology and associated malaria potential, and climate variability influences the intensity of transmission.

Over the next 50 years, these determinants are expected to change, but not necessarily predictably. If the early twenty-first century continues along the trends of the late twentieth century, then travel—whether for political, social, or economic reasons—will increase dramatically (Chapters 15 and 16), as will urbanization (Chapter 13). At this time, the direction of changes in rainfall quantity, timing, and intensity (Chapter 11) and vector habitat are not locally predictable into the twenty-first century with any confidence. Public health antimalaria activities are also difficult to predict much past the typical planning horizons of 10 years, because they are tied to other difficult-to-forecast local and global conditions such as freedom from armed conflict; local cooperation; the dominant malaria control philosophy; technological breakthroughs in vector control, treatment, and prevention (Chapter 12); and the prevailing economic situation (Chapter 14), which has implications for donor willingness and the adequacy of various infrastructures (transportation, administration, public health, energy, and communication).

Although many individual determinants of malaria may not be knowable in the decades ahead, there are some indications that, at least in the near term, the malaria situation should improve. For instance, if the goals of the Roll Back Malaria initiative1 are met, then the prospects for global malaria control in the twenty-first century are very encouraging. Yet-to-be-developed medical tools (Chapter 12) may contribute to the success of this and other programs. To succeed, the control strategies of the near future will have to contend with accelerated mixing of infected and susceptible populations, the degraded state of public health infrastructure in the less-industrialized world, economic development programs that may increase vector habitat or attract people to malarious areas, and population growth in places where the sanitary infrastructure is currently strained.

The Biggest Malaria Control Challenge

Africa south of the Sahara, where more than 90% of all malaria cases and fatalities occur (WHO 1998), stands out among other regions. The main malaria vectors in this region are efficient and widespread, and there are large areas of stable malaria where essentially everyone is repeatedly infected from infancy to death. In such areas, public health efforts are focused on saving lives, protecting the most vulnerable sectors of the population, and case management. Malaria control has remained largely outside the national public health systems (Chapter 17), which, coupled with inadequate transportation and health infrastructure, competing national interests, poverty, and government instability, contributes to slow progress in this region. This is not to say that there are no committed control programs doing excellent work within the confines of the resources available to them and the magnitude of the disease problem they face. Malaria control efforts have had a significant impact, notably, in Madagascar, South Africa, and Zimbabwe.

The importance of malaria in the rest of the world, where it causes much suffering and death, should not be dismissed. Many of the malarious areas in Asia and South and Central America also seem to be caught in a loop of partial malaria control followed by resurgence; these are regions where epidemics, drug resistance, and pesticide resistance are major problems.

Epidemics, Climate, Climate Change, and Climate Variability

Current Ability to Predict Future Climate and Climate Variability on Various Scales

To forecast the effects of the future climate on malaria risk, it is necessary to be able to predict climate change at a spatial scale relevant to vector ecology. Global climate models have some ability to predict average annual and seasonal temperature on global and continental scales (Chapter 11). However, there is little confidence in the details of their

---

1The goals of the Roll Back Malaria initiative, coordinated by the World Health Organization (WHO), include cutting the current malaria burden in half by 2010 and developing malaria-endemic countries' health systems to the point of being able to sustain antimalaria and other high-priority health programs. WHO's partners include malaria-endemic countries, the U.N. Development Programme, UNICEF, the World Bank, bilateral development agencies, development banks, nongovernmental organizations, and the private sector.

temperature predictions at the regional and local scales relevant to malaria transmission. Predictions of hydrological factors (total rainfall, time distribution of rainfall, and soil moisture) at such scales are even less confident.

However, evidence from climate models allows generalization about future changes in many climatic features relevant to malaria. On the global scale, some degree of warming is predicted for the twenty-first century, perhaps of several degrees, and it is likely that more hot days, fewer cold days, higher maximum temperatures, and higher minimum temperatures will accompany this warming. Larger year-to-year variation in precipitation and more intense precipitation are likely over some areas. Increased tropical cyclone peak winds and cyclone rainfall, increased drought occurrence in mid-latitude continental areas, and increased variability in Asian monsoon rainfall are also expected. The climate models have not resolved whether the basic El Niño–Southern Oscillation (ENSO) phenomenon (a natural episodic fluctuation of the global climate that arises from the interaction of the atmosphere with the tropical oceans; see Chapter 11) will change in response to global warming. However, even with little or no temperature change, more intense ENSO-related droughts and deluges probably will occur (IPCC 2001a).

Importance of Climate and Climate Variability to the Current Malaria Distribution

Some generalizations can be made about the importance of climate relative to the other determinants of malaria. Climate is an integral part of every ecosystem, which limits, in turn, the epidemiological types of malaria that can exist at a given location. Furthermore, climate extremes disallow malaria endemicity (but not malaria transmission) in very cold and very dry areas, where parasite and mosquito survival is brief or nil, although some malaria vectors and parasites have adapted to inhospitable climates by discovering amenable microhabitats or by taking advantage of resting states.

Thus, climate limits the epidemiological type of malaria transmission that can occur in a given location, modulates the seasonality of malaria transmission in some areas, and prevents transmission in extreme climates. However, climate does not determine whether malaria is transmitted. In other words, a climate amenable to malaria transmission is a necessary condition for malaria transmission, but not a sufficient one.

Malaria as a "Tropical" Disease. Although malaria is now geographically a tropical disease, it was truly a global scourge before the 1850s and was only completely eradicated in Europe and North America after the international eradication campaigns of the mid-twentieth century. Malaria flourished in chilly locales (Reiter 2000) and was transmitted as far north as Canada and Siberia in recent centuries. (The archetypal "tropical" malaria parasite, *Plasmodium falciparum*, was endemic in temperate parts of Europe and North America before the latter half of the twentieth century [Bruce-Chwatt and de Zulueta 1980; Faust 1941].) The current localization of malaria to tropical regions may contribute to the popular perception that temperature largely determines malaria risk. Just as cold temperatures did not prevent malaria transmission in North America and Europe in the recent past, cold temperatures cannot currently be responsible for the absence of malaria transmission in temperate regions. Analogously, future warming of temperate zones cannot remove the climatic barrier to malaria endemicity, because none currently exists (Reiter 2001).

Warming could accelerate malaria transmission in temperate regions if endemicity were established, as demonstrated by transmission potential calculations (Chapter 2), but this is a separate issue. Currently, there are numerous obstacles to the reestablishment of transmission in temperate regions—vector habitat reduction, medical and public health services, and reduced opportunities for exposure to mosquitoes. These would first have to be overcome. That said, the chapter on malaria in the Caucasus and Central Asia (Chapter 6) illustrates how easily and rapidly the current "barrier" to endemicity in temperate zones can vanish after societies lose their institutional ability to cope with the reintroduction of malaria via population movement.

Effects of Current Climate on Malaria Distribution. Climate (in its steady-state sense) as well as temperature and precipitation (as specific characteristics of climate) contribute to malaria risk, both directly and indirectly. However, they do not solely determine malaria distribution. On the broad regional scale, temperature and rainfall are currently first-order predictors of malaria distribution in (much of) only one region, sub-Saharan Africa. In the other regions, although temperature and rainfall contribute to malaria transmission intensity in some parts of the regions, malaria distribution varies within each region, less according to rainfall and temperature than to the presence or absence of the nonclimatic determinants. Furthermore, nonclimatic determinants are often identifiable as the proximate causes of the spread or containment of this disease.

Malaria had been temporarily eradicated from various areas of unstable transmission, only to be reintroduced after the suspension or radical abridgment of control programs (Mouchet 1998; Packard 1986; Mouchet et al. 1998). The massive increase in malaria in recent decades is attributed largely to nonclimatic factors: the spread of resistance of *Plasmodium* species to chloroquine and other drugs, frequent armed conflicts and civil unrest, rapid population growth, settlement of malarious areas, economically motivated migrations (and consequent mixing of infected and susceptible humans), water development projects, and changes in biting habits of the vectors (Chapters 4 and 6–10; Nchinda 1998). Nevertheless, climate (including its normal variability, particularly droughts and rainfall patterns) can correlate with transmission intensity (e.g., Mouchet et al. 1996; Craig, Snow, and le Sueur 1999; Bouma and Dye 1997).

Climate, as it shapes local ecology, greatly affects the success (or failure) of malaria control and eradication programs around the globe. For example, vector control can be less difficult in certain temperate regions (for instance, those with a single vector species) than in tropical ones, although this is not completely climatic. Malaria was eradicated in countries capable of mounting and maintaining the sophisticated effort required. Malaria eradication never really started in most of Africa south of the Sahara (except in Ethiopia, South Africa, and Zimbabwe [Trigg and Kondrachine 1998]) and is still considered too overwhelming a task—at least until this region achieves a higher level of socioeconomic development and stability.

Effects of Climate Phenomena Such as ENSO on Malaria. Climate anomalies and weather extremes associated with phenomena such as ENSO and the North Atlantic Oscillation have been dominant causes of year-to-year climatic variations over much of the globe since at least the late Pleistocene (17,500 years before the present) (Rittenour, Brigham-Grette, and Mann 2000). In malaria-endemic areas, both the regular seasonal rainfall pattern and climate anomalies correlate with the timing of malaria cases (Bouma and van der Kaay 1996; Bouma and Dye 1997; Bouma et al. 1997). ENSO events influence the timing and intensity of transmission during epidemics in areas of unstable malaria (Kovats 2000), although sometimes the effect is a reduction of transmission. Also, to the extent that ENSO leads to disastrous weather conditions such as floods and droughts, which may destroy infrastructure and interrupt the distribution of health-care services, it may have other effects on malaria. The impact would depend on the coping abilities of the affected population and the greater society. In places with inadequate antimalaria programs and emergency response capabilities, ENSO events and other climate features will doubtless continue to affect unstable malaria transmission in the future.

Effects of Climate Change on Malaria Distribution

Projections of Malaria Risk for the Twenty-First Century. Modeling of global transmission potential for future predicted climate scenarios (Chapter 2) has suggested that climate change could change malaria distribution in certain locations. For example, some regions of the world would become too dry for year-round malaria transmission, whereas other regions would become warm enough to support it. In other regions, existing transmission levels would intensify. The magnitude of the impact of global warming on malaria is still being debated (Martens et al. 1999; Rogers and Randolph 2000; Dye and Reiter 2000), but the general scientific consensus is currently that, depending on the evolution of the other contextual determinants of malaria, some of the effects of climate change will be of local significance to malaria risk (IPCC 2001b).

Effects of Recent Global Warming. There is some disagreement as to whether the recent small changes in global average temperature (about half a degree Celsius over the twentieth century) have had detectable effects on malaria transmission (Lindsay and Martens 1998; Mouchet et al. 1998; Reiter 1996, 1998a, 1998b; Kovats et al. 2001). There has been a resurgence of malaria in many less-industrialized countries since the 1970s, and the question that has not been answered quantitatively is how much is due to global warming and how much to other determinants.

It is argued that warmer temperatures speed up malaria transmission, based on known relationships between temperature and the development rates of mosquitoes and parasites. Dissenters counter that nonclimatic factors alone are enough to explain the observed increases in malaria, without invoking changes in biting rates or parasite maturation rates. In particular, they point to such factors as the mixing of infected with susceptible human populations in the presence of competent vectors coinciding with the cessation of vector control programs (Mouchet 1998; Mouchet et al. 1998; Reiter 1998a, 1998b, 2001; Sharma 1996).

The chapters in this volume richly illustrate the importance of nonclimatic variables in the resurgence of malaria around the world and the importance of climate in supporting malaria transmission. Overall, it seems that increased temperature may account for a minor fraction of malaria burden in some locations but not for the bulk of the rapid global resurgence of the past 30 years, the invasion of new territories, or the reinvasion of old ones.

Effects of Future Changes in Weather Extremes on Malaria. Global climate change may produce changes in the frequency and intensity of extreme events, such as droughts, floods, hurricanes, and typhoons (though not always for the worse; see for example, Risbey et al. forthcoming). Such events can influence malaria risk by placing people in health-compromising situations (e.g., lacking shelter, means of support, or medical care) and by increasing (or decreasing) vector habitat. It is especially true in less-industrialized countries, with their precarious economies, infrastructures, and ecosystems. The malaria risk from extreme events comes from the combination of malariogenic potential, the magnitude of the parasite reservoir in the human population, and the society's ability to cope with such emergencies.

In regions with extremely limited resources for risk management, extreme events such as prolonged droughts or severe storms could contribute to the overload and collapse of governmental antimalaria services (e.g., through loss of infrastructure, reduced tax revenues, and increased numbers of refugees). Such indirect effects of climate change, acting through extreme events, may also have significant effects on malaria risk.

Climate change science currently indicates that some changes in weather extremes are likely, but much remains unknown. Extreme events currently can influence malaria incidence in endemic areas, so it is safe to predict that they will continue to do so in the near future. Their impact in the twenty-first century will be influenced not only by their frequency and intensity but also by the evolution of other important contextual determinants, such as the success or failure of vaccine and drug development programs, population growth and geographic distribution, the level of economic progress in the currently less-industrialized world, and the success or failure of future antimalaria activities (Chapters 12–14 and 17, respectively).

The Human Dimension: Economics, Institutions, and Research

Programmatic Funding Shortfalls. Malaria cannot be controlled without adequate public health services, infrastructure, laboratory-based diagnostics and surveillance, trained personnel, and funding. The cost or difficulty of delivering health services is the major obstacle to malaria control in tropical areas. This concept has been repeatedly illustrated by the failure of public health systems composed of vertical, disease-specific, technology-dependent control programs inherited from colonial or postcolonial structures or from defunct totalitarian powers, in the latter half of the twentieth century. Without an economic base to sustain them, these programs collapsed (e.g., Pinheiro and Corber 1997; Vitek and Wharton 1998). The continued impoverishment of public health systems is a major determinant of malaria today.

Sometimes malaria control resources are diverted for private use. Sometimes, bribes are a condition of local consent to international public health programs. Such diversions increase the overall cost of control programs.

Governmental Functions and Dysfunction. Political incompetence, impotence, or indifference regarding the delivery of health services is a major determinant of malaria. Climate variability may precipitate environmental disasters, such as droughts and floods. However, the will and ability of the government to distribute services and supplies in the face of emergencies determines whether disaster increases malaria transmission.

Health policy and practices are not consistently effective around the globe. In many regions, national therapeutic drug policies are absent entirely or not enforced, leading to treatment anarchy. Certain government policies have contributed to the malaria problem both directly and indirectly and through errors of commission and omission. Policy decisions made to promote environmental protection, agricultural development, or economic development have had significant negative side effects on malaria incidence. For example, large-scale resource development projects have been undertaken without adequate consideration of their unintended effects on malaria. Some countries simply lack antimalaria programs and policies (Chapters 4, 6, and 8).

Even when public health programs are in place, they may be denied to marginalized minorities (e.g., ethnic groups and refugees). Disease surveillance and treatment programs often miss remote or transient populations, resulting in untreated, mobile, expanding foci of infection. Administrative and ecosystem boundaries usually do not coincide. They can create important problems for malaria control authorities and may give rise to important differences in the health status of communities that inhabit the same ecosystem but are separated by administrative boundaries (Chapter 6).

In some cases, inappropriate vector control strategies are used because antimalaria programs are implemented without adequate local preliminary assessment and postprogram performance audits. Budgetary constraints and lack of qualified personnel contribute to this problem.

Warfare, within a country's borders or in adjacent countries, can lead to the neglect or suppression of antimalaria programs. Warfare also encourages the export of malaria to other areas via troop and refugee movement (Chapters 6 and 7).

Resistance to Pesticides and Antimalaria Drugs. The rapid emergence of resistance to pesticides and drugs means that the medical community is losing tools for combating malaria faster than new tools are being developed.

Mosquito populations eventually develop resistance to the insecticides used to control them. For this reason, and for environmental and toxicological considerations, many insecticides are no longer used to combat malaria vectors.

Drug resistance in *P. falciparum* and, to a lesser extent, in *Plasmodium vivax* is now widespread in Asia, South America, and Africa, and multiple-drug resistance is increasing. Drug resistance enhances morbidity and increases mortality 5- to 15-fold and increases the cost of treating drug-resistant malaria by a factor of 10 to 40 in India (Chapter 8).

On the positive side, recent developments using recombinant technology of various antigens, including transmission blockers, DNA vaccines, and new adjuvants, give promise that one or more vaccines will be in place by 2050. New antimalaria drugs are now available or under development for the effective treatment of multiple-drug-resistant malaria. Unfortunately, as yet, none are sufficiently affordable for mass distribution in control programs. Malaria is receiving unprecedented attention from philanthropic, business, and scientific sectors (Chapter 12).

Economic Disincentives for Pesticide and Drug Research. Pesticide development has been driven by the needs of the agrochemical market, which is vastly larger than the public health market. Regulatory obstacles in industrialized countries slow pesticide registration and discourage the development of new pesticides.

Market forces alone are unlikely to stimulate the expansion of the antimalaria drug arsenal. Antimalaria drug development is not a high-return venture for drug companies, because malaria victims typically cannot afford high-profit, high-cost medicine. As a result, most such research is sponsored by international agencies, philanthropic organizations, and governments.

Economics and Individual Risk Behaviors. Poverty often exposes people to a greater risk of malaria. Poor people live in homes that are not screened from mosquitoes. They may not be able to afford methods of prevention or treatment. Poverty also leads people to undertake activities that put them at increased risk of malaria, such as participating in nocturnal forest enterprises (legal and illegal) or living in resource-extraction (e.g., mining or logging) labor camps where living conditions increase human–mosquito contact. People living in poverty often lack accurate information about disease-averting behaviors and available medical options (Chapters 7, 8, and 10), and, of course, poverty may make it impossible for people to obtain needed medical assistance.

Conclusion

Climate governs ecosystems, and malaria has adapted to various ecosystems in a range of climates. Thus, many of the patterns of malaria transmission are closely associated with geography and climate. However, climate and climate change will no more be first-order predictors of the spread of malaria to new territories in the future than they have been in the past, the strong predictors being factors such as the mixing of infected and susceptible human populations and the quality, stability, and ubiquity of public health services. Climate and climate change may complicate, facilitate, or have little effect on malaria control efforts, depending on local conditions. Extreme climatic events may put populations at increased risk of mosquito-borne infectious diseases by transiently increasing contact between vectors and humans. To the extent that global warming increases the intensity and frequency of such events, malaria risk may increase in some locations.

Controlling malaria is more difficult today than it was 50 years ago because of the resistance to the chemicals used to combat the malaria parasites and their vectors; accelerated mixing of infected and uninfected populations; rapid population growth, which is outpacing water supply and public health infrastructure expansion in many areas; and especially the enormously underfunded state of most malaria control programs.

Disclaimer

The opinions expressed by the authors are personal and do not necessarily reflect the policies of their employers.

References

Bouma, M.J., and C. Dye. 1997. Cycles of malaria associated with El Niño in Venezuela. *Journal of the American Medical Association* 278(21): 1772–1774.

Bouma, M.J., and H.J. van der Kaay. 1996. The El Niño Southern Oscillation and the historic malaria epidemics on the Indian subcontinent and Sri Lanka: An early warning system for future epidemics? *Tropical Medicine and International Health* 1(1): 86–96.

Bouma, M.J., G. Poveda, W. Rojas, D. Chavasse, M. Quinones, J. Cox, and J. Patz. 1997. Predicting high-risk years for malaria in Colombia using parameters of El Niño Southern Oscillation. *Tropical Medicine and International Health* 2(12): 1122–1127.

Bruce-Chawatt, L.J., and J. de Zulueta. 1980. *The Rise and Fall of Malaria in Europe*. Oxford, U.K.: Oxford University Press.

Craig, M.H., R.W. Snow, and D. le Sueur. 1999. A climate-based distribution model of malaria transmission in Sub-Saharan Africa. *Parasitology Today* 15(3): 105–111.

Dye, C., and P. Reiter. 2000. Climate change and malaria: Temperatures without fevers. *Science* 289(5485): 1697–1698.

Faust, E.C. 1941. The distribution of malaria in North America, Mexico, Central America, and the West Indies. In *A Symposium on Human Malaria, with Special Reference to North America and the Caribbean Region*. Washington, DC: American Association for the Advancement of Science, no. 15, 8–18.

IPCC (Intergovernmental Panel on Climate Change). 2001a. *Summary for Policy Makers: A Report of the Working Group I of the Intergovernmental Panel on Climate Change*. http://www.ipcc.ch (accessed Sept. 18, 2001).

———. 2001b. Technical summary. In *Climate Change 2001: Impacts, Adaptation, and Vulnerability.* A Report of Working Group II of the Intergovernmental Panel on Climate Change. http://www.ipcc.ch (accessed Sept. 18, 2001).

Kovats, R.S. 2000. El Niño and human health. *Bulletin of the World Health Organization* 78(9): 1127–1135.

Kovats, R.S., D.H. Campbell-Lendrum, A.J. McMichael, A. Woodward, and J. St. H. Cox. 2001. Early effects of climate change: Do they include changes in vector-borne disease? *Philosophical Transactions of the Royal Society of London, Series B* 656: 1057–1068.

Lindsay, S.W., and W.J.M. Martens. 1998. Malaria in the African highlands: Past, present and future. *Bulletin of the World Health Organization* 76(1): 33–45.

Martens, P., R.S. Kovats, S. Nijhof, P. De Vries, M.T.J. Livermore, D.J. Bradley, J. Cox, and A.J. McMichael. 1999. Climate change and future populations at risk of malaria. *Global Environmental Change* S9: 89–107.

Mouchet, J. 1998. Origin of malaria epidemics on the plateaus of Madagascar and the mountains of east and south Africa [in French]. *Bullétin de la Société de Pathologie Exotique* 91(1): 64–66.

Mouchet, J., O. Faye, J. Juivez, and S. Manguin. 1996. Drought and malaria retreat in the Sahel, West Africa. *Lancet* 348(9043): 1735–1736.

Mouchet J., S. Manguin, J. Sircoulon, S. Laventure, O. Faye, A.W. Onapa, P. Carnevale, J. Julvez, and D. Fontenille. 1998. Evolution of malaria in Africa for the past 40 years: Impact of climatic and human factors. *Journal of the American Mosquito Control Association* 14(2): 121–130.

Nchinda, T.C. 1998. Malaria: A reemerging disease in Africa. *Emerging Infectious Diseases* 4(3): 398–403.

Packard, M.R. 1986. Agricultural development, migrant labor, and the resurgence of malaria in Swaziland. *Social Science and Medicine* 22(8): 861–867.

Pinheiro, F.P., and S.J. Corber. 1997. Global situation of dengue and dengue haemorrhagic fever, and its emergence in the Americas. *World Health Statistics Quarterly* 50(3–4): 161–169.

Reiter, P. 1996. Global warming and mosquito-borne disease in the USA. *Lancet* 348(9027): 622.

———. 1998a. Global-warming and vector-borne disease in temperate regions and at high altitude. *Lancet* 351(9105): 839–480.

———. 1998b. Correspondence concerning "Global warming and vector-borne disease." *Lancet* 351(9117): 1737–1738.

———. 2000. From Shakespeare to Dafoe: Malaria in England in the Little Ice Age. *Emerging Infectious Diseases* 6(1): 1–11.

———. 2001. Climate change and mosquito-borne disease. *Environmental Health Perspectives* 109(Suppl. 1): 141–161.

Risbey, J.P. Kushner, M. Morgan, R. Miller, G. Roe, and P. Lamb. Forthcoming. Exploring the structure of regional climate scenarios by combining synoptic and dynamic guidance and GCM output. Accepted for publication in *Journal of Climate.*

Rittenour, T.M., J. Brigham-Grette, and M.E. Mann. 2000. El Niño-like climate teleconnections in New England during the late Pleistocene. *Science* 288(5468): 1039–1042.

Rogers, D.J., and S.E. Randolph. 2000. The global spread of malaria in a future, warmer world. *Science* 289(5485): 1763–1766.

Sharma, V.P. 1996. Re-emergence of malaria in India. *Indian Journal of Medical Research* 103(1): 26–45.

Trigg, P.I., and A.V. Kondrachine. 1998. Malaria control in the 1990s. *Bulletin of the World Health Organization* 79(1): 11–16.

Vitek, C.R., and M. Wharton. 1998. Diphtheria in the former Soviet Union: Reemergence of a pandemic disease. *Emerging Infectious Diseases* 4(4): 539–550.

World Bank Group. 1999. *World Development Indicators 1999.* Washington, DC: World Bank Group.

WHO (World Health Organization). 1998. *World Health Organization Information Factsheet.* http://www.who.int/inf-fs/en/fact094.html (accessed Aug. 1, 2000).

Index

References to tables are noted by *t*, figures by *f*, and color plates by *Pl*.

Canada
ENSO impacts, 193, 199
human population migration, 287
malaria status, 261
public health history, 351
Candau, Marcolino, 307
Cane, M.A., 200, 202–3, 205
Caucasus. *See* European Region; Newly independent states; *specific countries*
Celli, Angelo, 293
Centers for Disease Control (U.S.), 316
Central America. *See* Americas Region
Central Asia. *See* Eastern Mediterranean Region; European Region; *specific countries*
Central Institute of Hygiene (Yugoslavia), 301
Cerebral malaria
antimalaria drug research, 228
human population migration and, 274
Sub-Saharan Africa Region, 146, 168, 169
Chapin, Charles V., 299
Chicken malaria, 218–19, 225
Child health. *See* Fertility rates (in general); Maternal and child health
Children's Vaccine Trust Fund, 225, 230
Chile, malaria status, 44
China
antimalaria drug research, 227–28
climate change, climate variability, and malaria, 192
economic forecasting, 262
global population trends, 241, 254
human population migration, 288
malaria control and prevention, 338
malaria parasites, 337
malaria status, 94*t*, 99*f*, 102–5, 107, 127
malaria vectors, 142
public health history, 301
socioeconomic determinants, 338
Chinchona. See Cinchona (bark extract)
Chloroquine
Americas Region, 59, 64
drug research history, 219, 227–28, 229–31
Eastern Mediterranean Region, 138, 141, 156
European Region, 70
malaria control challenges, 352
Oceania and East Asia Region, 96
South East Asia Region, 118, 127, 129
Sub-Saharan Africa Region, 169–70, 179, 278, 343
WHO use of, 216
Cinchona (bark extract)
Americas Region, 59, 64
malaria control history, 294
Ciprofloxaxcin, 229
Climate change. *See also* Intergovernmental Panel on Climate Change; Malaria models
Americas Region, 195, 196
climate change, climate variability, and malaria, 4–5, 189–213, 332–34, 347, 349–54, 356
climate information services, 212
Eastern Mediterranean Region, 153, 158, 341
economic forecasting, 260, 265–67
European Region, 89–90, 157, 196
global population trends and, 240, 241*f*, 254–57, 354
health impact determination, 14–24, 190–91

Climate change—*continued*
historical dependence of determinants, 170
human population migration and, 272–73, 282
integrated assessment of risk, 332, 333–34, 341, 345, 347
natural variability, anthropogenic change, and models, 191–94
Oceania and East Asia Region, 96, 101, 102, 106–7
past and future global change, 190, 195–97, 211–13, 349–51, 353
regional scenarios, 189, 195–98
South East Asia Region, 121, 133
Sub-Saharan Africa Region, 157–58, 175, 182, 183
Climate Framework for Uncertainty Negotiation and Distribution, 17
Climatic and meteorological variables. *See also* El Niño–Southern Oscillation; *specific variables*
Americas Region, 38–43, 343, *Pl 4–3, Pl 4–6*
climate change, climate variability, and malaria, 4–5, 189–213, 347, 349–54, 356
climatic zone classifications, 40–41, 42*t*
Eastern Mediterranean Region, 141–42, 148–49, 153–54, 156–63, 341
European Region, 71, 79–83, 89–90, 152–53, 160
global population trends and, 245
health impact determination, 190–91
integrated assessment of risk, 332–38, 332–41, 343–44, 347
meteorological indicators in malariology, 159–62
modeling efforts, 15–16, 189, 191–94, 345–46
natural variability, anthropogenic change, and models, 191–94
Oceania and East Asia Region, 97–108, 338
South East Asia Region, 111–12, 116, 119–21, 133, 159, 336–37
Sub-Saharan Africa Region, 4, 16, 171–76, 179, 276, 343–44, 352, *Pl 10–1, Pl 10–2, Pl 10–3*
"weather" as short-term variability, 208–9
CLIMEX model, 16
Coastal areas. *See also specific regions*
Americas Region, 37, 39–40, 342, *Pl 4–4*
Oceania and East Asia Region, 95–99, 105–6, 337
South East Asia Region, 3, 115
Coffee plantations
Oceania and East Asia Region, 101
South East Asia Region, 125
Cohen, Sidney, 220, 221
Colombia
chloroquine resistance, 170
climate of, 38
human population migration, 277, 282, 342
malaria control and prevention, 53*f*
malaria modeling, 19
malaria status, 44
public health history, 305
Commonwealth of Independent States (CIS). *See also* Newly independent states; *specific countries*
malaria status, 76
Communicable Disease Center, 311
Complex models, description of, 23
Complicated models, description of, 23

About the Editors

Elizabeth A. Casman is currently a faculty member in the Department of Engineering and Public Policy at Carnegie Mellon University, where she works on a variety of projects aimed at quantifying the contribution of global change to the transmission of infectious disease, primarily malaria, cryptosporidiosis, and cholera. Her other current research interests include developing regulatory decisionmaking tools for genetically modified crops and evaluating the potential uses of biotechnology for bioterrorism surveillance.

Casman's background is in water quality modeling, microbiology, experimental design theory, and hydrology. After receiving a master's degree in microbiology from Northern Arizona University and a Ph.D. from the Department of Geography and Environmental Engineering at The Johns Hopkins University, she worked for more than a decade on eutrophication problems of the Chesapeake Bay and its tributaries, using numerical modeling techniques.

Hadi Dowlatabadi is Canada Research Chair in applied mathematics at the University of British Columbia, adjunct professor in Engineering and Public Policy at Carnegie Mellon University, and university fellow at Resources for the Future. He pursues interdisciplinary research focused on public policy at the intersection of technology, environment, and health.

Following his Ph.D. in physics from Cambridge University, Dowlatabadi took a postdoctoral position at Carnegie Mellon University to study the impact of acid rain regulations on the energy sector. In 1987, Dowlatabadi joined Resources for the Future for research on the control of air pollution. In 1989, he was awarded a Warren Weaver Fellowship at the Rockefeller Foundation where he codesigned LEAD (Leaders for Environment and Development). Dowlatabadi returned to Carnegie Mellon University in 1991 to coordinate and then direct a team focused on developing integrated assessments of climate change. In 1996, the National Science Foundation rewarded the team's accomplishments with support for an NSF Center of Excellence for research on the human dimensions of global change.

Dowlatabadi continued as director of the Center for the Integrated Study of the Human Dimensions of Global Change until 2001, when he joined the Sustainable Development Research Institute and the Liu Center for the Study of Global Issues at the University of British Columbia.